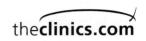

CLINICS IN CHEST MEDICINE

Cystic Fibrosis

GUEST EDITOR
Laurie A. Whittaker, MD

**For Internal Use ONLY.
Not for Distribution**

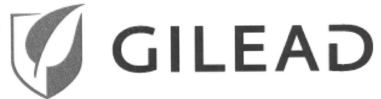

June 2007 • Volume 28 • Number 2

SAUNDERS

An Imprint of Elsevier, Inc.
PHILADELPHIA   LONDON   TORONTO   MONTREAL   SYDNEY   TOKYO

W.B. SAUNDERS COMPANY
A Division of Elsevier Inc.

Elsevier Inc. • 1600 John F. Kennedy Boulevard • Suite 1800 • Philadelphia, Pennsylvania 19103-2899

http://www.chestmed.theclinics.com

CLINICS IN CHEST MEDICINE
June 2007
Editor: Sarah E. Barth

Volume 28, Number 2
ISSN 0272-5231
ISBN-13: 978-1-4160-4286-0
ISBN-10: 1-4160-4286-5

Reprints: For copies of 100 or more, of articles in this publication, please contact the Commercial Reprints Department, Elsevier Inc., 360 Park Avenue South, New York, New York 10010-1710. Tel. (212) 633-3813; Fax: (212) 462-1935; e-mail: reprints@elsevier.com.

Clinics in Chest Medicine (ISSN 0272-5231) is published quarterly by Elsevier Inc., 360 Park Avenue South, New York, NY 10010-1710. Months of issue are March, June, September, and December. Business and Editorial Offices: 1600 John F. Kennedy Blvd., Suite 1800, Philadelphia, PA 19103-2899. Customer Service Office: 6277 Sea Harbor Drive, Orlando, FL 32887-4800. Periodicals postage paid at New York, NY and additional mailing offices. Subscription prices are $211.00 per year (US individuals), $330.00 per year (US institutions), $103.00 per year (US students), $232.00 per year (Canadian individuals), $396.00 per year (Canadian institutions), $135.00 per year (Canadian students), $270.00 per year (international individuals) $396.00 per year (international institutions), and $135.00 per year (international students). International air speed delivery is included in all *Clinics* subscription prices. All prices are subject to change without notice. **POSTMASTER:** Send address changes to *Clinics in Chest Medicine*, Elsevier Periodicals Customer Service, 6277 Sea Harbor Drive, Orlando, FL 32887-4800. Customer Service: 1-800-654-2452 (US). From outside of the US, call 1-407-345-4000.

Clinics in Chest Medicine is covered in *Index Medicus, Current Contents/Clinical Medicine, EMBASE/Excerpta Medica, Science Citation Index,* and *ISI/BIOMED.*

Printed in the United States of America.

GUEST EDITOR

LAURIE A. WHITTAKER, MD, Assistant Professor, Department of Medicine, University of Vermont; Director, Adult Cystic Fibrosis Program, Division of Pulmonary and Critical Care Medicine, The University of Vermont and Fletcher Allen Health Care, Burlington, Vermont

CONTRIBUTORS

JAMES F. CHMIEL, MD, MPH, Assistant Professor of Pediatrics, Division of Pediatric Pulmonology, Department of Pediatrics, Case Western Reserve University School of Medicine; Associate Director, LeRoy Mathews Cystic Fibrosis Center, Rainbow Babies and Children's Hospital, Cleveland, Ohio

PAMELA B. DAVIS, MD, PhD, Interim Dean and Vice President for Medical Affairs, Arline H. and Curtis F. Garvin, M.D. Research Professor, Professor of Pediatrics, Physiology and Biophysics and Molecular Biology & Microbiology, Case Western Reserve University School of Medicine, Cleveland, Ohio

AARON DEYKIN, MD, Assistant Professor of Medicine, Department of Medicine, Harvard Medical School, Boston, Massachusetts; Associate Physician, Division of Pulmonary and Critical Care Medicine, Brigham and Women's Hospital, Boston, Massachusetts

HILARY J. GOLDBERG, MD, Instructor in Medicine, Department of Medicine, Harvard Medical School; Associate Physician, Division of Pulmonary and Critical Care Medicine, Brigham and Women's Hospital, Boston, Massachusetts

MICHAEL W. KONSTAN, MD, Professor of Pediatrics, Division of Pediatric Pulmonology, Department of Pediatrics, Case Western Reserve University School of Medicine; Director, LeRoy Mathews Cystic Fibrosis Center, Rainbow Babies and Children's Hospital, Cleveland, Ohio

THOMAS LAHIRI, MD, Assistant Professor of Pediatrics, University of Vermont College of Medicine; and Director, Division of Pediatric Pulmonology, Vermont Children's Hospital at Fletcher Allen Health Care, Burlington, Vermont

JOHN R. McARDLE, MD, Director, Adult Cystic Fibrosis Program; and Assistant Professor of Medicine, Section of Pulmonary and Critical Care Medicine, Yale University School of Medicine, New Haven, Connecticut

CARLOS E. MILLA, MD, Associate Professor, Department of Pediatrics, Center for Excellence in Pulmonary Biology, Stanford University, Palo Alto, California

BRIAN M. MORRISSEY, MD, Associate Professor of Clinical Medicine, Division of Pulmonary/Critical Care Medicine, Department of Internal Medicine, School of Medicine, University of California-Davis, Sacramento, California

GERALD T. O'CONNOR, PhD, DSC, Associate Dean, Center for the Evaluative Clinical Sciences; and Professor of Medicine; and Professor of Community and Family Medicine, Dartmouth Medical School, Dartmouth-Hitchcock Medical Center, Lebanon, New Hampshire

H. WORTH PARKER, MD, Associate Professor of Medicine and Pediatrics; and New Hampshire Cystic Fibrosis Director, Dartmouth-Hitchcock Medical Center, Lebanon, New Hampshire

HEBE B. QUINTON, MS, Research Associate, Clinical Research Section, Department of Medicine, Dartmouth Medical School, Lebanon, New Hampshire

TERRY E. ROBINSON, MD, Assistant Professor, Department of Pediatrics, Center of Excellence in Pulmonary Biology (Pulmonary Division), Stanford University Medical Center, Palo Alto, California

MICHAEL J. ROCK, MD, Professor of Pediatrics, Division of Pediatric Pulmonology, University of Wisconsin Hospital and Clinics, Madison, Wisconsin

DAVID B. SEDER, MD, Instructor, Department of Medicine, The University of Vermont College of Medicine, Burlington, Vermont; Pulmonary Fellow, Division of Pulmonary and Critical Care, Maine Medical Center, Portland, Maine

STEVEN D. STRAUSBAUGH, MD, FCCP, Assistant Professor of Pediatrics and Medicine, Division of Pediatric Pulmonology; and Division of Adult Pulmonary Critical Care and Sleep Medicine; and Director, Adult Cystic Fibrosis Care Center, Rainbow Babies and Children's Hospital and University Hospitals at Case, Case Western Reserve University School of Medicine, Cleveland, Ohio

VIRANUJ SUEBLINVONG, MD, Clinical Instructor of Medicine, Division of Pulmonary and Critical Care Medicine, The University of Vermont and Fletcher Allen Health Care, Burlington, Vermont

BENJAMIN T. SURATT, MD, Assistant Professor of Medicine, Division of Pulmonary and Critical Care Medicine, The University of Vermont and Fletcher Allen Health Care, Burlington, Vermont

JAIDEEP S. TALWALKAR, MD, Associate Director, Adult Cystic Fibrosis Program; and Clinical Instructor, Department of Internal Medicine, and Department of Pediatrics, Yale University School of Medicine, New Haven, Connecticut

DANIEL J. WEISS, MD, PhD, Associate Professor of Medicine, Division of Pulmonary and Critical Care Medicine, The University of Vermont and Fletcher Allen Health Care, Burlington, Vermont

LAURIE A. WHITTAKER, MD, Assistant Professor, Department of Medicine, University of Vermont; Director, Adult Cystic Fibrosis Program, Division of Pulmonary and Critical Care Medicine, The University of Vermont and Fletcher Allen Health Care, Burlington, Vermont

JONATHAN B. ZUCKERMAN, MD, Associate Clinical Professor of Medicine, Department of Medicine, The University of Vermont College of Medicine, Burlington, Vermont; Director, Adult Cystic Fibrosis Program, Division of Pulmonary and Critical Care, Maine Medical Center, Portland, Maine

CONTENTS

> Improvements in outcomes for patients who have cystic fibrosis (CF) have been striking in the last 30 years. Median survival now approaches the fifth decade of life. Advances in the understanding of the basic defect and the pathobiology of CF have led to new treatments, some of which have undoubtedly contributed to this success. Improved understanding of the basic defect and the acquisition and maintenance of epidemiologic resources for the CF population in the United States have allowed us to determine predictors of survival and identify genetic, environmental, and therapeutic factors that may influence it. This article reviews some of the key epidemiologic and pathobiologic factors discovered thus far.

> Cystic fibrosis (CF) typically follows a more severe clinical course than non-CF bronchiectasis. Despite this recognized difference, the underpinnings of respiratory biology support a common pathogeneses of the anatomic deformations of bronchiectasis. This article reviews the observed manifestations among the related diseases of bronchiectasis and CF and discusses some of their similarities and differences. As more details of the mechanisms of bronchiectasis are unveiled, more parallels among the seemingly disparate causes of CF and non-CF bronchiectasis are recognized. With these insights, more opportunities to halt the vicious circle have become apparent.

> Newborn screening for cystic fibrosis (CF) was considered over 3 decades ago in 1970; however, the technology did not exist then for an accurate neonatal screening test. With the development of immunoreactive trypsinogen analysis, alone or coupled with DNA mutation analysis, the means were developed for CF newborn screening. Studies have demonstrated benefits of newborn screening in the areas of nutrition, cognitive function, pulmonary function, and survival.

FORTHCOMING ISSUES

RECENT ISSUES

THE CLINICS ARE NOW AVAILABLE ONLINE!

**Access your subscription at:
http://www.theclinics.com**

Clin Chest Med 28 (2007) xi

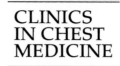

Erratum

Combination Therapy and New Types of Agents for Pulmonary Arterial Hypertension

Dermot S. O'Callaghan, MB, MRCPI
Sean P. Gaine, MD, PhD, FRCPI, FCCP

Department of Respiratory Medicine, Mater Misericordiae University Hospital,
University College Dublin, Eccles Street, Dublin 7, Ireland

In the above article, which was published in the March 2007 issue, Dr. O'Callaghan's full name should have appeared as Dermot S. O'Callaghan. Dr. O'Callaghan's middle initial was mistakenly omitted in the original publication. Dr. O'Callaghan's name is corrected in the title as it appears above.

ELSEVIER
SAUNDERS

Clin Chest Med 28 (2007) xiii–xiv

CLINICS
IN CHEST
MEDICINE

Preface

Cystic fibrosis (CF) is a common genetic disease that arises from mutations in the cystic fibrosis transmembrane conductance regulator (*CFTR*) gene. More than a thousand mutations in the gene encoding CFTR have been reported since it was first identified in 1989. It has been more than a decade since the publication of the last issue of *Clinics in Chest Medicine* dedicated to CF. In that time the understanding of CF disease pathogenesis has evolved, changing the landscape of CF care. Additionally, as the population of patients who have CF ages, clinicians have gained experience with the unique challenges of caring for adults who have CF. The goal of this issue of *Clinics in Chest Medicine* is to provide a "snapshot" of CF in 2007, highlighting what has been learned about disease pathogenesis and new therapies.

Major improvements in outcomes for patients who have CF have been made during the last several decades and result at least in part from improvements in the understanding of disease pathogenesis. Dr. Strausbaugh and Dr. Davis give an overview of CF and review key epidemiologic and pathobiologic factors discovered thus far. This information is followed up by a more in depth discussion by Dr. Morrissey on the pathogenesis of bronchiectasis.

Part of improving outcomes in CF requires early diagnosis and treatment. Newborn screening is an important first step in early diagnosis and has shown benefits in areas of nutrition, cognitive function, pulmonary function, and survival. The current approach to newborn screening and the experience of Wisconsin in this process is the topic of Dr. Rock's article. Once children who have CF are diagnosed, preservation of lung function is one of the most important goals and is closely associated with airway microbiology. Dr. Lahiri discusses the consequences of early *Pseudomonas*

aeruginosa colonization and the current approach to management including preliminary experience from an ongoing multicenter clinical trial.

Another important consideration in preservation of lung function in CF is nutritional support. Poor nutrition has long been associated with poor pulmonary and survival outcomes in CF, and aggressive nutritional support should be a fundamental component of any treatment regimen. Dr. Milla reviews the epidemiology and current literature that support a link between lung function and nutrition and discusses approaches to treatment.

In addition to aggressive nutritional support, treatment of airway infection and its associated inflammation is essential to preserving lung function in patients who have CF. Dr. Konstan and Dr. Chmiel provide an overview of the inflammatory response in the CF airway and the current understanding of anti-inflammatory therapies in CF. Dr. McArdle and Dr. Talwalkar then review the current data available for long-term macrolide therapy in CF and discuss the clinical benefits and potential host- and pathogen-related explanations for the positive therapeutic effect.

Although the treatment of airway infection and inflammation is the backbone of pulmonary-related CF care, other novel approaches are currently under investigation. Dr. Weiss, Dr. Sueblinvong, and Dr. Suratt review recent developments in gene and stem cell therapies including a discussion of the feasibility and limitations of these approaches.

Given the poor clinical outcomes associated with airway colonization with resistant organisms, infection-control practices to prevent patient-to-patient transmission of these bacteria are becoming increasingly important. Dr. Zuckerman and Dr. Seder outline some of the major historical events that signaled the need to understand better the mechanisms of infection in CF and discuss general principles of infection control. They then review the current literature on infection control practice, highlighting areas in which future investigation is needed.

As the understanding of CF lung disease pathogenesis has improved, so has the ability to image the chest. Dr. Robinson reviews current chest imaging modalities and discusses CT as a clinical and research tool and its potential to impact the management of CF lung disease.

A consequence of improved outcomes in CF is the aging population of patients who had CF. An important component of CF care now includes transition from a pediatric to an adult care program. Dr. Parker discusses the varied approaches to successful transition and offers advice for developing skills to help adult CF patients attain their best quality of life. Best quality of life for some adults who have CF includes starting a family. Dr. Sueblinvong and Dr. Whittaker review infertility in men and women who have CF and discuss key issues surrounding pregnancy. Once respiratory failure develops, quality of life may be improved by lung transplantation. Dr. Goldberg and Dr. Deykin review current issues in lung transplantation and special considerations for patients who have CF.

Although lung transplantation offers a treatment option and potentially meaningful, longer survival than the patient with CF's own lungs can provide, the best approach is a focus on delaying the need for lung transplant for as long as possible. Early diagnosis, aggressive nutritional support, and appropriate treatment of airway infection and inflammation are all important in improving outcomes. Despite the wide availability of tested therapies and CF centers that provide specialized multidisciplinary care by highly trained care givers, there is wide variability in outcomes across the United States. Drs. Quinton and O'Connor complete this issue by discussing quality improvement in CF treatment, including public reporting of CF patient registry data and the belief that providing better care using the currently available therapies is a powerful way to improve clinical outcomes.

The CF community can be proud of the great progress that has been made in the last decade, during which median survival has improved from 30 to 38 years of age. However, many opportunities exist to improve on prior successes, and further work is clearly needed. The CF Foundation has dedicated significant resources to promoting drug development and stimulating large-scale quality improvement efforts. With this support and the ongoing dedication of the CF community, helping patients who have CF live healthy and productive lives is more possible than ever before.

Laurie A. Whittaker, MD
Assistant Professor of Medicine
Department of Medicine
University of Vermont
149 Beaumont Avenue
Burlington, VT 05405, USA

Director
Adult Cystic Fibrosis Program
Division of Pulmonary and Critical Care Medicine
The University of Vermont and
Fletcher Allen Health Care
Burlington, VT 05405, USA

E-mail address: laurie.whittaker@uvm.edu

ELSEVIER
SAUNDERS

Clin Chest Med 28 (2007) 279–288

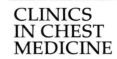
CLINICS
IN CHEST
MEDICINE

Cystic Fibrosis: A Review of Epidemiology and Pathobiology

Steven D. Strausbaugh, MD, FCCP[a,b,c,*],
Pamela B. Davis, MD, PhD[d]

[a]Division of Pediatric Pulmonology, Rainbow Babies and Children's Hospital and University Hospitals at Case,
Case Western Reserve University School of Medicine, 11100 Euclid Avenue, Cleveland, OH 44106-6006, USA
[b]Division of Adult Pulmonary Critical Care and Sleep Medicine, Rainbow Babies and Children's
Hospital and University Hospitals at Case, Case Western Reserve
University School of Medicine, 11100 Euclid Avenue, Cleveland, OH 44106-6006, USA
[c]Adult Cystic Fibrosis Care Center, Rainbow Babies and Children's Hospital and University Hospitals at Case,
Case Western Reserve University School of Medicine, 11100 Euclid Avenue, Cleveland, OH 44106-6006, USA
[d]Physiology and Biophysics and Molecular Biology & Microbiology, Case Western Reserve University
School of Medicine, Biomedical Research Building #113,
10900 Euclid Avenue, Cleveland, OH 44106-4915, USA

The infant that tastes of salt will surely die. This observation from ancient European folklore is probably the first recognition of cystic fibrosis (CF), a disease that is characterized by abnormal salt transport and, in early times, death in infancy. CF was first described as a separate disease entity in 1938 when pathologist Andersen [1] found mucous plugging of the glandular ducts of the pancreas in infants dying of malnutrition. She described this entity as "cystic fibrosis of the pancreas." Later, CF was characterized by fat and protein malabsorption, failure to thrive, and pulmonary disease, and the histologic picture of thick inspissated mucus that obstructs the ducts of mucous glands and was called "mucoviscidosis" [2]. CF was soon recognized to be inherited in a simple Mendelian autosomal recessive fashion [3]. The physiology of the basic defect in CF was first recognized by di Sant'Agnese [4]. During the 1948 heat wave in New York, he noticed that many of the infants presenting to the emergency room with heat

prostration and hyponatremic dehydration had CF. He subsequently discovered that the sweat in patients who had CF had abnormally high sodium and chloride. In 1983, working in the sweat duct, Quinton [5] identified defective cAMP-mediated regulation of chloride transport as the fundamental defect in CF. Shortly thereafter, the CF defect was localized to chromosome 7 [6], and in 1989 the gene was identified by positional cloning, one of the first genetic defects discovered this way [7–9]. More than 1500 specific mutations in the CF gene are recorded at http://www.genet.sickkids.on.ca/cftr/StatisticsPage/html. This article reviews the epidemiology of CF with an eye to new developments that focus on determinants of survival and identifies approaches likely to improve outcomes for patients who have CF.

Diagnosis

CF is among the most common lethal genetic diseases affecting Caucasians in the United States. There are approximately 30,000 patients who have CF in the United States. The incidence varies by ethnic group(Caucasians: 1:3200; African Americans: 1:15,000; and Asian Americans: 1:31,000) [10]. Diagnosis is made by clinical and laboratory evaluation. The criteria for diagnosis are evidence of chloride channel dysfunction (sweat chloride

---

* Corresponding author. Division of Pediatric Pulmonology, Rainbow Babies and Children's Hospital and University Hospitals at Case, Case Western Reserve University School of Medicine, 11100 Euclid Avenue, Cleveland, OH 44106-6006.

E-mail address: steven.strausbaugh@uhhs.com (S.D. Strausbaugh).

≥ 60 mEq/L or nasal potential difference consistent with CF), plus a family history of CF, sinopulmonary disease consistent with CF, or evidence of pancreatic insufficiency [11]. Genotyping is frequently done to aid in predicting pancreatic sufficiency and, to a lesser extent, severity of lung disease. This is feasible because nearly all patients who have CF have lesions in the same gene on chromosome 7, which encodes the CF transmembrane conductance regulator (CFTR), a cAMP-regulated chloride channel and a regulatory protein for other conductances.

Although investigation of symptoms is the most prevalent approach to diagnosis, newborn screening is becoming more prevalent in the United States. About half of the states are testing or are in the process of implementing a newborn screening program that uses blood spots from infant heel sticks. The initial screen is for immunoreactive trypsin level (IRT). Positive tests are repeated or subjected to a limited CFTR mutation screen. This series of tests yields a sensitivity of 87% for the IRT/IRT and 99% for the IRT/DNA test. Specificities are 99% for both [12]. Final diagnosis requires a sweat test or mutation analysis.

Several studies have evaluated the impact of newborn screening on various outcomes in CF. Using the Cystic Fibrosis Foundation registry data, Lai and colleagues [13] segregated patients into four diagnostic categories: (1) those diagnosed by newborn screening, (2) those diagnosed by meconium ileus (MI), (3) those diagnosed by symptoms other than MI, and (4) those diagnosed because of a family history of CF. She found that patients diagnosed due to MI or by symptoms had shorter survival (MI group: relative risk [RR], 1.8; 95% confidence interval [CI], 1.27–2.56; symptom group: RR, 1.76; 95% CI 1.24–2.48) compared with those diagnosed by screening. There was earlier pseudomonal acquisition and more patients who had a forced expiratory volume in 1 second (FEV_1) less than 70% predicted. In patients in the symptom group, those diagnosed by pulmonary and gastrointestinal (GI) symptoms had the highest risk of shortened survival compared with those without GI or pulmonary symptoms. The best outcomes were in patients who had other symptoms (not GI or pulmonary). Age at diagnosis was significantly associated with survival: For each year increase in age at diagnosis, the risk for shortened survival (3%; 95% CI, 2–4), acquisition of pseudomonas (5%; 95% CI, 3–7), or having and FEV_1 less than 70% predicted (3%; 95% CI, 1–5) decreased.

Assael and colleagues [14] did a population-based study in Italy where newborn screening has been in place since 1973. They found improved survival in patients diagnosed in the 1983 to 1992 cohort compared with the 1973 to 1982 cohort but no significant difference in survival in patients diagnosed in the 1993 to 2000 cohort compared with the 1983 to 1992 group. They found that calendar period of diagnosis is the best prognostic factor in CF (ie, patients diagnosed in more recent years live longer than those diagnosed earlier), even after newborn screening was in place. This observation strengthens the view that newer treatments and approaches to the disease, rather than early diagnosis, have improved survival in the last several years. The last period they describe (1993–2000) showed no improvement in survival. The authors postulate that perhaps CF-related complications such as CF-related diabetes or progressive liver disease, which tend to manifest more often in the second and third decades of life, balance the gains in survival from improved treatments. Based on these data, it is difficult to predict survival. Some studies do show benefits for newborn screening, including improved nutritional status in infancy and early childhood, lower rates of hospitalization, and better clinical scores in childhood. The extent to which early diagnosis influences long-term outcome is unclear [15–18].

Survival in CF has improved and may continue to improve. As patients live longer, it is possible that the complications that increase with advancing age will become more troublesome. On the other hand, new strategies for treatment may ameliorate these complications and their symptoms.

Clinical syndrome/treatment

The genetic and physiologic information obtained over the last two decades has led to an explosion of information on the structure and function of CFTR. This protein is expressed in several epithelia, including sweat duct, airway, pancreatic duct, intestine, biliary tree, and vas deferens. These discoveries provide a better understanding of epithelial cell biology and the pathogenesis of the CF disease and have led to new therapeutic approaches, including gene therapy, activation of alternative chloride channels, improving function of native CFTR, and correcting trafficking defects in native CFTR, which are now in clinical testing [19]. The level of functional CFTR is important in determining the manifestations of CF or may act as a disease modifier in other

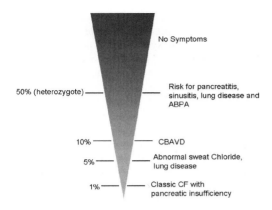

No Symptoms

50% (heterozygote) —— Risk for pancreatitis, sinusitis, lung disease and ABPA

10% —— CBAVD

5% —— Abnormal sweat Chloride, lung disease

1% —— Classic CF with pancreatic insufficiency

Fig. 1. CFTR activity and clinical manifestations. As the level of functional CFTR declines, more organ systems become involved. Once the functional level of CFTR is below approximately 5%, patients manifest the syndrome of CF. ABPA, allergic bronchopulmonary aspergillosis; CBAVD, congenital bilateral absence of the vas deferens. (*Data from* Davis PB. Cystic fibrosis since 1938. Am J Respir Crit Care Med 2006;173:475–82.)

disease states (Fig. 1). Therefore, even partial correction of the CF defect may produce significant clinical benefit.

Pulmonary disease

Lung disease is the primary cause of morbidity and mortality in CF. It is characterized by progressive cycles of infection and inflammation culminating in respiratory failure. At birth, the lungs of patients who have CF are nearly normal, although pathology specimens do show alterations in the submucosal glands consistent with glands that are already impacted with mucus [20]. The fact that the lungs are near normal at birth gives hope that early postnatal therapy directed at the basic defect might significantly reduce the morbidity and mortality in CF.

Infants who have CF contract the usual viral illnesses expected in infants but often have more symptoms with these episodes [21]. Infants who have CF, unlike healthy infants, develop bacterial pneumonias as well. These bacterial pneumonias clear with aggressive antibiotic treatment, but eventually permanent colonization of the airways occurs. Colonization probably occurs because of the thick, inspissated mucus in the airways, which traps inhaled microbes, and, because of a diminished periciliary fluid layer, mucociliary clearance in hindered. Because progressive lung disease is associated with bacterial colonization, strategies to prevent colonization are being tested in infants who have CF.

CF lung colonization and infection occurs with a distinctive spectrum of bacterial pathogens that are usually acquired in an age-dependent fashion (Fig. 2). Common organisms early in the course include *Staphylococcus aureus* and nontypable *Haemophilus influenzae* [22,23]. Later in the course of the disease, *Pseudomonas aeruginosa* is the most common pathogen, infecting approximately 80% of the population [24]. Acquisition of

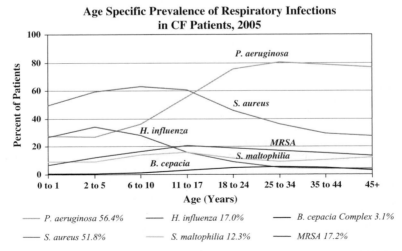

Age Specific Prevalence of Respiratory Infections in CF Patients, 2005

——— P. aeruginosa 56.4%   ——— H. influenza 17.0%   ——— B. cepacia Complex 3.1%
——— S. aureus 51.8%   ——— S. maltophilia 12.3%   ——— MRSA 17.2%

Fig. 2. Pulmonary colonization/infection follows an age-specific trend with respect to specific pathogens. (*From* 2005 Annual Data Report to the Center Directors. Cystic Fibrosis Patient Registry, Bethesda, MD; used with permission.)

Pseudomonas, especially mucoid strains, is associated with a more rapid clinical deterioration [23,25]. Other pathogens, such as *Stenotrophomonas maltophilia* or *Achromobacter xylosoxidans*, may be present but generally carry no worse prognosis. *Burkholderia cepacia* complex carries the worst prognosis. Some patients who have CF who acquire *B cepacia* develop a sepsis-like syndrome with severe necrotizing pneumonia called cepacia syndrome and have rapid deterioration, leading to death. Other patients who have *B cepacia* have a less dramatic course, though still with more rapid decline in lung function and higher mortality than those infected only with pseudomonas [26,27]. Of the nine genomovars within the cepacia complex of organisms, *B cenocepacia* (genomovar III) is the most frequently associated with cepacia syndrome [28].

Pulmonary fungal infection/colonization is common in CF. The most frequent fungal infection seen is *Candida* sp (50%–70% of patients), but this organism is generally considered commensal [29]. Aspergillus, on the other hand, is isolated from approximately 25% of patients [30] and can be associated with significant disease. Invasive aspergillosis, though rare, is often fatal. Allergic bronchopulmonary aspergillosis is fairly common, with an incidence of 3.2% for patients under 18 years of age and 5.2% for patients 18 years of age and older [24]. Allergic bronchopulmonary aspergillosis is caused by an exuberant allergic immunoglobulin E–mediated reaction to fungal antigens and is characterized by wheezing, pulmonary infiltrates, worsening bronchiectasis, and fibrosis [31].

About 13% of adults are colonized or infected by nontuberculous mycobacterium, most commonly the *Mycobacterium avium* complex (72%) or *M abscessus* (16%) [32]. Changes in high-resolution CT help distinguish between colonization and infection leading to progressive lung disease [33].

Airway infection leads to a marked, persistent neutrophilic inflammatory response that destroys small airways, leading to bronchiectasis. Inflammation has become an independent therapeutic target in CF. Angiogenesis in areas of intense inflammation predisposes patients to hemoptysis, which occurs in about 3.3% of adult patients per year. It is usually self-limiting, but occasionally embolization of a bronchial artery is required. The occurrence of hemoptysis does not alter life expectancy [34]. With continued inflammation, bronchial cysts and emphysema can develop. These areas are predisposed to pneumothorax.

Approximately 16% to 20% of adults who have CF have a pneumothorax at some point in their life, with an incidence of approximately 1% per year. Pneumothorax in CF is associated with a shortened survival (median survival 2 years after pneumothorax) [34].

Gastrointestinal disease

The presence of active CFTR in intestinal epithelium predicts that the GI tract will be a site of disease. Failure to secrete enough chloride and fluid into the gut can lead to reduced water content of the fecal stream, which results in the newborn period in meconium ileus (intestinal obstruction) in 11% to 20% of infants. It was previously associated with high mortality, but improved recognition and treatment strategies have reduced the mortality to under 10%, and long-term survival approaches that of the general CF population [35,36]. In older patients, distal intestinal obstruction syndrome, or "meconium ileus equivalent," can produce intermittent, recurrent episodes of partial small bowel obstruction, often near the ileo-cecal junction. Initially, obstruction may be incomplete, but, without treatment, it may progress to complete obstruction with vomiting and increasing abdominal distention. The incidence of distal intestinal obstruction syndrome is approximately 15% based on CFF registry data. Both genders seems to be affected equally, and all ages are affected. It is rarely fatal and is not associated with poorer prognosis. The CF abnormalities in the gut may lead, as they do in the lung, to excessive inflammation and contribute to the markedly increased incidence (12.5 fold) of Crohn's disease [37]. In addition, compared with age-matched control subjects, the odds ratio for GI malignancy in CF is 6.4 [38]. Therefor, rarer intestinal complications of CF can be severe.

Gastroesophageal reflux is common in CF. Over 20% of patients report heartburn or regurgitation-type symptoms [39]. Several factors likely contribute to gastroesophageal reflux disease, including large meals or large bolus tube feeds; head-down positions for airway clearance maneuvers; medications that reduce lower esophageal sphincter tone; and hyperexpansion of the lung, which flattens the diaphragm and impairs the physiologic sphincter [40]. Therapy with histamine receptor-2 blockers or proton pump inhibitors or even surgical intervention with a Nissen fundoplication may be required. The contribution of gastroesophageal reflux disease to the progression of pulmonary disease in CF is uncertain, but many physicians are vigorous in their treatment in part because of the possibility that there is some exacerbation associated with it.

Among the various GI organs affected by CF, exocrine pancreatic disease shows the strongest genotype/phenotype association. About 91% of patients are treated with pancreatic replacement therapy [24,40]. Frequently, destruction and loss of exocrine pancreatic function occurs at birth or in early infancy. Patients who have two severe mutations have pancreatic insufficiency; patients who have one or more mild mutations may be pancreatic sufficient. For patients who remain pancreatic sufficient, approximately 20% are at risk for developing acute or chronic pancreatitis [41]. There is a strong association with idiopathic pancreatitis and having one CFTR mutation [42]. Patients who have pancreatic insufficiency have worse prognosis than those who are pancreatic sufficient, but whether this is because of nutritional deficits or because the CFTR deficit is more severe is uncertain.

The liver is affected in CF in several ways. Most patients who have CF develop some level of liver disease, which may include elevated transaminases, hepatosteatosis, or biliary tract disease. Hepatic steatosis is common (20%–60% of patients) but is not correlated with outcome [43]. Cholelithiasis is also common, and 15% of adults have gallstones. A small number of patients who have CF develop frank liver disease with multilobar cirrhosis, portal fibrosis, cirrhosis, portal hypertension, and hypersplenism. This type of disease is usually diagnosed at median age 9 to 10 years [43,44] and progresses over time. No treatment has been shown to delay the progression of disease, but because it can be fatal, ursodeoxycholic acid, which improves the biochemical profile of liver disease, is often administered [45]. Liver disease was listed as the primary cause of death in 2.5% of deaths in patients who have CF, which places it as the second most common cause of death [24]. There were 11 liver transplants done in patients who had CF in 2005 [24].

Endocrine disease

As patients with CF live longer, CF-related diabetes (CFRD) is becoming more common. Patients who develop CFRD have an accelerated decline in clinical status, including lung function, and suffer higher mortality than those without CFRD [46–49]. The 2005 CFF registry data show that 14.3% of patients who have CF have CFRD or glucose intolerance, but intensive screening in one center showed a prevalence of CFRD of 11% over 5 years of age, and 17% had CFRD without fasting hyperglycemia [50].

The prevalence of CFRD increases with age. Moran [51] showed prevalence by age of 9% at 5 to 9 years, 26% at 10 to 19 years, 35% at 20 to 29 years, and 43% for over 30 years. As more patients survive into adulthood, the prevalence of CFRD is expected to increase. Microvascular complications of diabetes in CF can occur with increasing duration of diabetes and are likely to increase as the CF population ages [52]. Because of the impact of diabetes on the progression of lung disease and the potential for long-term diabetic complications, many centers treat aggressively, usually with insulin. The sulfonylureas, which increase insulin secretion, may delay the need for insulin therapy in some patients [53]. Peroxisome proliferator-activated receptor-γ agonists, which have been tested in type II diabetes as a means of delaying full-blown disease, have not been tested in CF, although they might confer a dual benefit because of their anti-inflammatory effect.

Bone disease is becoming a more prominent problem in CF, but its contribution to survival and symptomatology is not clear. CFF registry data for 2005 report 8.3% of patients over 18 years with osteopenia and 5% with frank osteoporosis, but only 0.4% have fractures [24]. The origins of bone disease are not fully understood but almost surely include steroid use, hypogonadism or delayed pubertal maturation, malabsorption of fat-soluble vitamins (especially vitamin K and D), poor nutritional status, inactivity, and chronic pulmonary inflammation, which causes elevated cytokine levels that increase bone resorption and suppress bone formation [54,55]. Bone mineral accrual is inadequate in CF, especially in late childhood and early adulthood, so there is reduced peak bone mineral density [56]. This, plus the accelerated bone losses, contributes significantly to bone diseases in CF [57]. Prevention of disease is crucial, with aggressive nutritional interventions, vitamin/mineral supplementation, and yearly screening. The data for the use of bisphosphonates in CF is minimal [54]; however, clinical trials are ongoing.

Changing demographics

Survival of patients who have CF has improved (Figs. 3 and 4) such that the median predicted

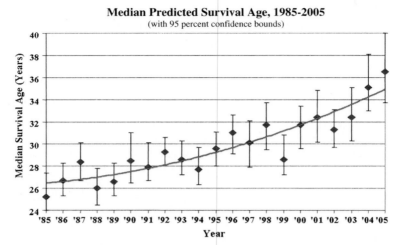

Fig. 3. As of August 2006, the median survival is 36.5 years for 2005. This represents the age by which half of the current CF registry population would be expected to be dead, given the ages of the patients in the registry and the mortality distribution of the deaths in 2005. The whiskers represent the 95% confidence intervals for the survival estimates, so the 2005 median predicted survival is between 33.7 and 40.0 years. (*From* 2005 Annual Data Report to the Center Directors. Cystic Fibrosis Patient Registry, Bethesda, MD; used with permission.)

survival for 2005 is 36.5 years [24]. Longitudinal cohort studies (epidemiologic study of cystic fibrosis) and national patient registries provide a tremendous resource that is available to all participating CF centers for studies of genetic, environmental, and therapeutic influences on CF survival. These resources place CF in the forefront of epidemiologic studies of genetic diseases [58]. Genetic factors, environmental factors, and treatment patterns influence the course of the disease.

Survival is influenced by the specific CF mutation. The more than 1500 mutations

described in the CFTR gene have been divided into classes based on the type of defect (Table 1) [59]. Class 1, 2, or 3 mutations are associated with more severe disease, worse pulmonary function, and pancreatic insufficiency. Class 4 or 5 mutations are associated with milder pulmonary disease and pancreatic sufficiency. McKone and colleagues [60], using standard mortality rates, showed that patients who have mutations in classes 1, 2, or 3 had higher mortality compared with patients who had class 4 or 5 mutations (RR, 2.25, 95% CI, 1.77–2.84; $P < .001$). Patients who have

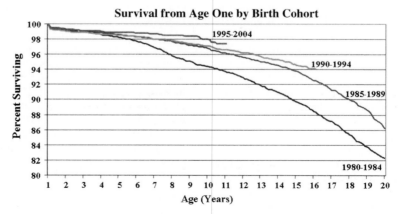

Fig. 4. Actual survival of patients in the registry has steadily improved since 1980. (*From* 2005 Annual Data Report to the Center Directors. Cystic Fibrosis Patient Registry, Bethesda, MD; used with permission.)

Table 1
Mutations in the CFTR gene based on type of defect

Class of mutation	CFTR production and function
Class 1 mutations	Defective protein production with premature termination of CFTR production
Class 2 mutations	Defective trafficking of CFTR so that it does not reach the apical surface membrane
Class 3 mutations	Defective regulation of CFTR despite the ability to reach the apical cell surface
Class 4 mutations	Defective channel conduction through CFTR despite reaching the apical surface
Class 5 mutations	Associated with reduced synthesis of functional CFTR
Class 6 mutations	CFTR reaches the apical surface but has more rapid turnover

class 4 or 5 mutations were also found to have increased FEV_1, better weight for height, and lower rates of Pseudomonas acquisition and pancreatic sufficiency, thus linking intermediate endpoints with the mortality data. The investigators caution that although there seems to be a difference in mortality when comparing classes of mutations, substantial phenotype variability exists. Recent studies on gene modifiers have indicated that some genetic variants significantly influence survival among patients who have the same CF mutations. The first of these to be confirmed in a large study is a genetic variant in the gene for transforming growth factor–β [61]. It is likely that the genetic makeup apart from CF accounts for at least some of the variability in disease severity.

Observations on survival trends show an improvement in survival in the 2- to 15-year age group. Between 1985 and 1999, mortality fell 61% (95% CI, 38–71) for patients 2 to 5 years of age, 70% (95% CI, 60–88) for patients 6 to 10 years of age, and 45% (95% CI, 32–66) for patients 11 to 15 years of age. Mortality rates improve only minimally for patients older than 15 years. Both genders showed this trend, but female survival was consistently lower than male survival between 2 and 20 years [62]. Potential contributors to

improved survival include improved nutritional intervention/management and the introduction of new therapies. Goss and Rosenfeld [58] also speculate that the minimal improvement in survival seen in adults may be because a result of the newly introduced therapies that impart less benefit for older individuals who have more advanced lung disease. Alternatively (or in addition), there is a potential survivor effect such that patients who have reached older ages survived without the new therapeutic interventions, so these treatments do not confer large benefit in this group. In the future, improved health in the younger population will allow more patients to approach adulthood in better health, thereby improving the survival of adults over time.

Using ESCF data, Johnson and colleagues [63] divided CF centers into quartiles based on patients' FEV_1 and assessed differences in treatment strategies for upper- compared with lower-quartile centers. The sites reporting highest median FEV_1 (upper quartile) had more frequent outpatient visits, had more frequent measurements of spirometry, and obtained sputum cultures more often. More patients were on inhaled cromolyn or nedocromil and oral corticosteroids in the upper-quartile centers. Upper-quartile centers used intravenous antibiotics more frequently and for longer durations. Upper-quartile centers also had a higher rate of multidrug-resistant micro-organisms, which may be related to increased antibiotic use, ascertainment bias (increased frequency of obtaining cultures), or both. The investigators concluded that there is a significant difference in intensity of care in centers with the best results compared with those with the poorest results (as defined by median FEV_1), with the middle two quartiles being intermediate. Thus, increased frequency of patient visits and aggressive interventions such as intravenous antibiotics could result in improved outcomes for patients who have CF.

There is a link between median household income and mortality rates. There is a 44% increased risk of death in patients who have a household income of less than $20,000/year, compared with those with household income of $50,000/year or more. The incidence of death decreased consistently across increasing household income strata. At each age, patients who had a higher median household income had better lung function and increased weight for height. There was no clear evidence of inadequate access to treatment modalities in the lower socioeconomic groups [64,65]. Other factors must contribute. One possibility is pollution in the environment, which may be greater in areas where patients in the lower socioeconomic strata reside. Goss and colleagues [66] showed that an increased exposure to particulate air pollution and ozone was linearly associated with an increased risk of pulmonary exacerbation. He also postulates that a significant proportion of the heterogeneity of CF lung disease may be attributable to factors that track with median household income and exposure to air pollution.

Improvements in outcomes for patients who have CF have been striking in the last 30 years. Median survival now approaches the fifth decade of life. Advances in the understanding of the basic defect and the pathobiology of CF have led to new treatments, some of which have contributed to this success. Improved understanding of the basic defect and the acquisition and maintenance of epidemiologic resources for the CF population in the United States have allowed us to determine predictors of survival and to identify genetic, environmental, and therapeutic factors that may influence it. Understanding the modifying genetic factors may lead to new therapeutic targets. Environmental factors can be changed, and new therapeutic agents and the overall aggressive approach to the disease can be better understood and implemented. Treatments directed at the basic defect, including drugs to activate mutant forms of CFTR and gene therapy, are now in and coming to clinical trial. There are many reasons for optimism today for patients who have CF.

References

[1] Andersen D. Cystic fibrosis of the pancreas and its relation to celiac disease. Am J Dis Child 1938;56: 344–99.

[2] Farber S. Pancreatic function and disease in early life v. pathologic changes associated with pancreatic insufficiency in early life. Arch Pathol 1944;37:238.

[3] Andersen D, Hodges R. Celiac syndrome v. genetics of cystic fibrosis of the pancreas with a consideration etiology. Am J Dis Child 1946;72:62.

[4] Di Sant'Agnese PA, Darling RC, Perera GA, et al. Abnormal electrolyte composition of sweat in cystic fibrosis of the pancreas: clinical significance and relationship to the disease. Pediatrics 1953;12(5): 549–63.

[5] Quinton PM. Chloride impermeability in cystic fibrosis. Nature 1983;301(5899):421–2.

[6] Tsui LC, Buchwald M, Barker D, et al. Cystic fibrosis locus defined by a genetically linked polymorphic DNA marker. Science 1985;230(4729):1054–7.

[7] Rommens JM, Iannuzzi MC, Kerem B, et al. Identification of the cystic fibrosis gene: chromosome walking and jumping. Science 1989;245(4922): 1059–65.

[8] Riordan JR, Rommens JM, Kerem B, et al. Identification of the cystic fibrosis gene: cloning and characterization of complementary DNA. Science 1989; 245(4922):1066–73.

[9] Kerem B, Rommens JM, Buchanan JA, et al. Identification of the cystic fibrosis gene: genetic analysis. Science 1989;245(4922):1073–80.

[10] Orenstein D, Rosenstein B, Stern R. Diagnosis of cystic fibrosis. In: Orenstein D, Rosenstein B, Stern R, editors. Cystic fibrosis medical care. Philidelphia: Lippincott Williams & WIlkins; 2000. p. 21–54.

[11] Rosenstein BJ, Cutting GR. The diagnosis of cystic fibrosis: a consensus statement. Cystic Fibrosis Foundation Consensus Panel. J Pediatr 1998; 132(4):589–95.

[12] Rock MJ, Hoffman G, Laessig RH, et al. Newborn screening for cystic fibrosis in Wisconsin: nine-year experience with routine trypsinogen/DNA testing. J Pediatr 2005;147(3 Suppl):S73–7.

[13] Lai HJ, Cheng Y, Cho H, et al. Association between initial disease presentation, lung disease outcomes, and survival in patients with cystic fibrosis. Am J Epidemiol 2004;159(6):537–46.

[14] Assael BM, Castellani C, Ocampo MB, et al. Epidemiology and survival analysis of cystic fibrosis in an area of intense neonatal screening over 30 years. Am J Epidemiol 2002;156(5):397–401.

[15] Dankert-Roelse JE, te Meerman GJ, Martijn A, et al. Survival and clinical outcome in patients with cystic fibrosis, with or without neonatal screening. J Pediatr 1989;114(3):362–7.

[16] Dankert-Roelse JE, te Meerman GJ. Long term prognosis of patients with cystic fibrosis in relation to early detection by neonatal screening and treatment in a cystic fibrosis centre. Thorax 1995;50(7): 712–8.

[17] Farrell PM, Kosorok MR, Laxova A, et al. Nutritional benefits of neonatal screening for cystic fibrosis. Wisconsin Cystic Fibrosis Neonatal Screening Study Group. N Engl J Med 1997; 337(14):963–9.

[18] Orenstein DM, Boat TF, Stern RC, et al. The effect of early diagnosis and treatment in cystic fibrosis: a seven-year study of 16 sibling pairs. Am J Dis Child 1977;131(9):973–5.

[19] Davis PB, Drumm M, Konstan MW. Cystic fibrosis. Am J Respir Crit Care Med 1996;154(5): 1229–56.

[20] Sturgess J, Imrie J. Quantitative evaluation of the development of tracheal submucosal glands in infants with cystic fibrosis and control infants. Am J Pathol 1982;106(3):303–11.

[21] Wang EE, Prober CG, Manson B, et al. Association of respiratory viral infections with pulmonary

deterioration in patients with cystic fibrosis. N Engl J Med 1984;311(26):1653–8.

[22] Armstrong DS, Grimwood K, Carlin JB, et al. Lower airway inflammation in infants and young children with cystic fibrosis. Am J Respir Crit Care Med 1997;156(4 Pt 1):1197–204.

[23] Rosenfeld M, Gibson RL, McNamara S, et al. Early pulmonary infection, inflammation, and clinical outcomes in infants with cystic fibrosis. Pediatr Pulmonol 2001;32(5):356–66.

[24] CFF Patient Registry. 2005 Annual Data Report to the Center Directors. Bethesda (MD): Cystic Fibrosis Foundation; 2006.

[25] Henry RL, Mellis CM, Petrovic L. Mucoid Pseudomonas aeruginosa is a marker of poor survival in cystic fibrosis. Pediatr Pulmonol 1992;12(3):158–61.

[26] Thomassen MJ, Demko CA, Klinger JD, et al. Pseudomonas cepacia colonization among patients with cystic fibrosis: a new opportunist. Am Rev Respir Dis 1985;131(5):791–6.

[27] Isles A, Maclusky I, Corey M, et al. Pseudomonas cepacia infection in cystic fibrosis: an emerging problem. J Pediatr 1984;104(2):206–10.

[28] Lipuma JJ. Update on the Burkholderia cepacia complex. Curr Opin Pulm Med 2005;11(6):528–33.

[29] Burns JL, Emerson J, Stapp JR, et al. Microbiology of sputum from patients at cystic fibrosis centers in the United States. Clin Infect Dis 1998;27(1):158–63.

[30] Bakare N, Rickerts V, Bargon J, et al. Prevalence of Aspergillus fumigatus and other fungal species in the sputum of adult patients with cystic fibrosis. Mycoses 2003;46(1–2):19–23.

[31] Greenberger PA. Allergic bronchopulmonary aspergillosis. J Allergy Clin Immunol 2002;110(5):685–92.

[32] Olivier KN, Weber DJ, Wallace RJ Jr, et al. Nontuberculous mycobacteria. I: multicenter prevalence study in cystic fibrosis. Am J Respir Crit Care Med 2003;167(6):828–34.

[33] Olivier KN, Weber DJ, Lee JH, et al. Nontuberculous mycobacteria. II: nested-cohort study of impact on cystic fibrosis lung disease. Am J Respir Crit Care Med 2003;167(6):835–40.

[34] Schidlow DV, Taussig LM, Knowles MR. Cystic Fibrosis Foundation consensus conference report on pulmonary complications of cystic fibrosis. Pediatr Pulmonol 1993;15(3):187–98.

[35] Kerem E, Corey M, Kerem B, et al. Clinical and genetic comparisons of patients with cystic fibrosis, with or without meconium ileus. J Pediatr 1989;114(5):767–73.

[36] Mabogunje OA, Wang CI, Mahour H. Improved survival of neonates with meconium ileus. Arch Surg 1982;117(1):37–40.

[37] Lloyd-Still JD. Crohn's disease and cystic fibrosis. Dig Dis Sci 1994;39(4):880–5.

[38] Neglia JP, FitzSimmons SC, Maisonneuve P, et al. The risk of cancer among patients with cystic fibrosis. Cystic Fibrosis and Cancer Study Group. N Engl J Med 1995;332(8):494–9.

[39] Scott RB, O'Loughlin EV, Gall DG. Gastroesophageal reflux in patients with cystic fibrosis. J Pediatr 1985;106(2):223–7.

[40] Ferry G, Klish W, Borowitz D, et al. Concensus conference for GI problems in CF. Presented at the Consensus Conference Gastrointestinal Problems in CF. Bethesda (MD), June 3–4, 1991.

[41] Couper RT, Corey M, Moore DJ, et al. Decline of exocrine pancreatic function in cystic fibrosis patients with pancreatic sufficiency. Pediatr Res 1992;32(2):179–82.

[42] Cohn JA, Friedman KJ, Noone PG, et al. Relation between mutations of the cystic fibrosis gene and idiopathic pancreatitis. N Engl J Med 1998;339(10):653–8.

[43] Sokol RJ, Durie PR. Recommendations for management of liver and biliary tract disease in cystic fibrosis. Cystic Fibrosis Foundation Hepatobiliary Disease Consensus Group. J Pediatr Gastroenterol Nutr 1999;28(Suppl 1):S1–13.

[44] Borowitz D, Durie PR, Clarke LL, et al. Gastrointestinal outcomes and confounders in cystic fibrosis. J Pediatr Gastroenterol Nutr 2005;41(3):273–85.

[45] Galabert C, Montet JC, Lengrand D, et al. Effects of ursodeoxycholic acid on liver function in patients with cystic fibrosis and chronic cholestasis. J Pediatr 1992;121(1):138–41.

[46] Lanng S, Thorsteinsson B, Nerup J, et al. Influence of the development of diabetes mellitus on clinical status in patients with cystic fibrosis. Eur J Pediatr 1992;151(9):684–7.

[47] Milla CE, Warwick WJ, Moran A. Trends in pulmonary function in patients with cystic fibrosis correlate with the degree of glucose intolerance at baseline. Am J Respir Crit Care Med 2000;162(3 Pt 1):891–5.

[48] Moran A, Hardin D, Rodman D, et al. Diagnosis, screening and management of cystic fibrosis related diabetes mellitus: a consensus conference report. Diabetes Res Clin Pract 1999;45(1):61–73.

[49] Marshall BC, Butler SM, Stoddard M, et al. Epidemiology of cystic fibrosis-related diabetes. J Pediatr 2005;146(5):681–7.

[50] Moran A, Doherty L, Wang X, et al. Abnormal glucose metabolism in cystic fibrosis. J Pediatr 1998;133(1):10–7.

[51] Moran A. Cystic fibrosis-related diabetes: an approach to diagnosis and management. Pediatr Diabetes 2000;1(1):41–8.

[52] Brennan AL, Geddes DM, Gyi KM, et al. Clinical importance of cystic fibrosis-related diabetes. J Cyst Fibros 2004;3(4):209–22.

[53] Rosenecker J, Eichler I, Barmeier H, et al. Diabetes mellitus and cystic fibrosis: comparison of clinical parameters in patients treated with insulin versus oral glucose-lowering agents. Pediatr Pulmonol 2001;32(5):351–5.

[54] Aris RM, Merkel PA, Bachrach LK, et al. Guide to bone health and disease in cystic fibrosis. J Clin Endocrinol Metab 2005;90(3):1888–96.

[55] Hecker TM, Aris RM. Management of osteoporosis in adults with cystic fibrosis. Drugs 2004;64(2):133–47.

[56] Bhudhikanok GS, Wang MC, Marcus R, et al. Bone acquisition and loss in children and adults with cystic fibrosis: a longitudinal study. J Pediatr 1998; 133(1):18–27.

[57] Haworth CS, Selby PL, Horrocks AW, et al. A prospective study of change in bone mineral density over one year in adults with cystic fibrosis. Thorax 2002;57(8):719–23.

[58] Goss CH, Rosenfeld M. Update on cystic fibrosis epidemiology. Curr Opin Pulm Med 2004;10(6): 510–4.

[59] Choo-Kang LR, Zeitlin PL. Type I, II, III, IV, and V cystic fibrosis transmembrane conductance regulator defects and opportunities for therapy. Curr Opin Pulm Med 2000;6(6):521–9.

[60] McKone EF, Emerson SS, Edwards KL, et al. Effect of genotype on phenotype and mortality in cystic fibrosis: a retrospective cohort study. Lancet 2003; 361(9370):1671–6.

[61] Drumm ML, Konstan MW, Schluchter MD, et al. Genetic modifiers of lung disease in cystic fibrosis. N Engl J Med 2005;353(14):1443–53.

[62] Kulich M, Rosenfeld M, Goss CH, et al. Improved survival among young patients with cystic fibrosis. J Pediatr 2003;142(6):631–6.

[63] Johnson C, Butler SM, Konstan MW, et al. Factors influencing outcomes in cystic fibrosis: a center-based analysis. Chest 2003;123(1):20–7.

[64] Schechter MS, Shelton BJ, Margolis PA, et al. The association of socioeconomic status with outcomes in cystic fibrosis patients in the United States. Am J Respir Crit Care Med 2001;163(6):1331–7.

[65] O'Connor GT, Quinton HB, Kneeland T, et al. Median household income and mortality rate in cystic fibrosis. Pediatrics 2003;111(4 Pt 1): e333–9.

[66] Goss CH, Newsom SA, Schildcrout JS, et al. Effect of ambient air pollution on pulmonary exacerbations and lung function in cystic fibrosis. Am J Respir Crit Care Med 2004;169(7):816–21.

ELSEVIER SAUNDERS

Clin Chest Med 28 (2007) 289–296

CLINICS IN CHEST MEDICINE

Pathogenesis of Bronchiectasis

Brian M. Morrissey, MD

Division of Pulmonary/Critical Care Medicine, Department of Internal Medicine, School of Medicine, University of California–Davis, 4150 V Street, Suite 3400, Sacramento, CA 95817, USA

Cystic fibrosis: pathogenesis of bronchiectasis

Despite improvements in childhood health—nutrition, immunizations, tuberculosis control, and improved access to antibiotics—chronic pulmonary infections and bronchiectasis remain significant clinical issues worldwide. Bronchiectasis manifests differently among patients, particularly in the areas of inciting pathology, causative organisms, and prognosis. Specifically, cystic fibrosis (CF) typically follows a more severe clinical course than non-CF bronchiectasis. Despite these and other recognized differences, the underpinnings of respiratory biology support a common pathogeneses of the anatomic deformations of bronchiectasis. This article reviews the observed manifestations among the related diseases of bronchiectasis and CF and discusses some of their similarities and differences.

Clinical features

Bronchiectasis refers to the anatomic distortion of conducting airways (thickening, herniation, or dilation) and is clinically characterized by chronic respiratory symptoms such as cough and sputum production. Pulmonary function testing in early or mild disease may be normal or reveal diminished late forced expiratory flow rates ($FEF_{25\%}$). A more obvious obstructive pattern develops that may be followed by a mixed pattern (obstructive/restrictive) as disease progresses. Most cases of bronchiectasis are attributable to previous childhood or prolonged pulmonary infections [1,2]. Less commonly, congenital disease, airway injuries, or toxic inhalational exposure may lead to bronchiectasis [3]. The incidence of non–CF-related bronchiectasis is difficult to determine [4]. The apparent decrease in non-CF bronchiectasis over the past decades is attributed to the increased use of antibiotics and improved overall childhood health [5]. Decreases in childhood respiratory illnesses (eg, measles, varicella, tuberculosis, influenza) and improved management of the occasional complicating bacterial infection have decreased the incidence of non-CF bronchiectasis [6]. Data available for CF, with an incidence of 1 in 2500 Caucasian births, suggest that CF is the largest single cause of chronic lung infection with resultant bronchiectasis in Western industrialized countries [7]. Childhood respiratory illnesses seem to be more severe or prolonged in children who have CF, suggesting a common vulnerability of the respiratory tract during youth. Although CF is a systemic genetic disorder appearing with prominent gastrointestinal, pulmonary, and reproductive manifestations, this article focuses on local mechanisms and does not fully address the systemic effects on the pulmonary disease.

Recognition of bronchiectasis

The anatomic changes of bronchiectasis are most clearly visualized by CT of the chest. In CF and non-CF bronchiectasis, early changes on CT identify disease even before the development of significant symptoms or pulmonary function abnormalities [8]. Early patterns of disease include air-trapping, bronchial wall thickening, and bronchiolitis [8]. CT findings of more severe disease include nontapering airways, increased ratio of airway to artery size, and nodules (representing mucus inspissation in airways).

Vicious circles

When bronchiectasis is established, the now-compromised clearance mechanisms of the

E-mail address: bnmorrissey@ucdavis.edu

0272-5231/07/$ - see front matter © 2007 Published by Elsevier Inc.
doi:10.1016/j.ccm.2007.02.014

airways result in repeated or prolonged respiratory infections; the chronic infections ensconced in the crypts and dilations of the distorted airways continue a self-perpetuating cycle of infection, which leads to more inflammation and further airway damage. Bronchiectasis names the essentially irreversible anatomic and histologic pathogenic changes to the respiratory airways—thickening, dilation, ectasia, and increased tortuosness. Histologic examination of areas of bronchiectasis shows that airways are grossly dilated (up to sixfold or more), with irregularly thickened bronchial walls and luminal strictures. The thickened walls may contain increased numbers of enlarged submucosal glands, increased collagen deposition, and areas of increased vascularity. Autopsies and examinations of explanted lungs reveal (within airways of nearly any size) mucus retention or mucus plugging, which are gross examples of impaired clearance. The mucus plugs contain high numbers of neutrophils and large amounts of mucin [9]. The epithelial surfaces show findings of bronchitis (intense neutrophil infiltration, increased goblet cells), desquamation, and patches of squamous metaplasia [10].

The anatomic changes of bronchiectasis disrupt various aspects of the normal airways' clearance mechanisms and represent an impairment of innate immunity. Thus, bronchiectasis impairs control, prevention, and resolution of respiratory tract disease. This vicious circle of bronchiectasis describes the recurrence or persistence of airway infection and inflammation, which leads to further structural damage that predisposes to prolonged infection; thus, it acts as a self-promoting cycle [11,12]. This pathologic paradigm implicates that the persistence and progression of bronchiectasis is due, at least in part, to positive feedback [11,13].

This autoprogressive airway pathology is present in patients who have CF-related and non-CF bronchiectasis. The abnormal airway physically and biochemically impairs restoration of normal airway biology. So far absent from this paradigm is the identification of the inciting event or trigger of bronchiectasis. Severe infections during childhood (a period of lung development) may explain some cases; however, unique exposures have not been identified among most of the individuals who have non-CF bronchiectasis. The typical presumed inciting events are more common than bronchiectasis itself. That is, more individuals have severe childhood respiratory infections than develop bronchiectasis. It remains to be fully explained why some of these individuals develop significant sequelae (chronic infections or bronchiectasis) and others do not. Likewise, we cannot yet predict why some patients who have CF fare better than others, even if they carry identical cystic fibrosis transmembrane regulator (CFTR) protein genotypes.

When the anatomic changes of bronchiectasis are present in an individual who has CF, the pattern of respiratory disease and progressive decline are well recognized: intermittent pulmonary exacerbations with increasing frequency and progressive pulmonary decline. This pattern mirrors the patterns seen in cases of severe non-CF bronchiectasis. The rate of this clinical decline is widely variable and depends on clinical, environmental, and genetic factors. What is the pathogenesis of the bronchiectasis and what are the mechanisms of positive feedback? Which of these deleterious positive feedbacks is due to a primary genetic abnormality or is secondary to induced phenotypic change. At times, it is unclear whether the changes are in response to the altered environment, subsequent infections, or other acquired changes? The following sections review and explore the pathogenesis and possible causes of CF-related bronchiectasis.

Hygiene disruption in the cystic fibrosis airway

In the normal human respiratory tract, several components of innate immunity protect the respiratory tract from constant environmental exposures (particulates, microorganisms, oxygen, and so forth). Fundamental among these protections within the lower respiratory tract are airway clearance (primarily the mucociliary elevator), physicochemical barriers (represented by the mucus-sol constituents of the airway surface liquid [ASL]), and cell-based innate defenses.

Mechanical clearance

Clearance in the normal lung has two major mechanisms, the mucociliary elevator (with cough) and phagocytic mechanisms. For clearance at the extremes of the lung anatomy—alveolar ducts and trachea—the movements of respiration and cough, respectively, contribute to normal pulmonary clearance. In the larger conducting airways, cough can effectively mobilize large quantities of mucus or foreign bodies. Effective cough is an explosive release of air at the release of expiration against an initially closed glottis. The high airflows in cough generate shearing forces within the airways. The shearing effect is increased by the anterior displacement of the pars flaccida. In severe cases of large airway bronchiectasis such as tracheobronchomegaly (Mounier-Kuhn's syndrome), clearance is less effective, in part due to the impairment of cough efficiency [14]. In CF, this condition is not typically seen except in the most severe and advanced stages.

Mucus's viscoelastic (ie, thixotropy or dilatant) physical properties facilitate centripetal propulsion and efficient globular clearance during cough. Dilatant substances are "stiffer" when greater energy is applied (eg, cough) and more pliable with low-energy manipulations; thixotropy substances exhibit the converse. Changes to these non-Newtonian properties are thought to impede ciliary movement or expectoration. Mucus in patients who have severe lung infection including CF may lose this characteristic [15]. Such a loss represents an impairment of sputum clearance and may not be unique to CF [16,17].

Beyond the columnar ciliated respiratory epithelium of the conducting airways, it is postulated that the ASL of the alveolar ducts is moved centripetally by the mechanical actions of normal respirations.

In the normal conducting airways, ciliated respiratory epithelium predominates, with a constituent surface liquid made of a periciliary lower-viscosity sol layer and a second, more luminal mucus layer of higher viscosity. Continuous centripetal movement of the ASL maintains an ever-renewing trap for exogenous substances to be transported up and away from the alveolar spaces, helping to maintain the normally pathogen-free lungs. In the most distal of airways, the mechanical changes associated with respiration support and foster the centripetal clearance of these less densely ciliated airways. Mucus production and ciliary beat are frequency stimulated by various stimuli and may range from minimal secretions in the healthy, unexposed individual to large quantities of secretions with chronic smoke or pathogen exposure [18]. Dramatic increases in mucus production can increase sputum transit times. In CF, mucociliary transit time (exclusive of cough) is for the most part (but not universally) found to be prolonged compared with normal subjects or other disease states [19].

The fundamental importance of ciliary motility to clearance of the respiratory tract is illustrated in part by primary ciliary dyskinesia (PCD). This group of syndromes describes individuals in whom ciliary function is impaired. In some cases, the cilia are immotile, whereas in others, the cilia are disorganized or have ineffective motility [20]. PCD, a genetic disorder of the cilia with a dysfunctional mucociliary elevator, leads to chronic sinopulmonary disease. The vast majority of individuals who have PCD develop bronchiectasis with lower-lobe predominance. Comparing PCD with CF, it is found that similar respiratory pathogens emerge and mucus velocity is impaired in both groups. Individuals who have PCD, however, develop bronchiectasis and infections at older ages. Also in contradistinction from CF, patients who have PCD can expect to live well into maturity. In PCD, cough, and respiratory hygiene mechanisms appear to provide effective adaptation to disordered ciliary function. Of interest, ultrastructural examination of the ciliated epithelial cells in chronically infected airways in CF or non-CF bronchiectasis reveal disrupted ciliary structure reminiscent of that seen in PCD [21]. Because these findings are seen only in areas of infection, these changes appear to be secondary to infection rather than a primary predisposing abnormality [22].

In the trachea and bronchi, submucosal mucus glands contribute most of the ASL. Within these glands, goblet cells are the primary mucus-producing cells, with serous cells contributing and controlling the water content [9]. In the conducting airways, ASL forms a mucus blanket layered atop a more proximate periciliary sol layer. Ordered and rhythmic beating of the cilia propel the mucus layer centripetally from the terminal airways toward the central airways [19]. The salt and water contents of the sol layer are also regulated at the apical membrane of epithelial cells. Within this sol layer, ciliary activity propels the mucus blanket centripetally. The cilia extend through the sol and, with clawlike extensions, engage and propel the mucus layer forward. Due to the defective CFTR function, the height and volumes of the periciliary sol layer are decreased in CF [23]. With the lowered height, no longer are just the tips of the cilia within in the mucus layer, but large portions of the cilia engage and thus frustrate the forward movement of flakes of mucus. Scanning electron micrographs show plaque-like formations that appear to entangle the cilia; thus, the effective clearance of the airways in CF is slowed in comparison to healthy airways [24].

Beyond the cartilaginous bronchi, mucus glands become less common and luminal goblet cells and clara cells start to predominate. At the level of bronchioles and the respiratory and terminal bronchioles, the ciliated epithelium transitions to primarily cuboid ciliated epithelial cells and clara cells. Finally, at the level of the alveolar duct, the airways are no longer ciliated.

Airway barriers

Constituents of the respiratory ASL, especially mucins, act as a protective physicochemical barrier [25]. Various mucins (eg, MUC5B, MUC5AC)—large complex molecules with carbohydrate side-chain moieties that are negatively charged and readily bind exogenous particles, organisms, and other molecules—form the bulk of the mucus layer [26]. The constituents of the mucus layer are largely products of submucosal glands. In CF, the mucin-producing cells and mucin products appear to be similar to the glands in non-CF airways; the identified changes in CF mucins (eg, suphonulruation) are likely due to post-translational and even postsecretory modification [27]. The larger glands in individuals who have CF expel their products more slowly, contain less water, and are possibly more viscous [28].

The periciliary sol portion of the ASL has an altered chemistry and is less abundant in CF. The decreased height of the sol layer decreases the buffer space between the mucus blanket with its exogenous constituents (eg, bacteria, fungi). It has been postulated that loss of this distance may allow bacteria trapped in the mucus layer easier access to the underlying epithelial cells, thus potentially stimulating epithelial cell inflammatory processes [29]. Indeed, several important pathogens (eg, *Pseudomonas aeruginosa*) possess receptor binding capacities to epithelial cells [30]. Although the precise constituents of the periciliary liquid are debated, whatever these changes are, they are likely to modify the chemistry of secondary defenses (eg, thiols, mucins, defensins). Among the nonmucin components of the ASL are small antibacterial peptides (eg, defensins) and various molecules that have antioxidant substances (eg, glutathione, ascorbic acid, glycoconjugates) known to play a role in overall respiratory tract defenses.

Inflammatory responses

Inflammation of CF airways is characterized by persistence and intensity. This inflammatory response may be primary or a result of persistent infection. Although diverse in etiology, cases of non-CF and CF-related forms of bronchiectasis share inflammatory pathways that are largely responsible for the destruction and remodeling of the respiratory tract that, in turn, are responsible for part of the pathobiology of bronchiectasis. Both forms manifest with neutrophil-dominant inflammation [31,32]. Their inflammatory profiles show increased and persistently elevated proinflammatory cytokines (eg, interleukin [IL]-1, IL-6, tumor necrosis factor [TNF]) with coincidently low anti-inflammatory cytokines (eg, IL-10) [12]. Systemic markers of inflammation such as elevated white blood cell counts, serum TNF-α levels, and serum C-reactive protein levels often remain chronically elevated [12,33]. Observations of lower levels of IL-10 and compromised antibacterial capacity contribute to the persistence of a proinflammatory state and may be heightened in CF [34] but remain controversial. Efforts to compare CF forms to non-CF forms suggest that the intensity of inflammation may be proportional to level of infection [35]. In CF, a controversy exists as to whether the proinflammatory state precedes infection [36] or is subsequent to infection [37]. In practice, the findings of airway inflammation and infection are present in most individuals who express the CF phenotype.

Overly exuberant inflammatory responses in cystic fibrosis

Whether the airway inflammatory response is extraordinarily robust or not, its presence is a primary feature in furthering the airway damage of bronchiectasis and compromising the resolution of infection, be it CF or non-CF bronchiectasis. Clinical markers of inflammation in patients who have CF are thought by some to be excessive relative to the degree of airway infection and remain elevated for long periods of time, especially during periods of exacerbation [38,39]. The presence of the exaggerated inflammatory response represents the most likely cause for the increased severity of bronchiectasis in CF [39]. A recent review outlines the potential mechanisms and laboratory evidence focused on the hypothesis that the CF airway has an overly exuberant inflammatory response [29].

Examinations of the airway mucus do not reliability demonstrate significant differences [40]. Certainly, the clinical data support higher levels in CF. What specific role the dysfunctional CFTR protein plays (as a primary cause or a secondary effect, as discussed earlier) is less certain.

It is important to note that the inflammatory response itself promotes release of proteases (eg, collagenase, elastase, trypsin) that are associated with further damage to the epithelium [41]. Activated airway neutrophils and their proteases have been strongly implicated in disrupting mucociliary clearances, inducing mucus secretion and potentiating epithelial injury [42].

Foreign-body aspiration

Foreign-body aspiration offers an example of combined disordered clearance and intense inflammation leading to bronchiectasis. Two characteristics of foreign-body aspiration in children alter the risk of resultant bronchiectasis: the time to removal and the proinflammatory characteristics of the aspirant [43]. In otherwise-healthy young children who aspirate foreign bodies, the likelihood that focal bronchiectasis develops is proportional to the length of time the foreign body remains blocking the airway. This example supports the idea that the fundamental need for clearance is an integral part of host hygiene, with time to clearance of the essence. In addition, proinflammatory objects such as peanuts or other organic material lead to more complications attributed to the provoked and secondary inflammation. Analogously, in CF and non-CF bronchiectasis, mucus plugging and proinflammatory elements (eg, aspergillus allergy) are associated with more exacerbations of disease [44].

Phagocyte functionality

The second method of clearing the respiratory tract of exogenous (eg, microorganisms, particulates) and endogenous (eg, apoptotic cells) debris is phagocytosis [45]. This cell-based clearance function is performed by numerous cellular constituents of the respiratory tract, particularly macrophages. Macrophage dysfunction is among the secondary effects of the altered milieu in the bronchiectatic airway. Clearance of apoptotic cells—efferocytosis—is a major role of the alveolar macrophage and is an important mechanism that controls and resolves inflammation. Proteolysis of opsins (including immune globulins) and cell receptors, oxidative protein damages, and generation of lipid peroxidation products contribute to disrupting the mechanisms [45,46]. Oxidation, depletion of antiproteases, receptor cleavage, and oxidant interference with signaling or impairment of aptoptic clearance have been found aberrant in CF. Specifically, cleavage of complement receptors (eg, phosphitidyl serine) in neutrophils and macrophages appears to hinder phagocytosis [42,47].

Infectious agent–mediated pathology

With chronic infection of the airway, be it saprophytic or invasive, the conditions in the airway may be directly influenced and altered by the infectious agent [48]. The infectious agent's interactions with the host may directly thwart host defense [48]. In the case of biofilm formation, the organisms may generate a colony within an alginate structure that offers a microenvironment that may impair antibiotic and cellular immune functions [49]. The presence of infection with *P aeruginosa* heralds a more severe clinical status and prognosis in the setting of bronchiectasis, be it CF or non-CF bronchiectasis [50]. This organism is particularly adapted to binding to injured epithelium, furthering a continued infection–injury cycle [51]. In addition, *P aeruginosa* impedes ciliary beating, in part by producing the pigment pyocyanin [52,53]. *P aeruginosa* may cause local cellular damage by producing proteases [42]. Saprophytic fungal infection in the airway associated with intense allergic-type inflammation is strongly associated with bronchiectasis. This syndrome, allergic bronchopulmonary mycosis (ABPM), is present in roughly 15% of individuals who have CF [54]. The fungus most commonly associated with ABPM, aspergillus, produces proteases. This fungus also acts as damaging proinflammatory stimuli, causes epithelial detachment, and disrupts ciliary beating [55–57].

Additional alterations of innate immunity

The alterations of the CF airway, whether they are inciting or resultant, interfere with control of inflammation. The recognized changes in the ASL of the CF respiratory tract relate to salt and water. Beyond the physical changes, this altered milieu may impart dysfunction and the altered chemistry on other constituents such as antimicrobial peptides, signaling capacity and cellular functions [58,59]. For example, β-defensin is secreted in airways and contributes to host defense but may be rendered less active by the altered ASL of CF airways [60].

Other altered cystic fibrosis lung defenses

Paradigms of bronchiectasis development, persistence, and promulgation are complex multiconstituent processes based on the interplay of environment, anatomy, and host immune system, among other genetic variables (eg, transforming growth factor β polymorphisms) [61]. Beyond the locally induced changes, mechanical and cellular clearance mechanisms of the lung systemic effects impact development. Gastrointestinal manifestations of CFTR dysfunctions may lead to relative systemic vitamin deficiencies (eg, vitamin E, beta carotene), which may impact respiratory tract oxidant defenses [62]. Concerns remain about epigenetic or other changes that may not solely relate to the CFTR dysfunction [63]. That is, the phenotype may engender further changes not primarily attributable to the primary defect but to the resultant condition, environment, or disease-related changes.

The idea that persistent inflammation is associated with the structural changes of bronchiectasis is supported by the strong association of the anatomic changes with the causative diseases of various forms and types of inflammation (eg, allergic bronchopulmonary apergillosis, CF, PCD, rheumatoid arthritis, childhood infection) [44]. Mechanistically, inflammation, with the attendant infiltration and migration of white blood cells, is associated with the dissolution of the extracellular matrix and supporting structure to allow for diapedesis and cell migration from the endovascular space through tight junctions, through the interstitium, and to the airway lumens [64,65]. With persistent inflammation in the airway, there is associated elevation of matrix metalloproteinases (MMPs) [66]. The roles of MMPs in the remodeling and repair associated with inflammation are recently coming to light [67]. Examinations of bronchiectatic airways, which revealed elevated concentrations of MMP-9 and MMP-8, support the role of MMPs in the pathogenesis of airway damage [68].

Summary

Outlined in this article are the primary and acquired abnormalities of the CF airway that stimulate the genesis of and promulgate the pathology of bronchiectasis. Inflammation and infection are central causative mechanisms of bronchiectasis. Their persistence appears to disrupt orderly reparative processes in the airway. Modulation of these processes and controlling the positive feedback of bronchiectasis afford some braking effects on the inexorable respiratory decline in patients who have CF and bronchiectasis. As more details of the mechanisms of bronchiectasis are

unveiled, more parallels among the seemingly disparate causes of CF and non-CF bronchiectasis are recognized. With these insights, more opportunities to halt the vicious circle have become apparent.

References

[1] Scala R, Aronne D, Palumbo U, et al. Prevalence, age distribution and aetiology of bronchiectasis: a retrospective study on 144 symptomatic patients. Monaldi Arch Chest Dis 2000;55(2):101–5.

[2] Tsao PC, Lin CY. Clinical spectrum of bronchiectasis in children. Acta Paediatr Taiwan 2002;43(5): 271–5.

[3] Barker AF. Bronchiectasis. N Engl J Med 2002; 346(18):1383–93.

[4] Morrissey BM, Harper RW. Bronchiectasis: sex and gender considerations. Clin Chest Med 2004;25(2): 361–72.

[5] Saynajakangas O, Keistinen T, Tuuponen T, et al. Bronchiectasis in Finland: trends in hospital treatment. Respir Med 1997;91(7):395–8.

[6] Saynajakangas O, Keistinen T, Tuuponen T, et al. Evaluation of the incidence and age distribution of bronchiectasis from the Finnish Hospital Discharge Register. Cent Eur J Public Health 1998;6(3):235–7.

[7] Nikolaizik WH, Warner JO. Aetiology of chronic suppurative lung disease. Arch Dis Child 1994; 70(2):141–2.

[8] Tiddens HA. Chest computed tomography scans should be considered as a routine investigation in cystic fibrosis. Paediatr Respir Rev 2006;7(3): 202–8.

[9] Burgel PR, Montani D, Danel C, et al. A morphometric study of mucins and small airway plugging in cystic fibrosis. Thorax 2007;62(2):153–61.

[10] Bedrossian CW, Greenberg SD, Singer DB, et al. The lung in cystic fibrosis. A quantitative study including prevalence of pathologic findings among different age groups. Hum Pathol 1976;7(2):195–204.

[11] Cole PJ. Inflammation: a two-edged sword—the model of bronchiectasis. Eur J Respir Dis Suppl 1986;147:6–15.

[12] Ionescu AA, Nixon LS, Luzio S, et al. Pulmonary function, body composition, and protein catabolism in adults with cystic fibrosis. Am J Respir Crit Care Med 2002;165(4):495–500.

[13] Angrill J, Agusti C, De Celis R, et al. Bronchial inflammation and colonization in patients with clinically stable bronchiectasis. Am J Respir Crit Care Med 2001;164(9):1628–32.

[14] Woodring JH, Howard RS 2nd, Rehm SR. Congenital tracheobronchomegaly (Mounier-Kuhn syndrome): a report of 10 cases and review of the literature. J Thorac Imaging 1991;6(2):1–10.

[15] Dawson M, Wirtz D, Hanes J. Enhanced viscoelasticity of human cystic fibrotic sputum correlates

with increasing microheterogeneity in particle transport. J Biol Chem 2003;278(50):50393–401.

[16] Bush A, Payne D, Pike S, et al. Mucus properties in children with primary ciliary dyskinesia: comparison with cystic fibrosis. Chest 2006;129(1):118–23.

[17] Lethem MI, James SL, Marriott C. The role of mucous glycoproteins in the rheologic properties of cystic fibrosis sputum. Am Rev Respir Dis 1990;142(5):1053–8.

[18] Widdicombe JH, Wine JJ. The basic defect in cystic fibrosis. Trends Biochem Sci 1991;16(12):474–7.

[19] Houtmeyers E, Gosselink R, Gayan-Ramirez G, et al. Regulation of mucociliary clearance in health and disease. Eur Respir J 1999;13(5):1177–88.

[20] Carlen B, Stenram U. Primary ciliary dyskinesia: a review. Ultrastruct Pathol 2005;29(3–4):217–20.

[21] Cornillie FJ, Lauweryns JM, Corbeel L. Atypical bronchial cilia in children with recurrent respiratory tract infections. A comparative ultrastructural study. Pathol Res Pract 1984;178(6):595–604.

[22] Bertrand B, Collet S, Eloy P, et al. Secondary ciliary dyskinesia in upper respiratory tract. Acta Otorhinolaryngol Belg 2000;54(3):309–16.

[23] Widdicombe JH. Regulation of the depth and composition of airway surface liquid. J Anat 2002;201(4):313–8.

[24] Doring G. Mechanisms of airway inflammation in cystic fibrosis. Pediatr Allergy Immunol 1996;7(9 Suppl):63–6.

[25] Finkbeiner WE. Physiology and pathology of tracheobronchial glands. Respir Physiol 1999;118(2–3):77–83.

[26] Lamblin G, Degroote S, Perini JM, et al. Human airway mucin glycosylation: a combinatory of carbohydrate determinants which vary in cystic fibrosis. Glycoconj J 2001;18(9):661–84.

[27] Schulz BL, Sloane AJ, Robinson LJ, et al. Mucin glycosylation changes in cystic fibrosis lung disease are not manifest in submucosal gland secretions. Biochem J 2005;387(Pt 3):911–9.

[28] Jayaraman S, Joo NS, Reitz B, et al. Submucosal gland secretions in airways from cystic fibrosis patients have normal [Na(+)] and pH but elevated viscosity. Proc Natl Acad Sci U S A 2001;98(14):8119–23.

[29] Machen TE. Innate immune response in CF airway epithelia: hyperinflammatory? Am J Physiol Cell Physiol 2006;291(2):C218–30.

[30] Zar H, Saiman L, Quittell L, et al. Binding of Pseudomonas aeruginosa to respiratory epithelial cells from patients with various mutations in the cystic fibrosis transmembrane regulator. J Pediatr 1995;126(2):230–3.

[31] Kubo K, Yamazaki Y, Hachiya T, et al. Mycobacterium avium-intracellulare pulmonary infection in patients without known predisposing lung disease. Lung 1998;176(6):381–91.

[32] Noone PG, Knowles MR. 'CFTR-opathies': disease phenotypes associated with cystic fibrosis transmembrane regulator gene mutations. Respir Res 2001;2(6):328–32.

[33] Ip M, Shum D, Lauder I, et al. Effect of antibiotics on sputum inflammatory contents in acute exacerbations of bronchiectasis. Respir Med 1993;87(6):449–54.

[34] Osika E, Cavaillon JM, Chadelat K, et al. Distinct sputum cytokine profiles in cystic fibrosis and other chronic inflammatory airway disease. Eur Respir J 1999;14(2):339–46.

[35] Dakin CJ, Numa AH, Wang H, et al. Inflammation, infection, and pulmonary function in infants and young children with cystic fibrosis. Am J Respir Crit Care Med 2002;165(7):904–10.

[36] Khan TZ, Wagener JS, Bost T, et al. Early pulmonary inflammation in infants with cystic fibrosis. Am J Respir Crit Care Med 1995;151(4):1075–82.

[37] Armstrong DS, Hook SM, Jamsen KM, et al. Lower airway inflammation in infants with cystic fibrosis detected by newborn screening. Pediatr Pulmonol 2005;40(6):500–10.

[38] Chmiel JF, Davis PB. State of the art: why do the lungs of patients with cystic fibrosis become infected and why can't they clear the infection? Respir Res 2003;4:8.

[39] Heeckeren A, Walenga R, Konstan MW, et al. Excessive inflammatory response of cystic fibrosis mice to bronchopulmonary infection with Pseudomonas aeruginosa. J Clin Invest 1997;100(11):2810–5.

[40] Barton AD, Ryder K, Lourenco RV, et al. Inflammatory reaction and airway damage in cystic fibrosis. J Lab Clin Med 1976;88(3):423–6.

[41] Mendis AH, Venaille TJ, Robinson BW. Study of human epithelial cell detachment and damage: effects of proteases and oxidants. Immunol Cell Biol 1990;68(Pt 2):95–105.

[42] Amitani R, Wilson R, Rutman A, et al. Effects of human neutrophil elastase and Pseudomonas aeruginosa proteinases on human respiratory epithelium. Am J Respir Cell Mol Biol 1991;4(1):26–32.

[43] Sirmali M, Turut H, Kisacik E, et al. The relationship between time of admittance and complications in paediatric tracheobronchial foreign body aspiration. Acta Chir Belg 2005;105(6):631–4.

[44] Morrissey BM, Evans SJ. Severe bronchiectasis. Clin Rev Allergy Immunol 2003;25(3):233–47.

[45] Vandivier RW, Henson PM, Douglas IS. Burying the dead: the impact of failed apoptotic cell removal (efferocytosis) on chronic inflammatory lung disease. Chest 2006;129(6):1673–82.

[46] Halliwell B, Cross CE. Oxygen-derived species: their relation to human disease and environmental stress. Environ Health Perspect 1994;102(Suppl 10):5–12.

[47] Berger M, Sorensen RU, Tosi MF, et al. Complement receptor expression on neutrophils at an inflammatory site, the Pseudomonas-infected lung in cystic fibrosis. J Clin Invest 1989;84(4):1302–13.

[48] Wilson R, Dowling RB, Jackson AD. The biology of bacterial colonization and invasion of the respiratory mucosa. Eur Respir J 1996;9(7):1523–30.

[49] Prince AS. Biofilms, antimicrobial resistance, and airway infection. N Engl J Med 2002;347(14):1110–1.

[50] Li Z, Kosorok MR, Farrell PM, et al. Longitudinal development of mucoid Pseudomonas aeruginosa infection and lung disease progression in children with cystic fibrosis. JAMA 2005;293(5):581–8.

[51] de Bentzmann S, Roger P, Puchelle E. Pseudomonas aeruginosa adherence to remodelling respiratory epithelium. Eur Respir J 1996;9(10):2145–50.

[52] Denning GM, Railsback MA, Rasmussen GT, et al. Pseudomonas pyocyanine alters calcium signaling in human airway epithelial cells. Am J Physiol 1998;274(6 Pt 1):L893–900.

[53] Hingley ST, Hastie AT, Kueppers F, et al. Effect of ciliostatic factors from Pseudomonas aeruginosa on rabbit respiratory cilia. Infect Immun 1986;51(1):254–62.

[54] Morrissey BM, Louie S. Allergic bronchopulmonary aspergillosis: an evolving challenge in asthma. In: Gershwin ME, Albertson TE, editors. Bronchial asthma, a guide for practical understanding and treatment. 5th edition. Totowa (NJ): Humana Press; 2006. p. 279–309.

[55] Knutsen AP, Bellone C, Kauffman H. Immunopathogenesis of allergic bronchopulmonary aspergillosis in cystic fibrosis. J Cyst Fibros 2002;1(2):76–89.

[56] Amitani R, Murayama T, Nawada R, et al. Aspergillus culture filtrates and sputum sols from patients with pulmonary aspergillosis cause damage to human respiratory ciliated epithelium in vitro. Eur Respir J 1995;8(10):1681–7.

[57] Robinson BW, Venaille TJ, Mendis AH, et al. Allergens as proteases: an Aspergillus fumigatus proteinase directly induces human epithelial cell detachment. J Allergy Clin Immunol 1990;86(5):726–31.

[58] Goldman MJ, Anderson GM, Stolzenberg ED, et al. Human beta-defensin-1 is a salt-sensitive antibiotic in lung that is inactivated in cystic fibrosis. Cell 1997;88(4):553–60.

[59] Chilvers MA, O'Callaghan C. Local mucociliary defence mechanisms. Paediatr Respir Rev 2000;1(1):27–34.

[60] Bals R, Wang X, Wu Z, et al. Human beta-defensin 2 is a salt-sensitive peptide antibiotic expressed in human lung. J Clin Invest 1998;102(5):874–80.

[61] Drumm ML, Konstan MW, Schluchter MD, et al. Genetic modifiers of lung disease in cystic fibrosis. N Engl J Med 2005;353(14):1443–53.

[62] Kelly FJ. Vitamins and respiratory disease: antioxidant micronutrients in pulmonary health and disease. Proc Nutr Soc 2005;64(4):510–26.

[63] Friedman KJ, Silverman LM. Cystic fibrosis syndrome: a new paradigm for inherited disorders and implications for molecular diagnostics. Clin Chem 1999;45(7):929–31.

[64] Huber AR, Weiss SJ. Disruption of the subendothelial basement membrane during neutrophil diapedesis in an in vitro construct of a blood vessel wall. J Clin Invest 1989;83(4):1122–36.

[65] Delclaux C, Delacourt C, D'Ortho MP, et al. Role of gelatinase B and elastase in human polymorphonuclear neutrophil migration across basement membrane. Am J Respir Cell Mol Biol 1996;14(3):288–95.

[66] Sepper R, Konttinen YT, Sorsa T, et al. Gelatinolytic and type IV collagenolytic activity in bronchiectasis. Chest 1994;106(4):1129–33.

[67] Reijerkerk A, Kooij G, van der Pol SM, et al. Diapedesis of monocytes is associated with MMP-mediated occludin disappearance in brain endothelial cells. Faseb J 2006;20(14):2550–2.

[68] Zheng L, Lam WK, Tipoe GL, et al. Overexpression of matrix metalloproteinase-8 and -9 in bronchiectatic airways in vivo. Eur Respir J 2002;20(1):170–6.

ELSEVIER SAUNDERS

Clin Chest Med 28 (2007) 297–305

CLINICS IN CHEST MEDICINE

Newborn Screening for Cystic Fibrosis

Michael J. Rock, MD

Division of Pediatric Pulmonology, University of Wisconsin Hospital and Clinics,
600 Highland Avenue, Room K4/946, Madison, WI 53792, USA

Cystic fibrosis (CF) is the most common, potentially lethal genetic disease in Caucasians, occurring with a frequency of approximately 1 in 3300 live births. The defective CF gene leads to abnormal CF transmembrane regulator protein, a protein that is expressed in the respiratory epithelial cells, gastrointestinal system including pancreatic and liver ductals, the vas deferens in male patients, mucous-secreting cervical cells of women, and sweat gland ductals. Involvement of these systems leads to various presentations including neonatal intestinal obstruction (meconium ileus), malabsorption of protein and fat leading to abnormal stools and failure to thrive, acute and chronic respiratory problems (ie, pneumonia, chronic cough, recurrent wheezing), and other signs or symptoms including electrolyte imbalance, nasal polyps and sinus disease, liver disease, and rectal prolapse.

The traditional method of diagnosis depends on a high index of suspicion for CF by the health care provider. Despite increased education of medical students and residents, the average age of diagnosis is 3.3 years, with a median age of diagnosis of 6 months [1]. There is a growing body of evidence demonstrating that there are nutritional, pulmonary and survival advantages of diagnosis through newborn screening. This article discusses the history of CF neonatal screening including technology employed for screening and the benefits of early diagnosis of CF.

History of cystic fibrosis newborn screening

The potential benefits of an early diagnosis of CF were first published by Shwachman and colleagues in 1970 [2]. In this report, there were 130 patients diagnosed under age 3 months who were subdivided into three categories: group A patients (n = 63) were diagnosed before symptoms; group B patients (n = 13) were diagnosed with mild symptoms; and group C patients (n = 54) were diagnosed during a hospitalization. In groups A and B combined, there were 11 deaths compared with 18 deaths in group C. Therefore, this article suggested that children younger than 3 months old who have CF diagnosed before symptoms or CF with mild symptoms had improved health outcomes compared with those who were symptomatic on diagnosis during a hospitalization. Another retrospective study further suggested benefits of an early diagnosis. In 1977, Orenstein and colleagues [3] published their 7-year study of 16 sibling pairs who had CF. The older child of the sibling pair was diagnosed after age 1 year, with a mean age of 48 months, and the younger sibling was diagnosed before age 1 year, with a mean age of 6 months. The younger siblings had significantly better chest radiograph scores, better total clinical scores, better residual volumes, and lower ratios of residual volume to total lung capacity.

Early attempts at CF neonatal screening used a test strip to measure increased protein (with albumin as the main constituent) in meconium [4,5]. This technology was problematic, including producing high numbers of false positives and false negatives, missing CF patients who had pancreatic exocrine sufficiency, and using a substance (meconium) that is not traditionally assayed in a population-based screening program. Mass

This work was supported by Grant No. R01 DK34108 from the National Institutes of Health/ National Institute of Diabetes and Digestive and Kidney Diseases.

E-mail address: mjrock@wisc.edu

newborn screening became possible in 1979, when Crossley and colleagues [6] demonstrated the elevation of immunoreactive trypsinogen (IRT) concentrations in children who had CF. The IRT level can be determined from dried blood spots on filter paper cards (Guthrie cards), which made this test amenable to mass newborn screening because Guthrie cards are already obtained from newborns for other tests such as congenital hypothyroidism and phenylketonuria.

Within 3 years of the discovery of IRT as a screening test for CF, the Cystic Fibrosis Foundation convened a task force to provide recommendations regarding neonatal screening for CF [7]. The Cystic Fibrosis Foundation task force recommendations are listed in Box 1. First and foremost, the value of early treatment on prognosis must be determined. There also needed to be extensive research on the IRT method, including standardization, sensitivity, and specificity. The ideal study to determine the value of newborn screening is to demonstrate the effectiveness of the program in a randomized trial. To this end, there have been two randomized controlled trials of neonatal screening for CF. In the United Kingdom, all babies born in Wales and the West Midlands during 1985 to 1989 were randomly allocated to be screened for CF by IRT on alternate weeks, thus generating a screened group and an unscreened group of CF patients [8]. In Wisconsin, the CF neonatal screening project randomly

assigned infants born during 1985 to 1994 to a screened group or a control group [9,10]. Infants in the screened group had their screening test fully completed and reported to the investigators, with a sweat test performed at age 4 to 6 weeks. Infants in the control group presented with symptoms or a family history (unless the family requested the result). For children in the control group who had not yet presented with symptoms, unblinding occurred at age 4 years to fully identify all cases of CF in the control group for comparison with all cases of CF in the screened group. These two randomized controlled trials and a number of historical-cohort, geographic-cohort, and observational studies have contributed to a wealth of information of the benefits of newborn screening.

Nutritional benefit of cystic fibrosis newborn screening

The nutritional benefit of newborn screening has been demonstrated by numerous trials. Investigators in Colorado commonly demonstrated low serum albumin levels and low levels of retinol and α-tocopherol at the initial evaluation of infants diagnosed by newborn screening [11–13]. These low levels of albumin and fat-soluble vitamins are easily corrected by the initiation of pancreatic enzymes and multivitamin therapy. A geographic-cohort study in France demonstrated significant differences for weight and height in screened patients compared with nonscreened patients [14]. Another geographic-cohort study in Italy showed a significant difference in weight and height z scores in a newborn-screened group compared with conventionally diagnosed patients [15]. Growth was near normal for the newborn-screened patients who had z scores close to zero. A historical-cohort study in Australia demonstrated that height and weight z scores were significantly lower in nonscreened patients than in screened patients at diagnosis [16]. Screened patients had significantly better weights than nonscreened patients at age 1 year; at age 5 years, screened patients were significantly taller than nonscreened patients. The most compelling evidence for nutritional benefits of newborn screening comes from the Wisconsin CF neonatal screening trial [17]. Fig. 1 demonstrates the height-for-age z score in pancreatic-insufficient patients diagnosed by newborn screening compared with control patients (excluding meconium ileus). In addition, the patients in the randomized controlled trial were compared with Cystic

---

Box 1. Cystic Fibrosis Foundation task force recommendations on neonatal screening

1. Determine the value of early treatment on prognosis.
2. Determine the reliability and validity of the screening method.
3. Determine the benefits and risks of early detection.
4. Define the incidence and preventability of stigmatization in families with false-positive and true-positive tests.
5. Determine the cost-effectiveness of mass screening.
6. Define the availability of competent counseling for families with false-negative, false-positive, and true-positive results.

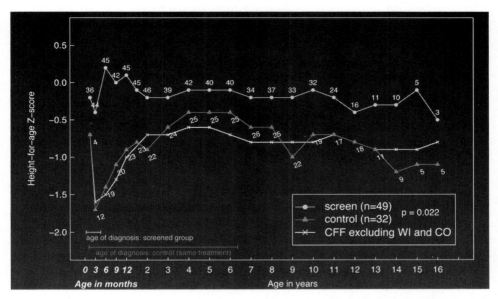

Fig. 1. Comparison of height-for-age *z* scores between patients who have CF diagnosed through neonatal screening ("screen," *yellow line*) or by standard methods ("control," *orange line*). Numbers of observations are provided adjacent to corresponding points. The white line represents mean values for 68,644 observations on 8381 CF pancreatic-insufficient (nonmeconium ileus) patients in the Cystic Fibrosis Foundation Patient Registry for United States birth cohort of 1985–1994, excluding patients born in Wisconsin (WI) and Colorado (CO). (*From* Farrell PM, Lai H, Li Z, et al. Evidence on improved outcomes with early diagnosis of cystic fibrosis through neonatal screening: enough is enough! J Pediatr 2005;147:S34; with permission.)

Fibrosis Foundation Patient Registry (CFFPR) data (excluding newborn-screened patients in Wisconsin and Colorado). The patients in the control group in the Wisconsin trial appear identical to the patients in the CFFPR. The screened patients had significantly better growth that persisted into the teen years. These studies challenge the dogma that there is "catch-up" growth in CF patients diagnosed due to failure to thrive. There appears to be permanent stunting of growth in CF patients diagnosed conventionally.

Pulmonary benefits of cystic fibrosis newborn screening

Unlike the near universal agreement among studies demonstrating a nutritional advantage of newborn screening, there have been variable outcomes of pulmonary function benefits of newborn screening. The randomized controlled trial in Wisconsin has not demonstrated a pulmonary function advantage of newborn screening to date [18]. Similarly, the geographic-cohort study in France did not demonstrate significant differences in pulmonary functions between patients diagnosed by newborn screening and patients

diagnosed conventionally [14]. An observational study in the Netherlands, however, demonstrated stable forced expiratory volume in 1 second (FEV_1) values in patients diagnosed by newborn screening compared with patients who did not have newborn screening, the latter group showing a statistically significant decrease in lung function with increasing age [19]. Likewise, the historical-cohort study in Australia demonstrated a significantly higher FEV_1 in the screened cohort, with an average difference of 9.4% of the predicted value [16]. More compelling evidence for a pulmonary function advantage of newborn screening comes from a recent analysis of CFFPR data [20]. As illustrated in Fig. 2, patients diagnosed by newborn screening had a significantly higher percent-predicted FEV_1 compared with patients diagnosed by symptoms or diagnosed by meconium ileus. This advantage was present in the 6- to 10-year-old age group and maintained in the 11- to 20-year-old age group.

Epidemiology of early lung disease

Although newborns have histologically normal lungs shortly after birth [21], there can be

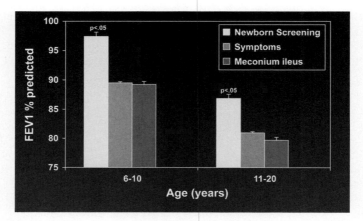

Fig. 2. Percent-predicted FEV₁ by diagnostic category and by age group for patients younger than 20 years from the CFFPR for the year 2002. (*From* Accurso FJ, Sontag MK, Wagener JS. Complications associated with symptomatic diagnosis in infants with cystic fibrosis. J Pediatr 2005;147:S40; with permission.)

inflammation in the lower airway, as reflected by increased neutrophils isolated from bronchoalveolar lavage fluid from young infants [22]. This evidence of inflammation can be present even in the absence of lower respiratory tract infection. The initial onset of respiratory tract infection can be challenging to diagnose. It has been demonstrated that oropharyngeal cultures can have poor sensitivity for the detection of pathogens in the lower airways. Bronchoalveolar lavage studies, however, have shown that lower respiratory cultures can be positive for *Pseudomonas aeruginosa* in 15% of patients by age 1 year and in 30% of patients by age 3 years [23]. In addition, when patients are diagnosed conventionally, up to one fourth have *Pseudomonas aerugonisa* present at their initial clinic visit. It has become clear more recently that chronic *Pseudomonas aeruginosa* infection is associated with poorer clinical outcomes, more rapid decline in lung function, and poorer survival. An analysis of CFFPR data demonstrated that respiratory infection with *Pseudomonas aeruginosa* was the major predictor of morbidity and mortality [24]. Patients aged 1 to 5 years from the 1990 CFFPR were studied for mortality and clinical outcomes in 1998. The 8-year risk of death was 2.6 times higher in patients who had respiratory cultures positive for *Pseudomonas aeruginosa* in 1990 than in children who did not have presence of *Pseudomonas aeruginosa*. These culture-positive patients also had a significantly lower percent-predicted FEV₁ and weight percentile at follow-up and they had an increased risk of continued respiratory infection with *Pseudomonas*

aeruginosa and need for hospitalization. It was initially believed that *Pseudomonas aeruginosa* could not be eradicated from CF patients; however, the initial colonization is with nonmucoid phenotypes that can potentially be eradicated with early aggressive treatment.

The randomized controlled trials and historical- and geographic-cohort studies began in the 1970 and 1980s, which was before the use of inhaled or oral antipseudomonal therapy for the first acquisition of *Pseudomonas aeruginosa* and before careful infection control (both of which are now standard of care in all CF centers). Newborn screening for CF provides the opportunity to diagnose patients before colonization with *Pseudomonas aeruginosa* and to intervene aggressively to forestall chronic colonization [25]. Therefore, it is likely that newborn screening has a pulmonary advantage.

Cognitive benefit of cystic fibrosis newborn screening

The randomized controlled trial of newborn screening in Wisconsin afforded the unique opportunity to investigate the effects of early malnutrition and fat-soluble vitamin deficiency as it related to subsequent cognitive function. Before the Wisconsin study, the cognitive development of children who had CF had not previously been studied systematically. In addition to the decreased length/height and weight of conventionally diagnosed patients compared with newborn-screened patients, the Wisconsin study also demonstrated a decreased head circumference in patients diagnosed conventionally [26]. The head circumference gradually recovered and equaled that of the newborn-screened group; however, this did not occur until age 2 years. The patients in the Wisconsin study were administered a test of cognitive skills, and the results of that test were correlated with the vitamin E level obtained previously at diagnosis. Conventionally diagnosed patients who had vitamin E deficiency at the time of diagnosis scored statistically significantly lower in the memory subsection and total composite cognitive skills index compared with patients in the newborn-screened group or with conventionally diagnosed patients who had normal vitamin E levels at diagnosis [27]. Vitamin E deficiency and nutritional insult early in life is thought to be associated with stunted cognitive development. Thus, newborn screening for CF appears to benefit the cognitive development of children with CF.

Survival benefit of cystic fibrosis newborn screening

Recently, a systematic review of the evidence on the association between newborn screening and CF-related child mortality was conducted [28]. This study demonstrated a statistically significantly decreased number of deaths of newborn-screened patients in a randomized controlled study in the United Kingdom, a historical-cohort study in Australia, a geographic-cohort study in Italy, and a geographic-cohort study in France. In addition, an analysis was performed of the CFFPR data as related to means of diagnosis [29]. In that analysis, early diagnosis through screening was associated with better survival compared with delayed diagnosis. Newborn screening provides the opportunity to prevent potentially fatal protein calorie malnutrition and electrolyte imbalance in infants, in addition to a probable overall survival advantage compared with symptomatic diagnosis.

Immunoreactive trypsinogen/immunoreactive trypsinogen and immunoreactive trypsinogen/DNA screening algorithms

There are two screening algorithms for CF newborn screening: IRT/IRT and IRT/DNA. In the IRT/IRT algorithm, a fixed cut-off for the IRT level is selected and obtained on the baby before discharge from the newborn nursery. If the initial IRT level is above the cut-off, then a second IRT is collected at age 2 weeks at a lower cut-off value. Infants are recalled for sweat testing if their second IRT is also elevated. In the IRT/IRT technique, there are a disproportionate number of African American babies and infants who have low Apgar scores who have elevated IRT levels [30]. In addition, the IRT/IRT technique requires a second specimen. This algorithm works best in states that routinely require a second newborn screening specimen. In the IRT/DNA algorithm, a lower cut-off for the initial IRT value from the newborn nursery can be selected [31]. Cut-off values vary from the highest 4% to 6% of IRT values. Infants who have an elevated IRT have cystic fibrosis transmembrane regulator mutation analysis performed on the original Guthrie card. Variable numbers of mutations can be analyzed. In most CF newborn screening programs with multimutation testing, 50% to 75% of patients can be identified as having CF directly from the newborn screening specimen by the identification of two CF mutations (although confirmation of CF is required with a sweat test; see later discussion). Infants who have one mutation must undergo sweat testing to ascertain CF status because of the possibility of a second mutation that was not on the newborn screening panel. The IRT/DNA algorithm detects infants who are CF carriers, and families require genetic counseling (see later discussion). Advantages of the IRT/DNA algorithm are that only one specimen is required and that there is a better sensitivity compared with the IRT/IRT algorithm due to a lower cut-off value used in the IRT/DNA algorithm. The State of California, which will begin CF newborn screening in July 2007, is further refining the IRT/DNA algorithm by performing CF gene sequencing on the Guthrie card specimen in infants who have an elevated IRT and only one mutation detected using a 38-mutation panel. If a second mutation is not detected from CF gene sequencing, then these infants are labeled as CF carriers and genetic counseling is provided. (Martin Kharrazi, PhD, MPH, California Department of Health Services Genetic Disease Branch, personal communication, 2006).

Regardless of choosing the IRT/IRT or the IRT/DNA screening algorithm, an important component of a CF newborn screening program is accurate sweat testing. The diagnosis of CF must be confirmed with a sweat test, which is true even for infants who have two identified mutations from the newborn screen, because the diagnosis of CF is a life-long, life-shortening disease. Although errors can be minimized by using bar codes on wrist/leg bands and bar codes on the Guthrie cards, such errors can never be completely eliminated in the newborn nursery or in the centralized testing laboratory. One must be completely sure that the abnormal newborn screening result for an infant actually belongs to that infant, and thus, the diagnosis must be confirmed by a sweat test. In the routine CF newborn screening program in Wisconsin, the author and colleagues initially performed a sweat test at age 4 weeks with the belief that an infant needed to be 1 month old to collect an adequate quantity of sweat. The infants' parents, however, were learning of the abnormal newborn screen at the infants' 7- or 10-day check-up and then needed to wait an additional 2 weeks until the sweat test was performed. This was a period of high anxiety for the parents. Therefore, in the year 2000, the author's institution no longer required infants to be 4 weeks of age for performance of a sweat test. In most infants, an adequate quantity of sweat can be obtained at less than 4 weeks of age, and infants are now scheduled for a sweat test as soon as possible [32,33].

As stated previously, the IRT/DNA algorithm detects infants who are CF carriers; therefore, at least one (and possibly both) of the parents must be a CF carrier. In turn, the aunts and uncles of the infant on at least one side of the family are at an increased risk (above the general population risk) of being a CF carrier. This complex genetic information, therefore, must be conveyed to the families through genetic counseling [34]. Although carrier detection is an unintended consequence of CF newborn screening, it can be considered a benefit of neonatal screening by identifying couples who are at high risk of having a child who has CF, by identifying CF carriers in the extended family, and by identifying previously undiagnosed siblings who have CF [35]. Neonatal screening for CF is viewed as favorable by families in which an infant has CF [36] and in families in which an infant is identified as a carrier [37].

Cost-effectiveness of cystic fibrosis newborn screening

Evidence is mounting that there is a potential cost savings through CF newborn screening

compared with the traditional method of diagnosis. An analysis was performed in Wisconsin examining the costs of sweat testing in the traditional method of disease presentation by clinical symptoms or family history compared with the program costs (IRT/DNA and sweat testing) of diagnosis through newborn screening [38]. The estimated annual cost per newly diagnosed CF infant using the traditional method was $4.97 per newborn infant compared with $4.58 per newborn infant by newborn screening diagnosis. This cost of diagnosis by newborn screening can be even less when one considers that the number of ordered sweat tests decreases in a newborn screening program. There has been an estimate in the past that in the traditional method of diagnosis, approximately 100 sweat tests are performed to diagnosis one CF patient. In a newborn screening program, care providers have a lower index of suspicion of CF and therefore order fewer sweat tests. Indeed, that was the case in Wisconsin in which the total annual number of sweat tests decreased from 1670 in 1991 (before routine CF neonatal screening) to 804 in 2000 [38]. If no additional sweat tests are ordered outside of the newborn screening program, then the estimated annual cost decreases to $2.66 per diagnosed infant. In addition, the level of savings from 866 fewer sweat tests accounts for 77% of the cost to operate Wisconsin's CF neonatal screening program. These costs were based on an IRT/DNA algorithm with analysis for the most common CF mutation, the ΔF508. More recently, a cost-effectiveness analysis was performed in the Netherlands comparing four strategies of neonatal screening: IRT/IRT, IRT/DNA, IRT/DNA/IRT, and IRT/DNA/extended mutation analysis by denaturing gradient gel electrophoresis (DGGE) [39]. The investigators concluded that IRT/IRT and IRT/DNA/DGGE were the most cost-effective strategies. As technology for multimutation analysis and gene sequencing is further refined, it is likely that costs will decrease and lead to more economical CF newborn screening.

Summary

In 1998, there were only three state-based CF newborn screening programs in the United States (Colorado, Wyoming, and Wisconsin). At of the end of 2006, newborn screening for CF was occurring in 22 states on a universal basis

Box 2. Opportunities to achieve more good than harm through CF neonatal screening

Opportunity to eliminate disparities associated with sex, race, and access associated with recognition deficiencies, economic limitations, and geographic factors

Opportunity to take advantage of informed reproduction after genetic risk communication and counseling

Opportunity to prevent potentially fatal salt depletion

Opportunity to prevent malnutrition after diagnosing pancreatic insufficiency
  Appropriate use of pancreatic enzyme supplements
  High-calorie diet with abundant essential fatty acids
  Fat-soluble vitamin supplements

Opportunity to prevent progressive lung disease
  Frequent, careful evaluation of pulmonary status
  Judicious use of oral antibiotics
  Protection of exposure to *Pseudomonas aeruginosa*
  Serologic and microbiologic monitoring for *Pseudomonas aeruginosa* acquisition and infection
  Aggressive antimicrobial therapy for *Pseudomonas aeruginosa*, as indicated, in efforts to prevent bronchopulmonary disease

From Farrell MH, Farrell PM. Newborn screening for cystic fibrosis: ensuring more good than harm. J Pediatr 2003;143:710; with permission.

required by law, in 3 states in which screening was offered to select populations or by request, in 2 states in which screening was universally offered but not yet required, and in 5 states in which testing was required but not yet implemented [40]. This rapid expansion of CF newborn screening has stemmed from the positive results of multiple studies and from recommendations from three health care organizations. The Centers for Disease Control and Prevention stated that "newborn screening for CF is justified" [41]. The Cystic Fibrosis Foundation stated that all states should routinely screen for CF in all newborns [42]. Lastly, the Maternal and Child Health Bureau of the Health Resources and Services Administration commissioned the American College of Medical Genetics (ACMG) to recommend a uniform panel of conditions to be included in state newborn screening programs. The ACMG recommended a panel of 29 core conditions for which screening should be mandated, and CF was one of these 29 disorders [43].

Box 2 illustrates opportunities to achieve more good than harm through CF neonatal screening [44]. Newborn screening for CF is the egalitarian method of diagnosis of CF and it eliminates disparities associated with sex and race. Neonatal screening for CF unequivocally provides an opportunity to prevent malnutrition through the appropriate use of pancreatic enzyme supplements, a high-calorie diet, and the immediate institution of fat-soluble vitamin supplements. This avoids prolonged vitamin E deficiency, which prevents cognitive deficits from occurring. Newborn screening for CF also provides the opportunity to prevent progressive lung disease through frequent careful evaluation of pulmonary status, monitoring for *Pseudomonas aeruginosa* acquisition and infection, and aggressive antimicrobial therapy as indicated. There appears to be a survival advantage and a pharmacoeconomic benefit of newborn screening. The neonatal lung in CF is histologically normal. As we look forward to improved therapies for the basic defect and to potentially direct therapies for treating the chloride channel defect, newborn screening will be crucial to diagnosing patients before irreversible lung disease. The patients who will benefit the most from these new therapies will be those diagnosed earliest through newborn screening.

Acknowledgments

The author thanks Cynthia Moodie for outstanding administrative support.

References

[1] Cystic Fibrosis Foundation Patient Registry. 2005 annual data report to the center directors. Bethesda (MD): Cystic Fibrosis Foundation; 2005.

[2] Shwachman H, Redmond A, Khaw K-T. Studies in cystic fibrosis: report of 130 patients diagnosed

under 3 months of age over a 20-year period. Pediatrics 1970;46:335–43.

[3] Orenstein DM, Boat TF, Stern RC, et al. The effect of early diagnosis and treatment in cystic fibrosis: a seven-year study of 16 sibling pairs. Am J Dis Child 1977;131:973–5.

[4] Stephan U, Busch EW, Kollberg H, et al. Cystic fibrosis detection by means of a test strip. Pediatrics 1975;55:35–8.

[5] Bruns WT, Connell TR, Lacey JA, et al. Test strip meconium screening for cystic fibrosis. Am J Dis Child 1977;131:71–3.

[6] Crossley JR, Elliott RB, Smith PA. Dried-blood spot screening for cystic fibrosis in the newborn. Lancet 1979;1:472–4.

[7] Taussig LM, Boat TF, Dayton D, et al. Ad hoc committee task force on neonatal screening, Cystic Fibrosis Foundation. Neonatal screening for cystic fibrosis: position paper. Pediatrics 1983;72:741–5.

[8] Chatfield S, Owen G, Ryley HC, et al. Neonatal screening for cystic fibrosis in Wales and the West Midlands: clinical assessment after 5 years of screening. Arch Dis Child 1991;66:29–33.

[9] Fost N, Farrell PM. A prospective randomized trial of early diagnosis and treatment of cystic fibrosis: a unique ethical dilemma. Clin Res 1989; 37:495–500.

[10] Farrell PM. Improving the health of patients with cystic fibrosis through newborn screening. Adv Pediatr 2000;47:79–115.

[11] Reardon MC, Hammond KB, Accurso FJ, et al. Nutritional deficits exist before 2 months of age in some infants with cystic fibrosis identified by screening test. J Pediatr 1984;105:271–4.

[12] Abman SH, Reardon MC, Accurso FJ, et al. Hypoalbuminemia at diagnosis as a marker for severe respiratory course in infants with cystic fibrosis identified by newborn screening. J Pediatr 1985; 107:933–5.

[13] Sokol RJ, Reardon MC, Accurso FJ, et al. Fat-soluble-vitamin status during the first year of life in infants with cystic fibrosis identified by screening of newborns. Am J Clin Nutr 1989;50:1064–71.

[14] Siret D, Bretaudea G, Branger B, et al. Comparing the clinical evolution of cystic fibrosis screened neonatally to that of cystic fibrosis diagnosed from clinical symptoms: a 10-year retrospective study in a French region (Brittany). Pediatr Pulmonol 2003; 35:342–9.

[15] Mastella G, Zanolla L, Castellani C, et al. Neonatal screening for cystic fibrosis: long-term clinical balance. Pancreatology 2001;1:531–7.

[16] Waters DL, Wilcken B, Irwig L, et al. Clinical outcomes of newborn screening for cystic fibrosis. Arch Dis Child Fetal Neonatal Ed 1999;80:F1–7.

[17] Farrell PM, Lai H, Li Z, et al. Evidence on improved outcomes with early diagnosis of cystic fibrosis through neonatal screening: enough is enough! J Pediatr 2005;147:S30–6.

[18] Farrell PM, Li Z, Kosorok, et al. Bronchopulmonary disease in children with cystic fibrosis after early or delayed diagnosis. Am J Respir Crit Care Med 2003;168:1100–8.

[19] Merelle ME, Schouten JP, Gerritsen J, et al. Influence of neonatal screening and centralized treatment on long-term clinical outcome and survival of CF patients. Eur Respir J 2001;18: 306–15.

[20] Accurso FJ, Sontag MK, Wagener JS. Complications associated with symptomatic diagnosis in infants with cystic fibrosis. J Pediatr 2005;147: S37–41.

[21] Tomashefski HF, Abramowsky CR, Dahms BB. The pathology of cystic fibrosis. In: Davis P, editor. Cystic fibrosis. New York: Marcel Dekker; 1993. p. 435–89.

[22] Khan TZ, Wagener JS, Bost T, et al. Early pulmonary inflammation in infants with cystic fibrosis. Am J Respir Crit Care Med 1995;151:1075–82.

[23] Rosenfeld M, Emerson J, Accurso F, et al. Diagnostic accuracy of oropharyngeal cultures in infants and young children with cystic fibrosis. Pediatr Pulmonol 1999;28:321–8.

[24] Emerson J, Rosenfeld M, McNamara S, et al. *Pseudomonas aeruginosa* and other predictors of mortality and morbidity in young children with cystic fibrosis. Pediatr Pulmonol 2002;34:91–100.

[25] Frederiksen B, Lanng S, Koch C, et al. Improved survival in the Danish center-treated cystic fibrosis patients: results of aggressive treatment. Pediatr Pulmonol 1996;21:153–8.

[26] Farrell PM, Kosorok MR, Laxova A, et al. Nutritional benefits of neonatal screening for cystic fibrosis. N Engl J Med 1997;337:963–9.

[27] Koscik RL, Lai HJ, Laxova A, et al. Preventing early, prolonged vitamin E deficiency: an opportunity for better cognitive outcomes via early diagnosis through neonatal screening. J Pediatr 2005;147: S51–6.

[28] Grosse SD, Rosenfeld M, Devine OJ, et al. Potential impact of newborn screening for cystic fibrosis on child survival: a systematic review and analysis. J Pediatr 2006;149:362–6.

[29] Lai HJ, Cheng Y, Farrell PM. The survival advantage of patients with cystic fibrosis diagnosed through neonatal screening: evidence from the United States Cystic Fibrosis Foundation registry data. J Pediatr 2005;147:S57–63.

[30] Rock MJ, Mischler EH, Farrell PM, et al. Immunoreactive trypsinogen screening for cystic fibrosis: characterization of infants with a false-positive screening test. Pediatr Pulmonol 1989;6:42–8.

[31] Gregg RG, Simantel A, Farrell PM, et al. Newborn screening for cystic fibrosis in Wisconsin: comparison of biochemical and molecular methods. Pediatrics 1997;99:819–24.

[32] Rock MJ, Hoffman G, Laessig RH, et al. Newborn screening for cystic fibrosis in Wisconsin: nine-year

experience with routine trypsinogen/DNA testing. J Pediatr 2005;147:S73–7.

[33] Parad RB, Comeau AM, Dorkin HL, et al. Sweat testing infants detected by cystic fibrosis newborn screening. J Pediatr 2005;147:S69–72.

[34] Ciske DJ, Haavisto A, Laxova A, et al. Genetic counseling and neonatal screening for cystic fibrosis: an assessment of the communication process. Pediatrics 2001;107:699–705.

[35] Wheeler PG, Smith R, Dorkin H, et al. Genetic counseling after implementation of statewide cystic fibrosis newborn screening: two years' experience in one medical center. Genet Med 2001;3(6): 411–5.

[36] Mérelle ME, Huisman J, Alderden-van der Vecht A, et al. Early versus late diagnosis: psychological impact on parents of children with cystic fibrosis. Pediatrics 2003;111:346–50.

[37] Parsons EP, Clarke AJ, Bradley DM. Implications of carrier identification in newborn screening for cystic fibrosis. Arch Dis Child Fetal Neonatal Ed 2003; 88:F467–71.

[38] Lee DS, Rosenberg MA, Peterson A, et al. Analysis of the costs of diagnosing cystic fibrosis with a newborn screening program. J Pediatr 2003;142: 617–23.

[39] van den Akker-van Marle ME, Dankert HM, Verkerk PH, et al. Cost-effectiveness of 4 neonatal screening strategies for cystic fibrosis. Pediatrics 2006;118(3):896–905.

[40] National Newborn Screening & Genetics Resource Center. Available at: http://genes-r-us.uthscsa.edu/. Accessed December 3, 2006.

[41] Grosse SD, Boyle CA, Botkin JR, et al. Newborn screening for cystic fibrosis: evaluation of benefits and risks and recommendations for state newborn screening programs. MMWR Recomm Rep 2004; 53(RR-13):1–36.

[42] Cystic Fibrosis Foundation-newborn screening. Available at: http://www.cff.org/AboutCF/Testing/NewbornScreening/. Accessed December 3, 2006.

[43] Watson MS, Mann MY, Lloyd-Puryear MA, et al. Newborn screening: toward a uniform screening panel and system—executive summary. Pediatrics 2006;117(5):S296–307.

[44] Farrell MH, Farrell PM. Newborn screening for cystic fibrosis: ensuring more good than harm. J Pediatr 2003;143:707–12.

ELSEVIER
SAUNDERS

Clin Chest Med 28 (2007) 307–318

CLINICS
IN CHEST
MEDICINE

Approaches to the Treatment of Initial *Pseudomonas aeruginosa* Infection in Children Who Have Cystic Fibrosis

Thomas Lahiri, MD[a,b,*]

[a]*University of Vermont College of Medicine, Burlington, VT 05401, USA*
[b]*Division of Pediatric Pulmonology, Vermont Children's Hospital at Fletcher Allen Health Care,
111 Colchester Avenue—Smith 556, Burlington, VT 05401, USA*

The preservation of lung function is foremost among the primary treatment goals for patients who have cystic fibrosis (CF). Of the many factors that influence the decline of pulmonary function, colonization or infection of the respiratory tract with bacterial pathogens is among the most important [1–3]. In young children, the most commonly recovered organisms from the airway are *Staphylococcus aureus* and *Haemophilus influenzae* [4]. Despite targeting these organisms with early antimicrobial therapy such as penicillins, the outcome for most patients who had CF in the 1950s was poor, with expected survival of only a year or two [5]. After decades of progress with regard to antibiotic development, the formerly dismal prognosis is in stark contrast to the present day median survival age of nearly 37 years in the United States [4].

The importance of *Pseudomonas aeruginosa* in pulmonary secretions of patients who have CF has long been recognized. It is difficult to treat or eradicate this pathogen, and its presence in respiratory secretions has been associated with increased pulmonary morbidity [6]. The clinical deterioration is most pronounced as the *P aeruginosa* phenotype shifts from a transient, nonmucoid one to a more chronic mucoid infection [6–8]. Today, the recovery of *P aeruginosa* from the respiratory tract of individuals who have CF is often regarded

as the sentinel medical event in their lives. The appropriate management of this first isolation has been debated over the past two decades without a clear consensus. In this article, the recovery of *P aeruginosa* in children who have CF is discussed, followed by a historical review of therapies directed against *P aeruginosa* in the CF-afflicted patient. Finally, the past and current treatment approaches to *P aeruginosa* colonization and infection are presented.

There has been much discussion over the use of "colonization" or "infection" to accurately describe the presence of *P aeruginosa* in CF respiratory cultures. The demonstration of elevated *Pseudomonas*-specific antibody levels in conjunction with recovery of *P aeruginosa* from respiratory culture is commonly referred to as an infection. To avoid further confusion, the term "infection" is used to describe any situation in which *P aeruginosa* is recovered from the airway of children who have CF.

Recovery of *P aeruginosa* from the pediatric airway

In patients who have CF, the sputum culture has been used to document infection and to follow the evolution of the infecting organisms. However, it is difficult to obtain sputum cultures from young children and infants who have CF. Even children who have a productive-sounding cough and more advanced disease may not expectorate sputum. The oropharyngeal (OP) or throat swab has become the routine manner in which surveillance respiratory cultures are obtained from (and

* Division of Pediatric Pulmonology, Vermont Children's Hospital at Fletcher Allen Health Care, 111 Colchester Avenue–Smith 556, Burlington, VT 05401.
E-mail address: thomas.lahiri@vtmednet.org.

0272-5231/07/$ - see front matter © 2007 Published by Elsevier Inc.
doi:10.1016/j.ccm.2007.02.003

chestmed.theclinics.com

often feared by) infants and young children. Although the OP culture is easy to perform, interpretation of the OP culture has been problematic. Oropharyngeal culture results may not accurately reflect the presence, absence, or specific microbiology of lower respiratory tract infection. With the use of bronchoscopy and bronchoalveolar lavage (BAL) as the gold standard for documenting lower respiratory infection, a number of investigators have studied the validity of OP cultures. Ramsey and colleagues [9] reported a positive predictive value (PPV) for the recovery of *P aeruginosa* of 83% and a negative predictive value (NPV) of 70% for OP cultures when compared with recovery of *P aeruginosa* from BAL. Other studies have revealed a much poorer PPV (41%–44%), especially in children less than 18 months of age, although the NPV was high (91%–97%) [6,10,11]. In one study of 40 patients who had CF, two consecutive OP cultures had a much better correlation with BAL results (PPV, 83%; NPV, 97%) [6]. Additionally, the use of hypertonic saline to induce sputum expectoration has been effectively accomplished in young children and may serve as a useful technique that does not require sedation [12–14].

The measurement of anti–*P aeruginosa* antibodies correlates with respiratory culture results and probably indicates infection. Microbiologic samples and immunologic studies have confirmed the relatively common occurrence of intermittent or transient *P aeruginosa* infection in infants and children who have CF [15]. Up to 29% of patients who have CF have evidence of *P aeruginosa* infection during the first year by respiratory culture [1,3]. By age 3, many have had infection by microbiologic or serologic evaluation [1,6]. In fact, there has been significant support for the use of levels of precipitating IgG antibodies to *P aeruginosa* by enzyme-linked immunosorbent assay to detect early infection. Several groups have discovered that in some cases, elevated titers may predate the recovery of *P aeruginosa* from sputum or OP cultures by over 1 year [15–23]. Others have found that antibody levels have not provided earlier information except in cases of patients who did not produce sputum [24]. Evidence exists that antibody levels have been useful in directing therapy and affecting patient outcome (eg, by imposing treatment for elevated titers until they return to the normal range) [15,25,26]. Anti–*P aeruginosa* IgA levels as a measure of the mucosal immune response has also been demonstrated to more closely follow infection with *P aeruginosa* compared with IgG levels [27].

The timing of first *P aeruginosa* infection in children is variable. Factors that increase the probability of recovery of *P aeruginosa* include the use of continuous antistaphylococcal suppressive therapy [28]. As a result, this previously popular practice has been largely abandoned. There is also a growing body of data from newborn screening programs that children who have CF who are conventionally diagnosed by the presence of symptoms are more likely to have pulmonary disease and *P aeruginosa* infection than those diagnosed by screening programs [29]. This, however, may reflect the older age at diagnosis.

The history of systemic antimicrobial therapy for *P aeruginosa*

The advent of effective antimicrobial therapy for patients who have CF emerged with the development of anti-staphylococcal agents. However, these agents were ineffective against *P aeruginosa*. Until the polymyxin antibiotic colistin was developed, there was no available parenteral antibiotic that could combat the inevitable *P aeruginosa* infections that plagued most patients who had CF and to which most eventually succumbed [30,31]. Although this represented a great step forward, intramuscular injections of colistin were associated with significant pain at the site of injection. To ease the pain of injection, Stern proposed intravenous antipseudomonal antibiotic treatments with a heparin lock system for intermittent infusions [32]. The efficacy of newer–generation, parenteral, antipseudomonal penicillins, such as carbenicillin, was demonstrated against *P aeruginosa* in patients who have CF as early as 1970 [33,34]. Combination antipseudomonal therapy, currently a mainstay, emerged at this time with the elimination of *P aeruginosa* from the sputum of 5 of 15 patients after treatment with intravenous tobramycin and inhaled and intravenous carbenicillin [35].

By the mid-1970s, the utility of aminoglycosides (eg, gentamicin and tobramycin) and β-lactam agents (eg, ticarcillin and carbenicillin) for the treatment of *P aeruginosa* respiratory tract infections in CF was well established. Attempts were made to learn if single agents or combinations of agents were more effective. The combination of intravenous tobramycin and ticarcillin resulted in improved clinical parameters for 11 patients who had CF despite failure to eradicate *P aeruginosa* from the sputum [36]. Intravenous gentamicin and ticarcillin therapy were later examined alone and in combination without significant difference. More than two thirds of patients receiving ticarcillin alone exhibited clinical improvement [37]. Amikacin, the aminoglycoside least susceptible to antimicrobial resistance via aminotransferases, was shown to be effective for the treatment of gentamicin-resistant mucoid *P aeruginosa* [38].

Regardless of the antimicrobial regimen, the development of resistance to antibiotics became problematic, particularly with respect to *P aeruginosa* isolates with a mucoid phenotype. It was recognized that mucoid isolates were a feature of chronic *P aeruginosa* infection and more severe pulmonary disease. Mucoid strains were and remain difficult to eradicate [39]. During the late 1970s, several studies carefully compared monotherapy with combination antibiotic therapy. Retrospective analyses revealed a better success rate for eradication of mucoid *P aeruginosa* with combination therapy but also found that for most the effect was not sustained [40]. Various combinations, such as tobramycin or gentamicin with carbenicillin, azlocillin, or piperacillin, have demonstrated efficacy in the management of acute CF pulmonary exacerbations [41–45].

The development of cephalosporins with broad-spectrum activity against gram-negative organisms in the 1980s led to further trials to evaluate their potential efficacy in patients who have CF. The rapid development of β-lactamase activity against ceftriaxone (as monotherapy or in combination with tobramycin) was observed in several *P aeruginosa* isolates during courses of treatment and served as a basis for avoiding the use of ceftriaxone in CF [46]. Ceftazidime and cefsulodin were substituted for penicillins with equivalent results with respect to *P aeruginosa* eradication and other clinical parameters [44,47–51]. The increasing use of third-generation cephalosporins such as ceftazidime was associated with the emergence of resistant and epidemic strains of *P aeruginosa* in some clinics [52]. Resistance was most pronounced when these agents were used alone [53,54]. Additionally, ceftazidime proved effective against some (*H influenzae*) [55] and ineffective against other (*Burkholderia*, formerly *Pseudomonas cepacia*) CF-associated bacteria [56]. Higher doses of ceftazidime (up to 320 mg/kg/d) were studied and were not found to be more effective than conventional doses [56,57]. The efficacy of continuous intravenous infusion of ceftazidime or cefepime has been demonstrated [58,59]. Widespread use of the regimen is not common because the benefit over conventional intermittent infusions remains unclear.

As newer β-lactam products were developed, they too were used in the battle against *P aeruginosa* infections in CF. The carbapenem antibiotic imipenem was initially highly effective, but monotherapy led to the rapid development of resistance [60–62]. The monobactam antibiotic aztreonam was effective against *P aeruginosa* and synergistically inhibited organisms when used with aminoglycosides [63,64]. The slower development of resistance to aztreonam (as opposed to imipenem or cephalosporins) was also an attractive benefit [65,66]. More recently, the effective use of meropenem and tobramycin for acute CF infections has been demonstrated [67].

In the mid-1980s, the development of the fluoroquinolone antibiotic ciprofloxacin, which possesses significant activity against *P aeruginosa* and *H influenzae*, dramatically changed anti-infective therapy. For the first time, an oral agent was available for the treatment of *P aeruginosa* in patients who had CF. Studies demonstrated that the efficacy of intravenous and oral ciprofloxacin-based antimicrobial regimens compared favorably with traditional parenteral aminoglycoside and β-lactam combinations [55,68,69]. Oral ciprofloxacin was extensively used in place of parenteral antibiotics in adolescents who had *P aeruginosa* infection [70]. Because of data in immature animals linking fluoroquinolones with joint arthropathy, many were concerned that fluoroquinolone use in children who had CF would lead to similar problems [71]. Fluoroquinolones have not been associated with joint arthropathy in patients who have CF. Based on the potential benefits of these agents, it has been deemed acceptable to use quinolones for CF infections, even in the very young [72]. As the resistance of some CF *P aeruginosa* isolates to ciprofloxacin and other fluoroquinolones has become more widespread, the efficacy of newer agents in this class, such as prulifloxacin, has been demonstrated [73].

More than 30 years of antimicrobial trials has shown that the use of any single antibiotic in patients who have CF has been associated with the rapid development of pseudomonal resistance to that antibiotic [66,74]. Combination therapy for the treatment of acute pulmonary exacerbations associated with nonmucoid and mucoid *P aeruginosa* isolates has become the mainstay of antimicrobial therapy for many years. More recently, checkerboard susceptibility testing has demonstrated that, in vitro, combinations of agents can act synergistically against even fairly resistant isolates [75]. Data are lacking to correlate in vitro susceptibilities and in vivo treatment efficacy [76,77]. This has further complicated the selection of appropriate antimicrobial agents for the treatment of CF pulmonary exacerbations.

Inhaled antimicrobial agents against *P aeruginosa*

Because of concerns over ototoxicity, nephrotoxicity, and discomfort associated with the administration of parenteral aminoglycosides, an attempt was made to administer intravenous formulations in aerosolized form to directly target the airways and lung. In 1989, there were two published trials of inhaled tobramycin in patients who have CF [78,79]. In both studies, those receiving inhaled tobramycin (80 mg twice [78] or three times [79] daily) exhibited an improved clinical status and an arrest of pulmonary function decline over a 2- to 3-year period compared with the control groups [79]. Another controlled trial of inhaled tobramycin at a dose of 80 mg twice daily for 12 months was examined in 22 patients. *P aeruginosa* infection was delayed in the treated group, but in this trial, there was no advantage in terms of lung function or other clinical parameters [80].

Further investigations were undertaken with a 12-week trial of tobramycin administered by aerosol in 22 patients who had CF. Although resistance to tobramycin developed over the course of treatment, it was felt to be transient. No appreciable neuro- or nephrotoxicity occurred in the study group [81]. The largest prospective, placebo-controlled trial of inhaled antibiotics examined the use of tobramycin solution for inhalation (TSI) (300 mg twice daily) administered on an alternate-month basis for 6 months in 520 patients who had CF. Higher forced expiratory volume in 1 second values, fewer hospitalizations, and decreased *P aeruginosa* density were found in the treatment group [82]. The effect of TSI was most pronounced in adolescents over a 2-year period, particularly with regard to forced expiratory volume in 1 second (14.3% higher compared with placebo) and body mass index [83]. The promising results in patients who had CF over 6 years of age led to another study to evaluate the safety and efficacy of TSI in 98 infants and children less than 6 years of age. The study was halted after 21 patients were enrolled because as eradication of *P aeruginosa* was observed in 8 out of 8 patients in the TSI group, compared with only 1 of 13 patients in the placebo group [84]. These TSI trials for patients who had CF have led to the

widespread use of this antibiotic in North America and elsewhere.

Nebulized colistin had been used for years in Denmark for the treatment of initial *P aeruginosa* isolation with success in delaying chronic infection [85]. Colistin has been further evaluated in a number of primarily European studies. The data published by Frederiksen, Høiby, and others have demonstrated the efficacy of colistin in patients who have CF and *P aeruginosa* infection [15,86–89]. A head-to-head comparison of inhaled colistin and tobramycin showed a suppressive antipseudomonal effect in both groups but showed a benefit only in the tobramycin group with regard to lung function [90]. The relatively low level of polymyxin-resistant *P aeruginosa* isolates has long been an argument in favor of the use of colistin. Although this remains the case, some polymyxin resistance has been described [91,92].

Inhaled gentamicin and amikacin have also been used as chronic inhaled therapy for CF airway infections. A study in 2002 compared the utility of continuous versus intermittent inhaled gentamicin therapy for delaying chronic *P aeruginosa* infection, favoring the latter [93]. Amikacin, via the inhaled route, has been investigated as an adjunct to parenteral therapy with some success [94]. Another promising feature of gentamicin and other aminoglycosides may be their ability to overcome premature termination codons in patients who have Class I mutations for the CF transmembrane conductance regulator [95,96]. Cephalosporins have also been investigated for possible use via the inhaled route. Ceftazidime has been used in patients who have CF and chronic *P aeruginosa* pulmonary infection [97], but this has not become standard therapy. Trials are underway to evaluate aerosolized aztreonam for patients who have CF and chronic *P aeruginosa*, and safety and antimicrobial properties have already been published [98]. The recent Cochrane database review of inhaled antibiotics concluded that aerosolized antibiotics were an effective modality for improving lung function in CF, although no single algorithm was advocated [99].

Early treatment strategies for the eradication of *P aeruginosa*

There is no uniform antimicrobial approach for an asymptomatic child who has CF from whom *P aeruginosa* has been recovered by respiratory culture for the first time. Physicians who care for patients who have CF have generally agreed that *something* should be done. Regional preferences for certain antibiotic regimens have driven practice patterns to some degree. The definition of "eradication" has been problematic. Earlier studies that assessed antibiotic efficacy against *P aeruginosa* described transient eradication as the absence of the organism from respiratory culture at the conclusion of a course of treatment. These studies primarily involved symptomatic patients who had chronic *P aeruginosa* infection [38,40–42,45,47], but the presence of *P aeruginosa* in respiratory cultures has negative prognostic implications. The use of *P aeruginosa* genotyping has been able to demonstrate eradication of certain strains and acquisition of different ones [87].

Some comment on the nature of early (hopefully transient) infection compared with chronic *P aeruginosa* CF infections is warranted. In most cases, nonmucoid susceptible isolates of *P aeruginosa* are recovered at the time of initial infection. Because *Pseudomonas* multiplies within the CF airway, there is a gradual change in the phenotype as a result of alginate production. This transition may take several years [3]. These organisms assume a rough, mucoid appearance and proceed with growth in a biofilm. These biofilms of mucoid *P aeruginosa* are most commonly associated with chronic infection because it is exceedingly difficult for antibiotics to penetrate the biofilm. Quorum sensing may play a role in biofilm development and the in virulence of *P aeruginosa* [100–102]. The development of multidrug resistance and discordance between in vitro susceptibilities and clinical efficacy can then be a consequence of chronic mucoid infections. Even oral decontamination with antibiotic rinses in conjunction with parenteral therapy has been attempted to no avail with regard to eradication of chronic *P aeruginosa* infections [103].

In the late 1980s, a small study of 28 children who had CF was undertaken to assess early treatment of *P aeruginosa*. These children were culture positive for *P aeruginosa* for an average of 5 months and received 2 weeks of parenteral therapy with tobramycin and azlocillin. Eradication was temporary (≤6 months) in most of the patients, although prolonged eradication (>14 months) was accomplished in 5 of 28 patients [104]. Littlewood and colleagues [105] described the efficacy of colistin for early *P aeruginosa* infection in seven patients who had CF. This experience served as further support for the early use of colistin.

It was the Danish experience with eradication after first isolation that became a model for aggressive early treatment. A 27-month trial randomized asymptomatic patients who had CF to receive no treatment or 3 weeks of oral ciprofloxacin and nebulized colistin each time *P aeruginosa* was isolated. The patients who were treated had significantly fewer chronic infections [85]. An observational analysis of aggressive early antipseudomonal therapy (a three-step protocol) compared with historical controls over a 3.5-year period was published in 1997 by Frederiksen and colleagues [86,106]. The group treated with 3 months of ciprofloxacin and colistin at the time of initial *P aeruginosa* discovery was afforded significant protection with regard to chronic *P aeruginosa* infections (78% fewer chronic infection) and maintenance of lung function (Fig. 1). This approach to eradication was confirmed with a study in which 47 patients who had CF with new *P aeruginosa* acquisition received ciprofloxacin and colistin. This group fared better than age-matched control subjects who had less chronic *P aeruginosa*, better preservation of lung function, and a lower long-term treatment cost [107].

The Danish experience has also demonstrated that aggressive treatment could be successfully extended to patients who have chronic *P aeruginosa*. Patients were treated on a quarterly basis with 2 weeks of parenteral therapy, regardless of symptoms, from 1976 to 1995. These strategies,

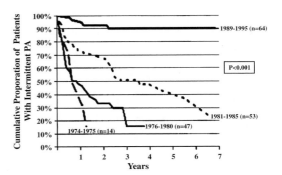

Fig. 1. Cumulative proportion of patients who have CF attending the Copenhagen CF Center from acquisition of first *Pseudomonas aeruginosa* (PA) colonization but who have not developed chronic PA infection (Kaplan-Meyer). *P* < .001 (log-rank test). N, number of patients with acquisition of first PA. (*From* Frederiksen B, Koch C, Høiby N. Changing epidemiology of Pseudomonas aeruginosa infection in Danish cystic fibrosis patients (1974–1995). Pediatr Pulmonol 1999;28(3):159–66; with permission.)

coupled with strict cohort isolation of patients with and without *P aeruginosa*, resulted in improved lung function and survival and in decreased chronic *P aeruginosa* in their patient population [106].

A comparison of nebulized tobramycin to placebo over a 1-year period achieved a delay of chronic infection, but lung function and inflammation were not improved in the treatment group [80]. Ratjen and colleagues [108] reported success in the eradication of *P aeruginosa* from 14 of 15 patients who had CF after 12 months of treatment with twice daily administration of 80 mg of nebulized tobramycin. The intermittent use of parenteral and inhaled antimicrobial therapy was found to be effective for the eradication of *P aeruginosa* by microbiologic and serologic parameters for 2 years in 15 of 17 patients who had CF [109]. The use of TSI for 28 days in patients 6 months and older with first *P aeruginosa* infection resulted in eradication for at least 56 days in the treatment group [84]. The early use of nebulized gentamicin was also examined in 28 children. Twelve of these received treatment (80 mg or 160 mg twice daily depending on age) for at least 3 years, and none developed chronic *P aeruginosa* infection. Of the remaining 16 patients who received interrupted or intermittent therapy, nearly half became chronically infected, and those children also had evidence of worse lung disease [93].

The studies mentioned in this article have served as the foundation for the current approach to the treatment of early *P aeruginosa* infection in CF (Table 1). Disagreement persists among physicians who treat the disease [110]. Treatment with TSI or colistin with or without ciprofloxacin has been officially supported by various groups [7,15,111–113]. The most recent Cochrane database review of *P aeruginosa* eradication in CF evaluated 15 published trials. Only three trials (including treatment with tobramycin or colistin/ciprofloxacin) were included in the final analysis. Although the methodology was thought to be problematic, the conclusion was that short-term eradication was possible, but the long-term benefit remained unclear [114].

Prevention of *P aeruginosa* infection

The potential for patient-to-patient transmission of *P aeruginosa* isolates is a concern for many CF care centers. Infection control practices have been carefully examined and may be important in the spread of certain transmissible *P aeruginosa* strains and many other common CF infections [115]. The cohorting of patients who have particular isolates may be beneficial [106,115]. Environmental acquisition also accounts for a significant proportion of new infections. The propensity of

Table 1
Studies that have evaluated *Pseudomonas aeruginosa* eradication in patients who have cystic fibrosis

Investigators	Year	Number of patients studied	Antipseudomonal intervention	Comparison group
Littlewood et al. [105]	1985	7	Inhaled colistin	None
Steinkamp et al. [78]	1989	14	Inhaled tobramycin	None
Steinkamp et al. [104]	1989	28	Parenteral tobramycin + azlocillin	None
Valerius et al. [85]	1991	26	Inhaled colistin + oral ciprofloxacin for 3 wk	Placebo
Frederiksen et al. [86]	1997	48	Inhaled colistin + oral ciprofloxacin for 3 mo	Historical
Wiesemann et al. [80]	1998	22	Inhaled tobramycin for 2 yr	Placebo
Ratjen et al. [108]	2001	15	Inhaled tobramycin for 1 yr	None
Griese et al. [109]	2002	17	Parenteral combination therapy and inhaled tobramycin	None
Heinzl et al. [93]	2002	28	Inhaled gentamicin: continuous versus intermittent treatment	None
Gibson et al. [84]	2003	21	TSI for 28 d	Placebo
Taccetti et al. [107]	2005	47	Inhaled colistin + ciprofloxacin	Historical

Abbreviation: TSI, tobramycin solution for inhalation.

P aeruginosa to adhere to and infect the CF airway results from properties of mutant CF transmembrane conductance regulator, airway surface liquid characteristics, increased mucus viscosity, and, as a result, impaired mucociliary clearance.

An effective vaccine against *Pseudomonas* has been under investigation for the past 30 years. The preliminary investigations, which were done in patients who have CF and in patients who have cancer, were not successful [116]. A prospective, controlled trial of a *Pseudomonas* CF vaccine was published in 1984 with discouraging microbiologic and clinical results [117]. Some promising clinical data surfaced when an octavalent O-polysaccharide-toxin A conjugate antipseudomonal vaccine was administered to 26 *P aeruginosa*–naive patients. Those patients who mounted a high-affinity antilipopolysaccharide antibody response were less likely to become infected or to have mucoid *P aeruginosa* strains. These patients were compared with historical control subjects and were discovered to have a lower rate of infection [118,119]. Larger studies are necessary to validate these results.

An oral vaccine to *P aeruginosa* was administered to human volunteers and was found to be safe and immunogenic, but no follow-up data are available [120]. A Cochrane review of antipseudomonal vaccine studies, published in 2000, reported only one trial that had long-term (10-year) follow-up and met criteria for review [121]. More recently, there has been increased interest in vaccine development [122]. In 2004, Lang and colleagues [123] reported the result of a new vaccine in 30 patients who had CF after 12 years of follow-up for 26 of 30 patients. The children immunized had no prior history of *P aeruginosa* infection and received booster immunization on an annual basis. Compared with matched control subjects, the immunized group had a lower rate of primary *P aeruginosa* infection, decreased chronic *P aeruginosa* infection, and decreased mucoid isolates. Furthermore, they had better lung function and nutritional status. Further larger studies are necessary to confirm these promising results. Work on passive immunity in patients who have CF and resistant *P aeruginosa* was published over 15 years ago. Adjunct therapy with *P aeruginosa* hyperimmune gamma globulin with conventional parenteral antibiotics conferred a treatment benefit in 10 patients [124]. No prospective studies of passive immunotherapy of patients who have CF without *P aeruginosa* have been reported, and this approach is not currently used.

Future directions

At the time of this writing, there is active research to evaluate the most efficacious regimen for *P aeruginosa* eradication in children. Ratjen and colleagues [125] have reported preliminary findings from the ELITE (Early Inhaled Tobramycin for Eradication) study. This study is in the process of examining the efficacy of TSI for the eradication of *P aeruginosa*. The patients were randomized to receive 28 or 56 days of TSI. Interim analysis has demonstrated safety and efficacy. A prospective randomized Australasian trial over a 5-year period is evaluating differences in outcome (radiographic score, lung function, quality of life, and BAL inflammation and culture) and eradication of *P aeruginosa* for patients who have CF who were diagnosed through newborn screening. One group of infants is receiving early BAL-directed therapy, with initial BAL at less than 6 months of age and subsequent BAL with pulmonary exacerbations that are unresponsive to nonpseudomonal antibiotics. The other group is receiving treatment for *P aeruginosa* on the basis of OP cultures (obtained as cough suction specimens) and will not undergo BAL during the study. In both groups, aggressive treatment is initiated for infants and children with positive *P aeruginosa* cultures: 2 weeks of parenteral antibiotics followed by prolonged inhaled and oral antipseudomonal therapy. *P aeruginosa* infection rates at the time of interim analysis were found to be high for both groups (>20%). Eradication of the majority of these isolates was also demonstrated [126].

In the United States, there are two complementary studies that are investigating risk factors for the acquisition of *P aeruginosa* and evaluating early treatment strategies. The EPIC (Early Pseudomonas Infection Control) Observational study has enrolled over 1700 patients who have CF who are under 13 years of age who have never had *P aeruginosa* or have not had *P aeruginosa* isolated over the previous 2 years. Microbiologic and serologic data and family questionnaires will be collected over 5 years (Bonnie Ramsey, MD, personal communication, 2006). The EPIC Clinical Trial has randomized ~190 of a planned 300 patients (1–12 years of age) who have cultured *P aeruginosa* for the first time or in the previous 6 months if there was no growth of *P aeruginosa* in the previous 2 years. All patients are treated at study enrollment with inhaled tobramycin (TSI) and placebo/oral ciprofloxacin. Patients are then randomized to cycle-based therapy (TSI + ciprofloxacin or placebo every 3 months) or culture-based therapy (antibiotics as mentioned previously only if a quarterly OP culture is *P aeruginosa* positive) for an 18-month period (Bonnie Ramsey, MD, personal communication, 2006). All patients in the EPIC clinical trial will be monitored in the EPIC observational study as part of the follow-up. The CF community eagerly awaits these results.

The outlook for children who have CF continues to improve in the 21st century. The implementation of early aggressive treatment strategies to target infection (*P aeruginosa* in particular) and inflammation has provided promising results. Because established infection with mucoid *P aeruginosa* is the reality for many patients who have CF, more attention to suppressive antimicrobial or maintenance anti-inflammatory therapies, the prevention of airways disease, and, ultimately, bronchiectasis are necessary to improve the quality and duration of life for these individuals.

Summary

P aeruginosa remains an important cause of pulmonary disease in patients who have CF. The development of antimicrobial therapy directed against this organism has resulted in the preservation of lung function and improved longevity. Efficacy has been demonstrated with agents administered via parenteral, inhaled, and oral routes. The optimal antibiotic regimen remains unclear. There is an active effort to use randomized, controlled clinical trials to rigorously test effective antibiotic for the eradication of *P aeruginosa* in young children or at least to delay the establishment of chronic infection.

Acknowledgments

The author thanks Drs. Barry Heath, Julie Adams, and William Raszka for their critical review of this chapter. The author acknowledges the assistance of Drs. Felix Ratjen, Claire Wainwright, Ron Gibson, and Bonnie Ramsey for providing data involving ongoing Pseudomonas treatment studies.

References

[1] Kerem E, Corey M, Gold R, et al. Pulmonary function and clinical course in patients with cystic fibrosis after colonization with Pseudomonas aeruginosa. J Pediatr 1990;116(5):714–9.

[2] Emerson J, Rosenfeld M, McNamara S, et al. Pseudomonas aeruginosa and other predictors of mortality and morbidity in young children with cystic fibrosis. Pediatr Pulmonol 2002;34(2):91–100.

[3] Li Z, Kosorok MR, Farrell PM, et al. Longitudinal development of mucoid Pseudomonas aeruginosa infection and lung disease progression in children with cystic fibrosis. JAMA 2005;293(5):581–8.

[4] Cystic Fibrosis Foundation Patient Registry. 2005 Annual Data Report to the Center Directors; 2006. Bethesda (MD), Cystic Fibrosis Foundation.

[5] Doershuk CF. The Matthews comprehensive treatment program: a ray of hope. In: Doershuk CF, editor. Cystic fibrosis in the 20th Century: people, events, progress. Cleveland (OH): AM Publishing, Ltd; 2001. p. 63–79.

[6] Burns JL, Gibson RL, McNamara S, et al. Longitudinal assessment of Pseudomonas aeruginosa in young children with cystic fibrosis. J Infect Dis 2001;183(3):444–57.

[7] Ratjen F. Treatment of early Pseudomonas aeruginosa infection in patients with cystic fibrosis. Curr Opin Pulm Med 2006;12(6):428–32.

[8] Henry RL, Mellis GM, Petrovic L. Mucoid Pseudomonas aeruginosa is a marker of poor survival in cystic fibrosis. Pediatr Pulmonol 1992;12: 158–61.

[9] Ramsey BW, Wentz KR, Smith AL, et al. Predictive value of oropharyngeal cultures for identifying lower airway bacteria in cystic fibrosis patients. Am Rev Respir Dis 1991;144(2):331–7.

[10] Armstrong DS, Grimwood K, Carlin JB, et al. Bronchoalveolar lavage or oropharyngeal cultures to identify lower respiratory pathogens in infants with cystic fibrosis. Pediatr Pulmonol 1996;21: 267–75.

[11] Rosenfeld M, Emerson J, Accurso F, et al. Diagnostic accuracy of oropharyngeal cultures in infants and young children with cystic fibrosis. Pediatr Pulmonol 1999;28(5):321–8.

[12] DeBoeck K, Alifer M, Vandeputte S. Sputum induction in young cystic fibrosis patients. Eur Respir J 2000;16:91–4.

[13] Suri R, Marshall LJ, Wallis C, et al. Safety and use of sputum induction in children with cystic fibrosis. Pediatr Pulmonol 2003;35(4):309–13.

[14] Ordonez CL, Kartashov AI, Wohl ME. Variability of markers of inflammation and infection in induced sputum in children with cystic fibrosis. J Pediatr 2004;145(5):689–92.

[15] Høiby N. Prospects for the prevention and control of pseudomonal infection in children with cystic fibrosis. Paediatr Drugs 2000;2(6):451–63.

[16] Brett MM, Ghoneim AT, Littlewood JM. Serum IgG antibodies in patients with cystic fibrosis with early Pseudomonas aeruginosa infection. Arch Dis Child 1987;62(4):357–61.

[17] Brett MM, Ghoneim AT, Littlewood JM. Prediction and diagnosis of early Pseudomonas aeruginosa infection in cystic fibrosis: a follow-up study. J Clin Microbiol 1988;26(8):1565–70.

[18] Abman SH, Ogle JW, Harbeck RJ, et al. Early bacteriologic, immunologic, and clinical courses of young infants with cystic fibrosis identified by neonatal screening. J Pediatr 1991;119(2):211–7.

[19] West SE, Zeng L, Lee BL, et al. Respiratory infections with Pseudomonas aeruginosa in children with cystic fibrosis: early detection by serology and assessment of risk factors. JAMA 2002; 287(22):2958–67.

[20] Pressler T, Frederiksen B, Skov M, et al. Early rise of anti-Pseudomonas antibodies and a mucoid phenotype of Pseudomonas aeruginosa are risk factors for development of chronic lung infection: a case control study. J Cyst Fibros 2006;5:9–15.

[21] Høiby N, Flensborg EW, Beck B, et al. Pseudomonas aeruginosa infection in cystic fibrosis: diagnostic and prognostic significance of Pseudomonas aeruginosa precipitins determined by means of crossed immunoelectrophoresis. Scand J Respir Dis 1977;58:65–79.

[22] Döring G, Høiby N. Longitudinal study of immune response to Pseudomonas aeruginosa antigens in cystic fibrosis. Infect Immun 1983;42:197–201.

[23] Pedersen SS, Espersen F, Høiby N. Diagnosis of chronic Pseudomonas aeruginosa infection in cystic fibrosis by means of enzyme linked immunosorbent assay. J Clin Microbiol 1987;25: 1830–6.

[24] Cordon SM, Elborn JS, Rayner RJ. IgG antibodies in early Pseudomonas aeruginosa infection in cystic fibrosis. Arch Dis Child 1992;67(6):737–40.

[25] Brett MM, Simmonds EJ, Ghoneim AT, et al. The value of serum IgG titres against Pseudomonas aeruginosa in the management of early pseudomonal infection in cystic fibrosis. Arch Dis Child 1992; 67(9):1086–8.

[26] Giordano A, Magni A, Filadoro F, et al. Study of IgG antibodies to Pseudomonas aeruginosa in early cystic fibrosis infection. New Microbiol 1998;21(4):375–8.

[27] DeBoeck K, Eggermont E, Smet M, et al. Specific decrease of anti-pseudomonal IgA after anti-pseudomonal therapy in cystic fibrosis. Eur J Pediatr 1995;154(2):157–60.

[28] Ratjen F, Comes G, Paul K, et al. Effect of continuous antistaphylococcal therapy on the rate of P aeruginosa acquisition in patients with cystic fibrosis. Pediatr Pulmonol 2001;31(1):13–6.

[29] Farrell PM, Li Z, Kosorok MR, et al. Bronchopulmonary disease in children with cystic fibrosis after early or delayed diagnosis. Am J Respir Crit Care Med 2003;168(9):1100–8.

[30] Koyama Y, Kurosawa A, Tsuchiya A, et al. A new antibiotic, colistin, produced by spore-forming soil bacteria. J Antibiot 1950;3:457.

[31] Nord NM, Hoeprich PD. Polymyxin B and colistin: a critical comparison. N Engl J Med 1964; 270:1030–5.

[32] Stern RC, Doershuk CF, Matthews LW. Use of a heparin lock to administer intermittent intravenous drugs. Clin Pediatr 1972;11:521–3.

[33] Boxerbaum B, Doershuk CF, Matthews LW. Use of carbenicillin in patients with cystic fibrosis. J Infect Dis 1970;122:S59–61.

[34] Phair JP, Tan TS, Watanakunakorn C, et al. Carbenicillin treatment of Pseudomonas pulmonary infection: use in children with cystic fibrosis. Am J Dis Child 1970;120(1):22–5.

[35] Crozier DN, Khan SR. Tobramycin in treatment of infections due to Pseudomonas aeruginosa in patients with cystic fibrosis. J Infect Dis 1976;134: S187–90.

[36] Parry MF, Neu HC. Tobramycin and ticarcillin therapy for exacerbations of pulmonary disease in patients with cystic fibrosis. J Infect Dis 1976;134: S194–7.

[37] Parry MF, Neu HC, Merlino M, et al. Treatment of pulmonary infections in patients with cystic fibrosis: a comparative study of ticarcillin and gentamicin. J Pediatr 1977;90(1):144–8.

[38] Lau WK, Young LS, Osher AB, et al. Amikacin therapy of exacerbations of Pseudomonas aeruginosa infections in patients with cystic fibrosis. Pediatrics 1977;60(3):372–7.

[39] Kulczycki LL, Murphy TM, Bellanti JA. Pseudomonas colonization in cystic fibrosis: a study of 160 patients. JAMA 1978;240(1):30–4.

[40] Friis B. Chemotherapy of chronic infections with mucoid Pseudomonas aeruginosa in lower airways of patients with cystic fibrosis. Scand J Infect Dis 1979;11(3):211–7.

[41] Moller NE, Høiby N. Antibiotic treatment of chronic Pseudomonas aeruginosa infection in cystic fibrosis patients. Scand J Infect Dis 1981; Supplement 29:87–91.

[42] Moller Ne, Eriksen KR, Feddersen C, et al. Chemotherapy against Pseudomonas aeruginosa in cystic fibrosis: a study of carbenicillin, azlocillin or piperacillin in combination with tobramycin. Eur J Respir Dis 1982;63(2):130–9.

[43] Grenier B, Gilly R. Azlocillin treatment of Pseudomonas aeruginosa bronchopulmonary infections in children with cystic fibrosis. Presse Med 1984; 13(13):815–8.

[44] Penketh A, Hodson ME, Gaya H. Azlocillin compared with carbenicillin in the treatment of bronchopulmonary infection due to Pseudomonas aeruginosa in cystic fibrosis. Thorax 1984;39(4): 299–304.

[45] Schaad UB, Desgrandchamps D, Kraemer R. Antimicrobial therapy of Pseudomonas pulmonary exacerbations in cystic fibrosis: a prospective evaluation of netilmicin plus azlocillin versus netilmicin plus ticarcillin. Acta Paediatr Scand 1986;75(1):128–38.

[46] Paull A, Morgan JR. Emergence of ceftriaxone-resistant strains of Pseudomonas aeruginosa in cystic fibrosis patients. J Antimicrob Chemother 1986; 18(5):635–9.

[47] Cabezudo I, Thompson RL, Selden RF, et al. Cefsulodin sodium therapy in cystic fibrosis patients. Antimicrob Agents Chemother 1984;25(1):4–6.

[48] Heilesen AM, Permin H, Koch C, et al. Treatment of chronic Pseudomonas aeruginosa infection in cystic fibrosis patients with ceftazidime and tobramycin. Scand J Infect Dis 1983;15(3):271–6.

[49] Moller NE, Koch C, Vesterhauge S, et al. Treatment of pulmonary Pseudomonas aeruginosa infection in cystic fibrosis with cefsulodin. Scand J Infect Dis 1982;14(3):207–11.

[50] Caplan DB, Buchanan CN. Treatment of lower respiratory tract infections due to Pseudomonas aeruginosa in patients with cystic fibrosis. Rev Infect Dis 1984;6 Suppl 3:S705–10.

[51] DeBoeck K, Smet M, Eggermont E. Treatment of Pseudomonas lung infection in cystic fibrosis with piperacillin plus tobramycin versus ceftazidime monotherapy: preliminary communication. Pediatr Pulmonol 1989;7(3):171–3.

[52] Pedersen SS, Koch C, Høiby N, et al. An epidemic spread of multiresistant Pseudomonas aeruginosa in a cystic fibrosis centre. J Antimicrob Chemother 1986;17(4):505–16.

[53] Watkins J, Francis J, Kuzemko JA. Does monotherapy of pulmonary infections in cystic fibrosis lead to early development of resistant strains of Pseudomonas aeruginosa? Scand J Gastroenterol 1988;Suppl 143:81–5.

[54] Dalzell AM, Sunderland D, Hart CA, et al. Ceftazidime treatment in cystic fibrosis: resistant organisms in sputum and faeces. Thorax 1991;46(4): 239–41.

[55] Govan JR, Doherty C, Glass S. Rational parameters for antibiotic therapy in patients with cystic fibrosis. Infection 1987;15(4):300–7.

[56] Reed MD, Stern RC, O'Brien CA, et al. Randomized double-blind evaluation of ceftazidime dose ranging in hospitalized patients with cystic fibrosis. Antimicrob Agents Chemother 1987; 31(5):698–702.

[57] DeBoeck K, Breysem L. Treatment of Pseudomonas aeruginosa lung infections in cystic fibrosis with high or conventional doses of ceftazidime. J Antimicrob Chemother 1998;41(3):407–9.

[58] Rappaz I, Decosterd LA, Bille J, et al. Continuous infusion of ceftazidime with a portable pump is as effective as thrice-a-day bolus in cystic fibrosis children. Eur J Pediatr 2000;159(12):919–25.

[59] Bernard E, Breilh D, Bru JP, et al. Is there a rationale for the continuous infusion of cefepime? A multidisciplinary approach. Clin Microbiol Infect 2003;9(5):339–48.

[60] Pedersen SS, Pressler T, Høiby N, et al. Imipenem/cilastatin treatment of multiresistant Pseudomonas aeruginosa lung infection in cystic fibrosis. J Antimicrob Chemother 1985;16(5):629–35.

[61] Pedersen SS, Pressler T, Jensen T, et al. Combined imipenem/cilastatin and tobramycin therapy of multiresistant Pseudomonas aeruginosa in cystic fibrosis. J Antimicrob Chemother 1987;19(1):101–7.

[62] Strandvik B, Malmborg AS, Bergan T, et al. Imipenem/cilastatin, an alternative treatment of pseudomonas infection in cystic fibrosis. J Antimicrob Chemother 1988;21(4):471–80.

[63] Bosso JA, Saxon BA, Matsen JM. In vitro activity of aztreonam combined with tobramycin and gentamicin against clinical isolates of Pseudomonas aeruginosa and Pseudomonas cepacia from patients with cystic fibrosis. Antimicrob Agents Chemother 1987;31(9):1403–5.

[64] Bosso JA, Saxon BA, Matsen JM. In vitro activities of combinations of aztreonam, ciprofloxacin, and ceftazidime against clinical isolates of Pseudomonas aeruginosa and Pseudomonas cepacia from patients with cystic fibrosis. Antimicrob Agents Chemother 1990;34(3):487–8.

[65] Allen JE, Bosso JA, Saxon BA, et al. Absence of rapidly developing resistance during treatment of cystic fibrosis patients with aztreonam. Diagn Microbiol Infect Dis 1987;8(1):51–5.

[66] Bosso JA, Allen JE, Matsen JM. Changing susceptibility of Pseudomonas aeruginosa isolates from cystic fibrosis patients with the clinical use of newer antibiotics. Antimicrob Agents Chemother 1989; 33(4):526–8.

[67] Blumer JL, Saiman L, Konstan MW, et al. The efficacy and safety of meropenem and tobramycin vs ceftazidime and tobramycin in the treatment of acute pulmonary exacerbations in patients with cystic fibrosis. Chest 2005;128(4):2336–46.

[68] Rubio TT, Shapiro C. Ciprofloxacin in the treatment of Pseudomonas infection in cystic fibrosis patients. J Antimicrob Chemother 1986;18 Suppl D:147–52.

[69] Rubio TT. Ciprofloxacin in the treatment of Pseudomonas infection in children with cystic fibrosis. Diagn Microbiol Infect Dis 1990;13(2):153–5.

[70] Lebel M. Fluoroquinolones in the treatment of cystic fibrosis: a critical appraisal. Eur J Clin Microbiol Infect Dis 1991;10(4):316–24.

[71] von Kreutz E, Ruhl-Fehlert C, Drommer W, et al. Effects of ciprofloxacin on joint cartilage in immature dogs immediately after dosing and after a 5-month treatment free period. Arch Toxicol 2004; 78(7):418–24.

[72] Grady R. Safety profile of quinolone antibiotics in the pediatric population. Pediatr Infect Dis J 2003; 22(12):1128–32.

[73] Roveta S, Schito AM, Marchese A, et al. Microbiological rationale for the utilization of prulifloxacin, a new fluoroquinolone, in the eradication of serious infections caused by Pseudomonas aeruginosa. Int J Antimicrob Agents 2005;26(5):366–72.

[74] Bauernfeind A, Emminger G, Horl G, et al. Bacteriological effects of anti-Pseudomonas aeruginosa chemotherapy in cystic fibrosis. Infection 1987; 15(5):403–6.

[75] Weiss K, Lapointe JR. Routine susceptibility testing of four antibiotic combinations for improvement of laboratory guide to therapy of cystic fibrosis infections caused by Pseudomonas aeruginosa. Antimicrob Agents Chemother 1995;39(11): 2411–4.

[76] Wolter JM, Bowler SD, McCormack JG. Are antipseudomonal antibiotics really beneficial in acute respiratory exacerbations of cystic fibrosis? Aust N Z J Med 1999;29(1):5–7.

[77] Smith AL, Fiel SB, Mayer-Hamblett N, et al. Susceptibility testing of Pseudomonas aeruginosa isolates and clinical response to parenteral antibiotic administration: lack of association in cystic fibrosis. Chest 2003;123(5):1495–502.

[78] Steinkamp G, Tummler B, Gappa M, et al. Long-term tobramycin aerosol therapy in cystic fibrosis. Pediatr Pulmonol 1989;6(2):91–8.

[79] MacLusky IB, Gold R, Corey M, et al. Long-term effects of inhaled tobramycin in patients with cystic fibrosis colonized with Pseudomonas aeruginosa. Pediatr Pulmonol 1989;7(1):42–8.

[80] Wiesemann HG, Steinkamp G, Ratjen F, et al. Placebo-controlled, double-blind, randomized study of aerosolized tobramycin for early treatment of Pseudomonas aeruginosa colonization in cystic fibrosis. Pediatr Pulmonol 1998;25(2): 88–92.

[81] Smith AL, Ramsey BW, Hedges DL, et al. Safety of aerosol tobramycin administration for 3 months to patients with cystic fibrosis. Pediatr Pulmonol 1989;7(4):265–71.

[82] Ramsey BW, Pepe MS, Quan JM, et al. Intermittent administration of inhaled tobramycin in patients with cystic fibrosis. N Engl J Med 1999; 340(1):23–30.

[83] Moss RB. Long-term benefits of inhaled tobramycin in adolescent patients with cystic fibrosis. Chest 2002;121(1):55–63.

[84] Gibson RL, Emerson J, McNamara S, et al. Significant microbiological effect of inhaled tobramycin in young children with cystic fibrosis. Am J Respir Crit Care Med 2003;167(6):841–9.

[85] Valerius NH, Koch C, Høiby N. Prevention of chronic Pseudomonas aeruginosa colonization in cystic fibrosis by early treatment. Lancet 1991; 338(8769):725–6.

[86] Frederiksen B, Koch C, Høiby N. Antibiotic treatment of initial colonization with Pseudomonas aeruginosa postpones chronic infection and prevents deterioration of pulmonary function in cystic fibrosis. Pediatr Pulmonol 1997;23(5):330–5.

[87] Munck A, Bonacorsi S, Mariani-Kurkdjian P, et al. Genotypic characterization of Pseudomonas aeruginosa strains recovered from patients with cystic fibrosis after initial and subsequent colonization. Pediatr Pulmonol 2001;32(4):288–92.

[88] Beringer P. The clinical use of colistin in patients with cystic fibrosis. Curr Opin Pulm Med 2001; 7(6):434–40.

[89] Høiby N, Frederiksen B, Pressler T. Eradication of early Pseudomonas aeruginosa infection. J Cyst Fibros 2005;4:49–54.

[90] Hodson ME, Gallagher CG, Govan JR. A randomized clinical trial of nebulised tobramycin or colistin in cystic fibrosis. Eur Respir J 2002; 20(3):658–64.

[91] Tamm M, Eich C, Frei R, et al. Inhaled colistin in cystic fibrosis. Schweiz Med Wochenschr 2000; 130(39):1366–72.

[92] Brannon MK, Pier M, Yeung L, et al. Highly colistin-resistant Pseudomonas aeruginosa as an emerging pathogen in cystic fibrosis. Pediatr Pulmonol 2006; Suppl 29:314.

[93] Heinzl B, Eber E, Oberwaldner B, et al. Effects of inhaled gentamicin prophylaxis on acquisition of Pseudomonas aeruginosa in children with cystic fibrosis: a pilot study. Pediatr Pulmonol 2002;33(1): 32–7.

[94] Schaad UB, Wedgwood-Krucko J, Suter S, et al. Efficacy of amikacin as adjunct to intravenous combination therapy (ceftazidime and amikacin) in cystic fibrosis. J Pediatr 1987;111(4):599–605.

[95] Kerem E. Mutation specific therapy in cystic fibrosis. Paediatr Respir Rev 2006;7 Suppl: S166–9.

[96] Du M, Kelling KM, Fan L, et al. Clinical doses of amikacin provide more effective suppression of the human CFTR-G542X stop mutation than gentamicin in a CF transgenic mouse model. J Mol Med 2006;84(7):573–82.

[97] Stead RJ, Hodson ME, Batten JC. Inhaled ceftazidime compared with gentamicin and carbenicillin in older patients with cystic fibrosis infected with Pseudomonas aeruginosa. Br J Dis Chest 1987; 81(3):272–9.

[98] Gibson RL, Retsch-Bogart GZ, Oermann C, et al. Microbiology, safety and pharmacokinetics of aztreonam lysinate for inhalation in patients with cystic fibrosis. Pediatr Pulmonol 2006;41(7): 656–65.

[99] Ryan G, Mukhopadhyay S, Singh M. Nebulised anti-pseudomonal antibiotics for cystic fibrosis. Cochrane Database Syst Rev 2003;3:CD001021, 2003.

[100] Koch C. Early infection and progression of cystic fibrosis lung disease. Pediatr Pulmonol 2002; 34(3):232–6.

[101] Høiby N. Understanding bacterial biofilms in patients with cystic fibrosis: current and innovative approaches to potential therapies. J Cyst Fibros 2002;1(4):249–54.

[102] VanDevanter DR, Van Dalfsen JM. How much do Pseudomonas biofilms contribute to symptoms of

pulmonary exacerbation in cystic fibrosis? Pediatr Pulmonol 2005;39(6):504–6.

[103] Dalzell AM, van Saene HK, Heaf DP. Cystic fibrosis, Pseudomonas aeruginosa, and selective decontamination. Arch Dis Child 1990;65(12):1365–7.

[104] Steinkamp G, Tummler B, Malottke R, et al. Treatment of pseudomonas aeruginosa colonization in cystic fibrosis. Arch Dis Child 1989;64(7):1022–8.

[105] Littlewood JM, Miller AG, Ghoneim AT. Nebulised colomycin for early pseudomonas colonization in cystic fibrosis. Lancet 1985;1(8433):865.

[106] Frederiksen B, Koch C, Høiby N. Changing epidemiology of Pseudomonas aeruginosa infection in Danish cystic fibrosis patients (1974–1995). Pediatr Pulmonol 1999;28(3):159–66.

[107] Taccetti G, Campana S, Festini F, et al. Early eradication therapy against Pseudomonas aeruginosa in cystic fibrosis patients. Eur Respir J 2005;26(3): 458–61.

[108] Ratjen F, Döring G, Nikolaizik WH. Effect of inhaled tobramycin on early Pseudomonas aeruginosa colonization in patients with cystic fibrosis. Lancet 2001;358(9286):983–4.

[109] Griese M, Muller I, Reinhardt D. Eradication of initial Pseudomonas aeruginosa colonization in patients with cystic fibrosis. Eur J Med Res 2002;7(2): 79–80.

[110] Steinkamp G, Ullrich G. Different opinions of physicians on the importance of measures to prevent acquisition of Pseudomonas aeruginosa from the environment. J Cyst Fibros 2003;2(4):199–205.

[111] Banerjee D, Stableforth D. The treatment of respiratory pseudomonas infection in cystic fibrosis: what drug and which way? Drugs 2000;60(5): 1053–64.

[112] Canton R, Cobos N, de Garcia J, et al. Antimicrobial therapy for pulmonary pathogenic colonization and infection by Pseudomonas aeruginosa in cystic fibrosis patients. Clin Microbiol Infect 2005;11(9):690–703.

[113] Döring G, Taccetti G, Campana S, et al. Eradication of Pseudomonas aeruginosa in cystic fibrosis patients. Eur Respir J 2006;27(3):653.

[114] Wood DM, Smyth AR. Antibiotic strategies for eradicating Pseudomonas aeruginosa in people with cystic fibrosis. Cochrane Database Syst Rev 2006;1:CD004197, 2006.

[115] Saiman L, Siegel T. Infection control in cystic fibrosis. Clin Microbiol Rev 2004;17(1):57–71.

[116] Pennington JE. Preliminary investigations of Pseudomonas aeruginosa vaccine in patients with leukemia and cystic fibrosis. J Infect Dis 1974;130 (Suppl 0):S159–62.

[117] Langford DT, Hiller J. Prospective, controlled study of a polyvalent pseudomonas vaccine in cystic fibrosis: three year results. Arch Dis Child 1984;59(12):1131–4.

[118] Lang AB, Schaad UB, Rudeberg A, et al. Effect of high-affinity anti-Pseudomonas aeruginosa lipopolysaccharide antibodies induced by immunization on the rate of Pseudomonas aeruginosa infection in patients with cystic fibrosis. J Pediatr 1995;127(5):711–7.

[119] Cryz SJ Jr, Lang A, Rudegerg A, et al. Immunization of cystic fibrosis patients with a Pseudomonas aeruginosa O-polysaccharide-toxin A conjugate vaccine. Behring Inst Mitt 1997;98:345–9.

[120] Cripps AW, Dunkley ML, Clancy RL, et al. Vaccine strategies against Pseudomonas aeruginosa infection in the lung. Behring Inst Mitt 1997;98: 262–8.

[121] Keogan MT, Johansen HK. Vaccines for preventing infection with Pseudomonas aeruginosa in people with cystic fibrosis. Cochrane Database Syst Rev 2000;2:CD001399, 2000.

[122] Zuercher AW, Horn MP, Que JU, et al. Antibody responses induced by long-term vaccination with an octovalent conjugate Pseudomonas aeruginosa vaccine in children with cystic fibrosis. FEMS Immunol Med Microbiol 2006;47(2): 302–8.

[123] Lang AB, Rudeberg A, Schoni MH, et al. Vaccination of cystic fibrosis patients against Pseudomonas aeruginosa reduces the proportion of patients infected and delays time to infection. Pediatr Infect Dis J 2004;23(6):504–10.

[124] Van Wye JE, Collins MS, Baylor M, et al. Pseudomonas hyperimmune globulin passive immunotherapy for pulmonary exacerbations in cystic fibrosis. Pediatr Pulmonol 1990;9(1):7–18.

[125] Ratjen F, Munck A, Campello V. Inhaled tobramycin nebuliser solution for treatment of early Pseudomonas aeruginosa infection: first results from the ELITE study. Pediatr Pulmonol 2006; Suppl 29:318.

[126] Wainwright C, Carlin J, Cooper P, et al. Australasian cystic fibrosis BAL study interim analysis. Pediatr Pulmonol 2006; Suppl 29:317.

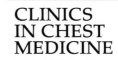

CLINICS
IN CHEST
MEDICINE

Clin Chest Med 28 (2007) 319–330

Nutrition and Lung Disease in Cystic Fibrosis

Carlos E. Milla, MD

Department of Pediatrics, Center for Excellence in Pulmonary Biology, Stanford University,
770 Welch Road, Suite 350, Palo Alto, CA 94304, USA

It is well recognized that among patients who have cystic fibrosis (CF), lung disease is a significant reason for morbidity and pulmonary function is the primary predictor of death [1]. Consequently, the rate at which pulmonary function is lost is the most important variable predicting mortality [2]. To this day, despite the importance given to pulmonary cares and the multiple advances in this aspect of the disease, the long-term preservation of lung function remains difficult to accomplish. Long-term preservation of lung function is likely a multifactorial process whereby the factors with the strongest influence remain unclear or difficult to control. Nutritional status is clearly recognized as a factor that is tightly intertwined in this process, and the temporality of this association has long been debated. Still, from the time when the first effective therapeutic strategies for the management of CF were described [3,4], aggressive nutritional support has been a fundamental component of the recommended treatment regimens.

Magnitude of the problem

The most recent consensus statements on nutritional management for patients who have CF [5,6] introduced important changes in the assessment parameters and categorization schemes recommended for the classification of nutritional status (Table 1) [7,8]. With the availability of the Centers for Disease Control and Prevention body mass index (BMI) percentiles and the increased familiarity of adult care providers with this parameter, BMI is now favored over percentage ideal body weight (%IBW) as the preferred

assessment parameter for children and adults. Added to the fact that the calculation of %IBW remains cumbersome, comparative studies have demonstrated a better discriminatory ability of BMI percentile over %IBW for the detection of underweight malnutrition [9,10]. Further, recent reviews of the US Cystic Fibrosis Foundation Patient Registry (CFFPR) have revealed that BMI percentile in children and BMI values in adults are directly and strongly correlated with pulmonary function parameters such as forced expiratory volume in 1 second (FEV_1) (Fig. 1). In view of this finding, the current recommendation is to aim for a BMI at the 50th percentile for children and a BMI of 22 kg/m^2 for adult women or 23 kg/m^2 for adult men [11]. In addition, added emphasis is given to the assessment of linear growth in children not only in terms of height-for-age percentile but also by interpreting this percentile in relation to the child's growth potential as determined by the target adult height percentile.

Epidemiologic studies

Given that many early studies showed good correlation between the degree of malnutrition and the severity of pulmonary disease, this finding has been taken as indirect evidence for the influence that nutrition has on the course of the lung disease and subsequent mortality [12]. Despite these observations, malnutrition continues to be one of the main clinical manifestations of CF across the age span, regardless of the time from diagnosis. The most recent estimates in the United States continue to indicate that inadequate weight gain and linear growth retardation are highly prevalent among children who have CF. Data reported by the CFFPR show that 22% of children who have CF

E-mail address: cmilla@stanford.edu

Table 1
Consensus criteria for the assessment of nutritional status in patients who have cystic fibrosis

Status	Height %ile[a] 2–20 y	%IBW[b] All ages	W/H %ile 0–2 y	BMI %ile 2–20 y	BMI (kg/m^2) >20 y
Adequate	At or above genetic potential	≥90%	>25th %ile	>25th %ile	22 (women) 23 (men)
At risk	Not at genetic potential	≥90% but weight loss or plateau	10th–25th %ile	10th–25th %ile	19–22 (women) 19–23 (men)
Malnutrition	<5th %ile	<90%	<10th %ile	<10th %ile	<19

Values are taken from the Centers for Disease Control and Prevention 2000 normative data.

Abbreviations: BMI, body mass index; %IBW, percentage ideal body weight; %ile, percentile; W/H, weight-for-height.

[a] For height %ile, genetic potential is estimated by first calculating the target adult height (TAH) from the parents' heights and then obtaining the percentile that will correspond to that height at age 20 years. TAH can be obtained by calculating the midparental height (MPH) and then applying the formulas proposed by Luo and colleagues [7]:

Females: TAH (cm) = 37.85 + 0.75 × MPH

Males: TAH (cm) = 45.99 + 0.78 × MPH

[b] %IBW is calculated by dividing the actual weight by the IBW and multiplying by 100. The IBW in children can be estimated by obtaining first the height %ile and then estimating the weight that will correspond to the same percentile in the growth curve. Alternatively, the IBW formulas proposed by Budd and colleagues [8] can be employed, which apply across the age span:

Females: IBW (kg) = $e^{(-0.3198 \times Ln(Ht^4) + 7.5767 \times Ln(Ht^3) - 63.306 \times Ln(Ht^2) + 222.74 \times Ln(Ht) - 299.6)}$

Males: IBW (kg) = $e^{(-1.0504 \times Ln(Ht^4) + 20.689 \times Ln(Ht^3) - 151.4 \times Ln(Ht^2) + 490.3 \times Ln(Ht) - 592.49)}$,

where Ht is height in centimeters and Ln is natural logarithm.

fall below the 10th percentile for weight and that 14% fall below the fifth percentile for height [11]. In addition, and not surprising given its high prevalence in childhood, as age increases, so does the prevalence of malnutrition among adult patients. According to the most recent estimates available, on average, 60.8% of adults who have CF have a BMI below the recommended levels [11], and the rate of nutritional failure (BMI < 19 kg/m^2) is estimated to be 38.5% [13].

In contrast, over 2 decades ago, the Toronto Cystic Fibrosis Center reported that their patient population had growth parameters that did not differ from the available normative data [14]. Their data showed, on average, fairly normal height percentiles in male and female patients. In addition, although weight percentiles were lower in female patients, underweight rates were lower than those reported from other centers. This report was followed by the classic Boston–Toronto comparison study. The study demonstrated clear-cut differences in the median survival of the two cohorts of patients: 21 years in Boston versus 30 years in Toronto. There was also a sharp contrast in the average growth parameters observed at each clinic, with the children in Toronto being ahead in their

percentiles, particularly for height. Most interesting was the fact that pulmonary function parameters were comparable between the two groups. Given the differences noted in growth parameters, the survival advantage of the Toronto cohort was ascribed to their better nutritional status [15].

A second important finding of this study was that the main difference between the treatment programs was the approach to dietary intervention, with the Toronto site being unrestrictive in terms of fat intake [16]. A second look 10 years later at the United States and Canadian data revealed that although there were still differences in the nutritional parameters, the gap noted on the previous study had already narrowed [17], probably as a reflection of the adoption of the Canadian nutritional support approach by United States centers [18].

Multiple previous longitudinal and cross-sectional studies that have looked at the relationship between morbidity and nutritional status concur that in CF patients, growth abnormalities and development of lung disease are linked [19–21]. Further, there is also evidence that interventions to establish weight gain are associated with improvements in pulmonary function [22–24]. In

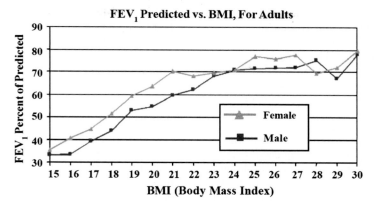

Fig. 1. Average percentage of predicted FEV_1 plotted against BMI (in kg/m^2) by sex. Increasing levels of BMI correlate with increasing levels of FEV_1, and this relationship starts to plateau at BMI levels between 22 and 23. (*From* 2004 Annual Data Report to the Center Directors. Cystic Fibrosis Patient Registry, Bethesda, MD; used with permission.)

addition, in agreement with the findings of the Toronto group, a review of the CFFPR data revealed that children who had a height percentile below the fifth percentile at age 5 or 7 years had a higher risk of death from the disease, with the risk estimates ranging from 3 to 6 times higher and without significant differences between boys and girls [25]. These results are in concordance with the assertion that growth, particularly linear growth, is intimately connected to the evolution of lung health in children who have CF.

From a clinical perspective, regardless of disease entity, the link between malnutrition and lung dysfunction is well established. The lung disease seen in patients who have CF primarily involves the airways and produces obstructive changes. Severe obstructive lung disease increases energy expenditure from the high demands of the work of breathing [26], and this is prominent in CF patients who have more advanced stages of lung disease [27–31]. The causal relationship between malnutrition and pulmonary dysfunction, however, particularly in terms of its temporality, remains unclear in CF. In the early, presymptomatic stages of lung disease during infancy and childhood, it is intuitive to assume that because this stage is crucial for lung growth and development, any nutritional derangements may affect the rate at which the lungs grow. This decreased growth, in turn, becomes a strong determinant for the development of lung disease [32,33]. There is some support for this possibility in the observation that CF patients who do not suffer from pancreatic insufficiency not only have better

nutritional parameters but also a lower rate of pulmonary deterioration [34,35].

Perhaps the interrelations between nutrition and lung disease could become clearer if studied in infants, because 85% have digestive manifestations even in the newborn period, and lung disease is not apparent in many young infants. Clarifying these interrelations, however, might not be so simple because studies on infants diagnosed by newborn screening [36,37] and studies with CF fetal airways [38] have demonstrated that there is an active inflammatory process present in the airways even before chronic infection and a symptomatic stage are reached.

Several longitudinal and prospective observational studies have provided mounting evidence for the temporal and potential causal relationship between malnutrition and pulmonary dysfunction in CF. Thomson and colleagues [33], in a prospective evaluation of their CF patient population, were able to identify important relationships between changes in growth and pulmonary function. In this study of CF patients who had pancreatic insufficiency, growth was assessed by conventional anthropometric parameters and accretion of body cell mass was assessed by total body potassium. Potassium is the main intracellular cation, and the change in its total content in the body is an accurate surrogate for the change in the cell mass [39]. Children who kept their cell mass accrual within the expected range experienced a decline in FEV_1 at a rate of less than half of that observed in children who were not able to accrue at an acceptable rate. Thus, this finding suggests that the lack of adequate growth also affected the growth and preservation of the lung tissue mass.

At a larger population level, information from longitudinal studies has also suggested that the presence of malnutrition precedes the development of lung dysfunction. In a report from the German CF Quality Assurance database, malnourished patients had significantly lower pulmonary function parameters, independent of the presence of infection with *Pseudomonas aeruginosa* [40]. More important, during childhood, patients who had good nutrition kept stable levels of FEV_1. In addition, a negative trend in weight-for-height over a 3-year period was associated with a decline in FEV_1, suggesting that maintaining weight was an important determinant of stability in lung function.

The author and colleagues [41] further investigated the effect of changes in growth parameters at a younger age on pulmonary function. A retrospective analysis of the Minnesota Cystic Fibrosis Database, a large repository of prospectively collected clinical data, revealed important associations between the rate of weight gain and changes in FEV_1. Children who maintained an adequate rate of weight gain between ages 6 and 8 years experienced significantly higher gains in FEV_1 during the same period. By repeated-measures regression analysis, sex and age at diagnosis did not play a role in the longitudinal trends in pulmonary function. Weight at first observation, however, had a strong effect, with a 55-mL difference in FEV_1 for every kilogram of difference in the initial weight ($P < .0001$). More important, weight gain during the 2-year follow-up was also strongly associated with change in FEV_1. An increase in weight of 1 kg was associated with a 32-mL increase in FEV_1 ($P < .0001$). Height and change in height from first observation were not significantly associated with FEV_1 values ($P = .08$ and $P = .20$, respectively). These results could be interpreted as reflecting better lung growth among children who experienced adequate rates of body mass accrual.

A larger study of the data prospectively collected in the Epidemiologic Study of Cystic Fibrosis on children who had their clinical information collected at ages 3 and 6 years demonstrated important effects of growth parameters on pulmonary function [42]. Significant differences were noted in the pulmonary function measurements at age 6 years according to the percentiles recorded at age 3 years. These differences were more pronounced for the relationship between weight-for-age

and FEV_1, in which there was a difference of 15 points between children in the highest and lowest percentile categories. In addition, changes in weight-for-age between ages 3 and 6 years were directly associated with changes in FEV_1.

Insights into mechanisms

From a developmental and mechanistic perspective, multiple animal and human studies have provided mounting evidence for a causal association between malnutrition and pulmonary abnormalities. Studies conducted in populations in which nutritional deprivation in early childhood is highly prevalent have shown important deficits in lung function. A study with Indian children showed significant associations between low BMI and differences in FEV_1, in addition to relationships between head circumference and lung function [43]. The differences noted increased with age, suggesting that as the child grows older, the differences in lung capacities become more profound, possibly because of differential rates of lung growth. Further, peak expiratory flow rate corrected for height was affected to a much lesser degree, suggesting that a reduction in airway caliber was unlikely to be responsible for the differences in pulmonary function. This finding was taken to be consistent with a reduction in lung volumes from impaired lung alveolar growth during postnatal life. A second study with children in Africa confirmed important pulmonary function deficits in a group of stunted and underweight children [44]. In addition to confirming the findings of previous, similar studies, this study found a direct relationship between fat-free mass (FFM) and lung function. Although forced vital capacity and FEV_1 were lower in the malnourished group compared with control subjects, the spirometric pattern that was noted was of an obstructive process. This finding was not further investigated to see whether it represented airway disease, but the enrolled children were free from respiratory disease and had a negative respiratory history. These findings were interpreted as indicative of the limited energy expenditure associated with malnutrition hampering lung development and function.

The potential mechanisms behind these associations can be drawn out from animal studies. Animal models of caloric deprivation have shown significant changes in the terminal airspaces, with consequent changes in the lung mechanical properties [45]. Investigations that have focused on the effects of nutritional deprivation in the early stages of postnatal lung development have demonstrated immediate and long-term alterations in the lung structure. In rats, intermittent food deprivation in the first week of life leads to the development of enlarged alveoli from defective septation, with thicker walls and decreased deposition of elastin [46]. In addition, early nutritional deprivation induces disruption of epithelial differentiation in bronchioles; this effect seems permanent because it persists after re-establishing adequate food intake [47]. At later stages in life, malnutrition also has important effects on lung structure and function. Increases in surface forces with a decrease in tissue elasticity are noted in excised lungs, perhaps reflecting changes in surfactant properties and remodeling of the connective tissue support. Of interest, with refeeding, surface forces return to normal, but the elastic forces only partially recover [45]. Evidence for alveolar remodeling with expansion of the terminal airspaces has been demonstrated in multiple animal studies [48–50], which concurs with the lung findings in anorectic humans [51,52]. Of interest, air trapping is a common finding in CF patients, being noted in young asymptomatic infants [53–55] and correlating with the degree of malnutrition [56]. Further, Massaro and colleagues [57] identified an up-regulation in caspases and granzymes in association with the development of emphysematous changes in the lungs of starved mice, suggesting activation of cytotoxic T lymphocytes and natural

killer cells. As a corollary to this finding, it could be proposed that on the background of the heightened inflammatory response typical of CF, malnutrition could provide an additional mechanism for immune activation. In addition, vitamins and other nutrients seem to have a strong influence on respiratory health [58]; their deficiencies are known to have deleterious effects on lung defense mechanisms such as ciliary activity, antioxidant balance, and innate immunity [59].

Together, these different deleterious effects have important implications for CF. As summarized in Fig. 2, these effects are likely to compound the airway surface defects that are known in the pathophysiology of CF lung disease. More important, these effects likely play a role during crucial periods of lung development early in life and may condition the rate at which the lung disease progresses.

Pancreatic insufficiency and the resultant chronic malabsorption is a major determinant of malnutrition in patients who have CF. This state is compounded by the added effects of chronic infection and inflammation with poor appetite and the development of comorbidities like CF-related diabetes mellitus (CFRD) and other gastrointestinal pathology. Given that these factors affect the intake and retention of nutrients, the nutritional problems in CF patients can be best understood if seen as the end result of an unfavorable energy balance as proposed by Pencharz and Durie [60]. Thus, to maintain growth rates and a nutritional status comparable to healthy controls, it has

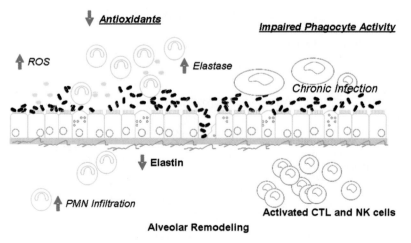

Fig. 2. Interactions in the lung (beyond abnormal mucus clearance) between the presence of CF (*italic letters*) and the effects of malnutrition (*bold letters*); effects likely to be conditioned by both are underlined. CTL, cytotoxic T lymphocytes; NK, natural killer; PMN, polymorphonuclear leukocyte; ROS, reactive oxygen species.

long been recommended that children who have CF should reach 120% to 150% of the typical recommended daily caloric intake [5,61]. Studies have shown, however, that the actual dietary intake of CF patients frequently falls short of these recommendations [62]. This deficit in energy balance will certainly be aggravated as the lung disease reaches a symptomatic stage and the repeated episodes of infection further promote a catabolic process. Many patients then fall into a vicious spiral that over time contributes to lung disease progression and overall health decline, as summarized in Fig. 3.

Data on resting energy expenditure (REE) in children who have CF consistently show increases compared with control children, children in preclinical stages [63,64], and children who have different degrees of disease severity [65]. This information has been taken as evidence for a phenotypic primary defect in the metabolism of these children leading to an increase in energy requirements. At the basic level, some studies show supporting evidence for a disruption in the intracellular energy use associated with the presence of a defective cystic fibrosis transmembrane conductance regulator, leading to increases in energy expenditure [66,67]. Bronstein and colleagues [68], however, reported a normal REE in a group of CF infants who did not have clinical signs or symptoms of the disease. This finding was confirmed by Bines and colleagues [69], establishing that REE in CF infants is comparable to that in healthy controls. Further, the growth deficits noted can be explained solely on the basis of pancreatic insufficiency and malabsorption, thereby arguing against a genetically determined alteration in energy metabolism. What is important is that the presence of even mild lung disease is associated with elevations in REE, suggesting that REE could be a sensitive marker of clinical status before lung disease becomes clinically apparent [70], although there seems to be a differential response between boys and girls [71]. Certainly, the development and progression of the lung disease determines increases in REE, which in turn adds to the energy imbalance [72], and the presence of chronic infection with *Pseudomonas*, with its consequent exuberant inflammatory state, magnifies this effect [73].

The nutritional status of a CF patient can be seen as the result of a very dynamic process influenced by energy intake and the presence of all of the factors known to influence the energy balance against the metabolic demands imposed by the lung disease. The body weight at any point in time reflects the status of this balance. Weight by itself can be interpreted as an indirect marker of protein mass and energy stores, and changes in body weight measured serially in patients who do not have fluid problems reflect changes in the protein mass, energy content, or both [74]. Body weight can be seen as reflecting the amounts of two basic components: fat mass and FFM. The main components of the FFM are skeletal muscle,

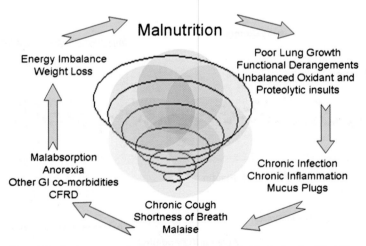

Fig. 3. The role of malnutrition in the progression of lung disease and health decline in CF. Although likely a multifactorial process with complex interactions, malnutrition can be best understood if viewed as a vicious spiral that is incrementally affected by the development of nutritional deficiencies from early in life. As malnutrition develops, the effects and rate of progression of the process is magnified with each cycle. GI, gastrointestinal.

water, and bone mass, with muscle constituting the largest component. These components of body mass can be estimated from calculations based on anthropometric measurements or more directly from isotope studies or by dual-energy x-ray absorptiometry, among other methods [74].

Studies that have specifically looked at the different components of body mass in patients who have CF compared with control subjects have been inconsistent in their findings, with some studies finding important differences [75,76] and others finding small, nonsignificant differences [77,78]. The only long-term longitudinal study reported to date that has looked at body composition changes in children who have CF [70,79] reported significant relationships between FFM and REE and a divergence over time in the accrual of FFM between children who have CF and control subjects. In adults who have CF, important associations between FFM and circulating inflammatory mediators have been noted [28]. In addition, patients who have an already compromised FFM had higher markers of catabolism and inflammation during pulmonary exacerbations and showed a lower response in these markers after therapy for the exacerbation [80].

These findings could have important implications for the possible role of FFM in the progression of CF lung disease. Although weight gain per se is important, maintenance of normal muscle mass may be intimately connected with normal growth and with good pulmonary function in patients who have CF. There are several reports of increased protein catabolism in poorly growing children who have CF [81–84]. The presence of a delay in the accrual of an adequate FFM implies lower development of the skeletal muscle, including the respiratory muscles. Previous studies using measures such as the maximum inspiratory and expiratory pressures and the maximum voluntary ventilation have shown abnormalities in the performance of the respiratory pump in CF patients who have different degrees of pulmonary dysfunction, particularly with respect to their respiratory muscle strength [85–87]. Respiratory muscle weakness, however, was not found in children who have CF and normal pulmonary function compared with control subjects, implying that the loss of muscle mass or strength precedes the development of lung disease [88]. In addition, studies on the effect of nutritional intervention for malnourished CF patients have shown that although gains in pulmonary function may not be consistently achieved, positive changes in the

respiratory muscle function can be achieved [89]. Also of interest, one study showed that the improvement in FEV_1 seen with nocturnal gastrostomy tube supplementation was correlated to change in lean body mass rather than to change in body fat [90]. In addition, reversal of protein catabolism stabilizes pulmonary function and decreases the number of hospitalizations for acute pulmonary exacerbation [83].

Nutritional intervention in cystic fibrosis

With the clear recognition of the important role that nutrition plays in the clinical course of CF, current guidelines recommend considering aggressive intervention in the presence of malnutrition despite an appropriate nutritional regimen [5,91]. This intervention usually entails the institution of enteral supplementation through the use of tube feedings. Several interventional studies have been conducted to look at the benefits of aggressive nutritional support [22,83,90,92]. A meta-analysis of the interventions available classified them into behavioral, oral supplements, enteral supplements, and parenteral nutrition [93]. All of the reported interventions, regardless of class, were found to be effective at inducing weight gain and to comparable degrees. Although most studies were small and of relatively short duration, of interest is that less aggressive interventions like behavioral modification were as efficacious as more aggressive interventions, particularly when applied early.

Most studies, however, have looked only at the effects of regimens aimed at the nutritional rescue of the most severely affected patients. A recent Cochrane review of enteral feedings in CF concluded that despite the wide acceptance of this treatment modality, its efficacy has not been fully evaluated and the available data are limited [94]. The studies found in the literature have reported on interventions in the clinical setting using different strategies for enteral supplementation, which makes interpretation and generalization of results difficult. Most of these studies have shown modest but significant gains in weight and other nutritional markers. At the same time, positive gains in pulmonary function were not consistently achieved, and mortality did not seem to be influenced by the intervention [95–97]. These results should be interpreted with caution because most studies were small and did not include an appropriate control group to be able to draw more firm conclusions. It is likely, however, that in a severely compromised patient population, a control group with no intervention may experience worst outcomes and may be ethically unfeasible. It must also be taken into account that these interventions are not free from complications. Problems such as gastroesophageal reflux and formula intolerance [97], hyperglycemia [98], stoma infections, and equipment malfunction can frequently be encountered. There is also a potential trade-off between the gains to be obtained from the intervention and the deleterious effects that could be induced. Certainly, in the sickest patients, it is likely that this risk–benefit balance needs careful consideration and close monitoring for complications is required. This risk of failure also implies that after the patient has reached a stage where there is severe lung damage already present, the potential gains may not have an effect strong enough to offset the disease progression. In a report on the long-term outcomes of a group of patients who had severely compromised lung function, Milla and Warwick [2] noted that nutritional status did not seem to influence the risk of mortality. It is therefore intuitive to assume that it is the earlier stages of the disease in which interventions are more likely to have a stronger positive influence.

Controlled trials on other interventions to improve nutrition have included the use of appetite stimulants and growth hormone. Small randomized controlled trials of megestrol acetate as an appetite stimulant have noted significant gains in weight and pulmonary function during treatment [99,100]. In one of the studies, however, only half of the subjects completed the trial and some lost the gains during the washout phase [100]. By body composition analysis, the main component of the weight gain was in fat mass. The caveat to this intervention is that such gains seem to be short-lived given that most of the weight gained represents water and fat, and there is the risk of important side effects such as glucose intolerance and adrenal suppression [100,101]. A small trial with cyproheptadine as an appetite stimulant has shown a better safety profile and more sustained weight gains [102]. Two small controlled trials with growth hormone given for 1 year have shown improvements in respiratory status in association with significant gains in lean body mass [103,104]. The study by Hardin and colleagues [103] demonstrated a significant improvement in forced vital capacity and improvements in measures of respiratory muscle strength and hospitalization rates in the treated group. Schibler

and colleagues [104] did not find any improvements in pulmonary function but found important gains in exercise capacity in the group randomized to active treatment.

Given the high prevalence of glucose metabolism abnormalities in CF [105] and the impact that the development of CFRD has in disease progression [106,107], early identification of CFRD though screening and aggressive management of this complication have been clearly recognized as important components of the management of CF patients [108]. Because insulin deficiency is one of the key pathophysiologic features of CFRD, insulin is the currently recommended standard treatment. Although there is a lack of randomized trials supporting this recommendation, previous small observational studies suggest that aggressive insulin therapy for CFRD might have a beneficial effect on CF pulmonary disease [109]. A large long-term multicenter study is currently underway in the United States and Canada to more formally evaluate the benefits of chronic insulin therapy in the management of CFRD [110]. The management of patients who only have glucose intolerance remains controversial. Case series reports point toward a benefit of starting early insulin therapy with small doses [111,112]. In some of these patients, however, the diabetic condition might be temporary and often related to their overall health status, with great fluctuations over time. A recommendation for long-term insulin therapy is therefore difficult to justify, and more studies are needed in this area given the potential implications for maintaining an adequate nutritional status and long-term preservation of pulmonary health.

Summary

A large body of data provides significant evidence for a link between nutritional status and lung health in CF. In addition, adequate growth plays a role in the development of lung function in children who have CF. More important, these studies suggest that the development of lung function abnormalities can be influenced by changes in nutritional status. Based on this information, it could be argued that aggressive nutritional support needs to start before significant nutritional derangements are noted. Not only it is likely that such an early intervention should have better chances of success but it also has the potential to decelerate or even prevent lung function deterioration and to positively affect survival. Because the nutritional deficiency frequently seen early in life is primarily related to pancreatic insufficiency and malabsorption [69], aggressive nutritional support and adequate pancreatic replacement management should lead to normal growth and to lung function preservation. Further, the relationship between protein and energy metabolism that is present in patients who have CF may have important prognostic and therapeutic implications; however, the relative importance of these factors in determining pulmonary function deterioration remains unknown. It is also not clear whether this relationship is due to inadequate growth of the lung or from an inability of the respiratory pump to efficiently meet the requirements imposed by the airway disease.

Nutritional intervention for CF patients is predicated on the hypothesis that improved nutritional status improves pulmonary function, which in some small studies seems to be the case. Which interventions will be of most value and have sustained gains is not completely clear from the available data. It is possible that the most effective interventions will have to include multiple components and go beyond the simple addition of caloric supplementation. Taking into account that several factors condition the deficits that lead to malnutrition in CF, multidisciplinary interventions are likely to give the best results. A comprehensive individualized management program should involve optimizing pancreatic enzyme use, addressing gastrointestinal comorbidities, identifying CFRD, maximizing caloric intake, addressing behavioral maladaptive responses, and controlling lung disease. More research is certainly needed not only to better dissect the nutritional factors involved in the lung disease but also (and perhaps more important) to identify effective and safe interventions through systematic controlled trials.

References

[1] Kerem E, Reisman J, Corey M, et al. Prediction of mortality in patients with cystic fibrosis. N Engl J Med 1994;326:1187–91.

[2] Milla CE, Warwick WJ. Risk of death in cystic fibrosis patients with severely compromised lung function. Chest 1998;113(5):1230–4.

[3] Matthews LW, Doerschuk C, Wise M, et al. A therapeutic regimen for patients with cystic fibrosis. J Pediatr 1964;65(4):558–75.

[4] Doershuk CF, Matthews LW, Tucker AS, et al. Evaluation of a prophylactic and therapeutic program for patients with cystic fibrosis. Pediatrics 1965;36(5):675–8.

[5] Borowitz D, Baker RD, Stallings VA. Consensus report on nutrition for pediatric patients with cystic fibrosis. J Pediatr Gastroenterol Nutr 2002;35(3): 246–59.

[6] Yankaskas JR, Marshall BC, Sufian B, et al. Cystic fibrosis adult care: consensus conference report. Chest 2004;125(1):1S–39S.

[7] Luo ZC, Low LC, Karlberg J. A comparison of target height estimated and final height attained between Swedish and Hong Kong Chinese children. Acta Paediatr 1999;88:248–52.

[8] Budd JR, Warwick WJ, Wielinski CL, et al. A medical information relational database system (MIRDS). Comput Biomed Res 1988;21:419–33.

[9] Lai HC, Kosorok MR, Sondel SA, et al. Growth status in children with cystic fibrosis based on the National Cystic Fibrosis Patient Registry data: evaluation of various criteria used to identify malnutrition. J Pediatr 1998;132(3 Pt 1):478–85.

[10] Zhang Z, Lai HC. Comparison of the use of body mass index percentiles and percentage of ideal body weight to screen for malnutrition in children with cystic fibrosis. Am J Clin Nutr 2004;80:982–91.

[11] Cystic Fibrosis Foundation Patient Registry. 2005 annual data report to the center directors. Bethesda (MD): Cystic Fibrosis Foundation; 2006.

[12] Borowitz D. The interrelationship of nutrition and pulmonary function in patients with cystic fibrosis. Curr Opin Pulm Med 1996;2(6):457–61.

[13] Cystic Fibrosis Foundation Patient Registry. 2004 annual data report to the center directors. Bethesda (MD): Cystic Fibrosis Foundation; 2005.

[14] Corey M. Longitudinal studies in cystic fibrosis. In: Sturgess JM, editor. Perspectives in cystic fibrosis. Proceedings of the 8th International Congress on cystic fibrosis. Toronto: Canadian Cystic Firbrosis Foundation; 1980. p. 246–55.

[15] Corey M, McLaughlin FJ, Williams M, et al. A comparison of survival, growth and pulmonary function in patients with cystic fibrosis in Boston and Toronto. J Clin Epidemiol 1988;41(6): 583–91.

[16] Parsons HG, Beaudry PH, Dumas A, et al. Energy needs and growth in children with cystic fibrosis. J Pediatr Gastroenterol Nutr 1983;2(1):44–9.

[17] Lai HC, Corey M, Fitz-Simmons SC, et al. Comparison of growth status of patients with cystic fibrosis between the United States and Canada. Am J Clin Nutr 1999;69:531–8.

[18] Ramsey BW, Farrell PM, Pencharz PB. Nutritional assessment and management in cystic fibrosis: a consensus report. Am J Clin Nutr 1992;55:108–16.

[19] Kraemer R, Rudeberg A, Hadorn HB, et al. Relative underweight in cystic fibrosis and its prognostic value. Acta Paediatr Scand 1978;76:33–7.

[20] Nir M, Lanng S, Johansen HK, et al. Long term survival and nutritional data in patients with cystic fibrosis treated in a Danish centre. Thorax 1996;51: 1023–7.

[21] Zemel BSP, Jawad A. Longitudinal relationship among growth, nutritional status, and pulmonary function in children with cystic fibrosis: analysis of the Cystic Fibrosis Foundation National CF Patient Registry. J Pediatr 2000;137(3):374–80.

[22] Levy LD, Durie PR, Pencharz PB, et al. Effects of long-term nutritional rehabilitation on body composition and clinical status in malnourished children and adolescents with cystic fibrosis. J Pediatr 1985;107(2):225–30.

[23] Dalzell AM, Shepherd RW, Dean B, et al. Nutritional rehabilitation in cystic fibrosis: a five year follow up study. J Pediatr Gastroenterol Nutr 1992; 15:141–7.

[24] Schoni MH, Casaulta C. Nutrition and lung function in cystic fibrosis patients: review. Clin Nutr 2000;19(2):79–85.

[25] Beker LT, Russek-Cohen E, Fink RJ. Stature as a prognostic factor in cystic fibrosis survival. J Am Diet Assoc 2001;101(4):438–42.

[26] Wilson DO, Rogers RM, Hoffman RM. State of the art: nutrition and chronic lung disease. Am Rev Respir Dis 1985;132:1347–65.

[27] Vaisman N, Pencharz PB, Corey M, et al. Energy expenditure of patients with cystic fibrosis. J Pediatr 1987;111(4):496–500.

[28] Elborn JS, Cordon SM, Western PJ, et al. Tumour necrosis factor-alpha, resting energy expenditure and cachexia in cystic fibrosis. Clin Sci 1993;85(5): 563–8.

[29] Bell SC, Saunders MJ, Elborn JS, et al. Resting energy expenditure and oxygen cost of breathing in patients with cystic fibrosis. Thorax 1996;51(2): 126–31.

[30] Wilson DC, Pencharz PB. Nutrition and cystic fibrosis. Nutrition 1998;14(10):792–5.

[31] Sharma R. Wasting as an independent predictor of mortality in patients with cystic fibrosis. Thorax 2001;56(10):746–50.

[32] Elborn JS, Bell SC. Nutrition and survival in cystic fibrosis. Thorax 1996;51:971–2.

[33] Thomson MA, Quirk P, Swanson CE, et al. Nutritional growth retardation is associated with defective lung growth in cystic fibrosis: a preventable determinant of progressive pulmonary dysfunction. Nutrition 1995;11(4):350–4.

[34] Gaskin K, Gurwitz D, Durie PR, et al. Improved respiratory prognosis in patients with cystic fibrosis with normal fat absorption. J Pediatr 1982;100: 875–82.

[35] Gaskin KJ, Waters DL, Soutter VL, et al. Body composition in cystic fibrosis. Basic Life Sci 1990; 55:15–21.

[36] Kirchner KK, Wagener JS, Khan T, et al. Increased DNA levels in bronchoalveolar lavage fluid obtained from infants with cystic fibrosis. Am J Respir Crit Care Med 1996;154:1426–9.

[37] Armstrong DS, Grimwood K, Carlin JB, et al. Lower airway inflammation in infants and young children with cystic fibrosis. Am J Respir Crit Care Med 1997;156(4 Pt 1):1197–204.

[38] Tirouvanziam R, de Bentzmann S, Hubeau C, et al. Inflammation and infection in naive human cystic fibrosis airway grafts. Am J Respir Crit Care Med 2000;23(2):121–7.

[39] Shepherd RW, Holt TL, Greer R, et al. Total body potassium in cystic fibrosis. J Pediatr Gastroenterol Nutr 1989;9(2):200–5.

[40] Steinkamp G, Wiedenmann DE. Relationship between nutritional status and lung function in cystic fibrosis: cross sectional and longitudinal analyses from the German CF quality assurance (CFQA) project. Thorax 2002;57(7):596–601.

[41] Peterson ML, Jacobs DR, Milla CE. Longitudinal changes in growth parameters are correlated with changes in pulmonary function in children with cystic fibrosis. Pediatrics 2003;112(3):588–92.

[42] Konstan MW, Butler SM, Wohl MEB, et al. Growth and nutritional indexes in early life predict pulmonary function in cystic fibrosis. J Pediatr 2003;142(6):624–30.

[43] Mukhopadhyay S, Macleod KA, Ong TJ, et al. "Ethnic" variation in childhood lung function may relate to preventable nutritional deficiency. Acta Paediatr 2001;90:1299–303.

[44] Glew RH, Brock HS, VanderVoort J, et al. Lung function and nutritional status of semi-nomadic Fulani children and adolescents in Northern Nigeria. J Trop Pediatr 2004;50(1):20–1.

[45] Sahebjami H. Nutrition and lung structure and function. Exp Lung Res 1993;19(2):105–24.

[46] Das RM. The effects of intermittent starvation on lung development in suckling rats. Am J Pathol 1984;117(2):326–32.

[47] Massaro GD, McCoy L, Massaro D. Postnatal undernutrition slows development of bronchiolar epithelium in rats. Am J Physiol Regul Integr Comp Physiol 1988;255(24):521–6.

[48] Sahebjami H, Wirman JA. Emphysema-like changes in the lungs of starved rats. Am Rev Respir Dis 1981;124(5):619–24.

[49] Kerr JS, Riley DJ, Lanza-Jacoby S, et al. Nutritional emphysema in the rat. Influence of protein depletion and impaired lung growth. Am Rev Respir Dis 1985;131:644–50.

[50] Karlinsky JB, Goldstein RH, Ojserkis B, et al. Lung mechanics and connective tissue levels in starvation-induced emphysema in hamsters. Am J Physiol Regul Integr Comp Physiol 1986;251: 282–8.

[51] Cook VJ, Coxson HO, Mason AG, et al. Bullae, bronchiectasis and nutritional emphysema in severe anorexia nervosa. Can Respir J 2001;8:361–5.

[52] Coxson HO, Chan IHT, Mayo JR, et al. Early emphysema in patients with anorexia nervosa. Am J Respir Crit Care Med 2004;170:748–52.

[53] Ljungberg H, Hulskamp G, Hoo AF, et al. Estimates of plethysmographic FRC exceed those by

gas dilution in infants with cystic fibrosis but not in healthy controls. Thorax 2002;57(S3):23.

[54] Castile RG, Iram D, McCoy K. Gas trapping in normal infants and in infants with cystic fibrosis. Pediatr Pulmonol 2004;37:461–9.

[55] Davis SD, Kerby GS, Acton JD, et al. Feasibility, sensitivity and variability of adult-type pulmonary function tests in infants with CF in a multicenter, longitudinal trial. Pediatr Pulmonol 2006; 29(Suppl):334.

[56] Kraemer R, Aebi C, Casaulta Aebischer C, et al. Early detection of lung disease and its association with the nutritional status, genetic background and life events in patients with cystic fibrosis. Respiration 2000;67(5):477–90.

[57] Massaro D, Massaro GD, Baras A, et al. Calorie-related rapid onset of alveolar loss, regeneration, and changes in mouse lung gene expression. Am J Physiol Lung Cell Mol Physiol 2004;286:896–906.

[58] Kelly Y, Sacker A, Marmot M. Nutrition and respiratory health in adults: findings from the Health Survey for Scotland. Eur Respir J 2003;21:664–71.

[59] Harding R, Cock ML, Albuquerque CA. Role of nutrition in lung development before and after birth. In: Harding R, Pinkerton KE, Plopper CG, editors. The lung: development, aging and the environment. London: Elsevier Academic Press; 2004. p. 253–66.

[60] Pencharz PB, Durie PR. Pathogenesis of malnutrition in cystic fibrosis, and its treatment. Clin Nutr 2000;19(6):387–94.

[61] Roy CC, Darling P, Weber AM. A rational approach to meeting macro and micronutrient needs in cystic fibrosis. J Pediatr Gastroenterol Nutr 1984;3(S1):154–62.

[62] Wootton SA, Murphy JL, Bond SA, et al. Energy balance and growth in cystic fibrosis. J R Soc Med 1991;84(S18):22–7.

[63] Girardet JP, Tounian P, Sardet A, et al. Resting energy expenditure in infants with cystic fibrosis. J Pediatr Gastroenterol Nutr 1994;18(2):214–9.

[64] Thomson MA, Wilmott RW, Wainwright C, et al. Resting energy expenditure, pulmonary inflammation, and genotype in the early course of cystic fibrosis. J Pediatr 1996;129(3):367–73.

[65] Lucas A, Prentice AM, Shepherd RW. Energy expenditure and cystic fibrosis. Lancet 1988;2(8613):737.

[66] Fiegel RJ, Shapiro BL. Mitochondrial calcium uptake and oxygen consumption in cystic fibrosis. Nature 1979;278:276–7.

[67] Bell CL, Quinton PM. Regulation of CFTR Cl− conductance in secretion by cellular energy levels. Am J Physiol 1993;264(4 Pt 1):C925–31.

[68] Bronstein MN, Davies PS, Hambidge KM, et al. Normal energy expenditure in the infant with presymptomatic cystic fibrosis. J Pediatr 1995;126(1):28–33.

[69] Bines JE, Truby H, Armstrong DS, et al. Energy metabolism in infants with cystic fibrosis [article]. J Pediatr 2002;140(5):527–33.

[70] Zemel BS, Kawchak DA, Cnaan A, et al. Prospective evaluation of resting energy expenditure, nutritional status, pulmonary function and genotype in children with cystic fibrosis. Pediatr Res 1996;40: 578–86.

[71] Allen JR, McCauley JC, Selby AM, et al. Differences in resting energy expenditure between male and female children with cystic fibrosis. J Pediatr 2003;142(1):15–9.

[72] Fried M, Durie PR, Tsui LC, et al. The cystic fibrosis gene and resting energy expenditure. J Pediatr 1991;119:913–6.

[73] Vinton NE, Padman R, Davis M, et al. Effects of Pseudomonas colonization on body composition and resting energy expenditure in children with cystic fibrosis. JPEN J Parenter Enteral Nutr 1999; 23(4):233–6.

[74] Heymsfield SB, Baumgartner RN, Pan S. Nutritional assessment of malnutrition by anthropometric methods. In: Shils ME, Olson JA, Shike M, et al, editors. Modern nutrition in health and disease. 9th edition. Baltimore (MD): Williams & Wilkins; 1999. p. 903–21.

[75] Henderson RC, Madsen CD. Bone mineral content and body composition in children and young adults with cystic fibrosis. Pediatr Pulmonol 1999;27(2): 80–4.

[76] Spicher V, Roulet M, Schaffner C, et al. Bio-electrical impedance analysis for estimation of fat-free mass and muscle mass in cystic fibrosis patients. Eur J Pediatr 1993;152(3):222–5.

[77] Tomezsko JL, Scanlin TF, Stallings VA. Body composition of children with cystic fibrosis with mild clinical manifestations compared with normal children. Am J Clin Nutr 1994;59(1):123–8.

[78] Allen JR, Humphries IR, McCauley JC, et al. Assessment of body composition of children with cystic fibrosis (CF). Appl Radiat Isot 1998;49(5–6): 591–2.

[79] Stettler N, Kawachak DA, Boyle LL, et al. A prospective study of body composition changes in children with cystic fibrosis. Ann N Y Acad Sci 2000; 904:406–9.

[80] Ionescu AA, Nixon LS, Evans WD, et al. Bone density, body composition, and inflammatory status in cystic fibrosis. Am J Respir Crit Care Med 2000; 162(3 Pt 1):789–94.

[81] Holt TL, Ward L, Francis PJ, et al. Whole body protein turnover in malnourished cystic fibrosis patients and its relationship to pulmonary disease. Am J Clin Nutr 1985;41:1061–6.

[82] Miller M, Ward L, Thomas BJ, et al. Altered body composition and muscle protein degradation in nutritionally growth-retarded children with cystic fibrosis. Am J Clin Nutr 1982;36(3):492–9.

[83] Shepherd RW, Holt TL, Thomas BJ, et al. Nutritional rehabilitation in cystic fibrosis: controlled studies of effects on nutritionally growth-retarded children with cystic fibrosis. J Pediatr 1986;109:788–94.

[84] Shepherd RW, Holt TL, Johnson LP, et al. Leucine metabolism and body cell mass in cystic fibrosis. Nutrition 1995;11(2):138–41.

[85] Asher MI, Pardy RL, Coates AL, et al. The effects of inspiratory muscle training in patients with cystic fibrosis. Am Rev Respir Dis 1982;126: 855–9.

[86] Szeinberg A, England S, Mindorff C, et al. Maximal inspiratory and expiratory pressures are reduced in hyperinflated, malnourished, young adult male patients with cystic fibrosis. Am Rev Respir Dis 1985;132:766–9.

[87] Lands L, Desmond KJ, Denizo D, et al. The effects of nutritional status and hyperinflation on respiratory muscle strength in children and young adults. Am Rev Respir Dis 1990;141:1506–9.

[88] Hanning RM, Blimkie CJ, Bar-Or O, et al. Relationships among nutritional status and skeletal and respiratory muscle function in cystic fibrosis: does early dietary supplementation make a difference? Am J Clin Nutr 1993;57(4):580–7.

[89] Mansell AL, Andersen JC, Muttart CR, et al. Short-term pulmonary effects of total parenteral nutrition in children with cystic fibrosis. J Pediatr 1984;104:700–5.

[90] Steinkamp G, von der Hardt H. Improvement of nutritional status and lung function after long-term nocturnal gastrostomy feedings in cystic fibrosis. J Pediatr 1994;124:244–9.

[91] Sinaasappel M, Stern M, Littlewood JM, et al. Nutrition in patients with cystic fibrosis: a European consensus. J Cyst Fibros 2002;1:51–75.

[92] Pencharz P, Hill R, Archibald E, et al. Energy needs and nutritional rehabilitation in undernourished adolescents and young adult patients with cystic fibrosis. J Pediatr Gastroenterol Nutr 1984; 3(Suppl 1):S147–53.

[93] Jelalian E, Stark LJ, Reynolds L, et al. Nutrition intervention for weight gain in cystic fibrosis: a meta analysis. J Pediatr 1998;132(3 Pt 1):486–92.

[94] Conway SP, Morton A, Wolfe S. Enteral tube feeding for cystic fibrosis. Cochrane Database Syst Rev 1999;3:CD001198.

[95] Levy LD, Durie PR, Pencharz PB, et al. Prognostic factors associated with patient survival during nutritional rehabilitation in malnourished children and adolescents with cystic fibrosis. J Pediatr Gastroenterol Nutr 1986;5:97–102.

[96] O'Loughlin E, Forbes D, Parsons H, et al. Nutritional rehabilitation of malnourished patients with cystic fibrosis. Am J Clin Nutr 1986;43:732–7.

[97] Oliver MR, Heine RG, Ng CH, et al. Factors affecting clinical outcome in gastrostomy-fed children with cystic fibrosis. Pediatr Pulmonol 2004; 37:324–9.

[98] Milla CE, Doherty L, Raatz S, et al. Glycemic response to dietary supplements in cystic fibrosis is dependent on the carbohydrate content of the formula. JPEN J Parenter Enteral Nutr 1996;20(3): 182–6.

[99] Eubanks VMR, Koppersmith NMR, Wooldridge NMR, et al. Effects of megestrol acetate on weight gain, body composition, and pulmonary function in patients with cystic fibrosis. J Pediatr 2002; 140(4):439–44.

[100] Marchand V, Baker SS, Stark TJ, et al. Randomized, double-blind, placebo-controlled pilot trial of megestrol acetate in malnourished children with cystic fibrosis. J Pediatr Gastroenterol Nutr 2000;31(3):264–9.

[101] McKone EF, Tonelli MR, Aitken ML. Adrenal insufficiency and testicular failure secondary to megestrol acetate therapy in a patient with cystic fibrosis. Pediatr Pulmonol 2002;34(5):381–3.

[102] Homnick DN, Marks JH, Hare KL, et al. Long-term trial of cyproheptadine as an appetite stimulant in cystic fibrosis. Pediatr Pulmonol 2005; 40(3):251–6.

[103] Hardin DSM, Ellis K, Dyson M, et al. Growth hormone improves clinical status in prepubertal children with cystic fibrosis: results of a randomized controlled trial. J Pediatr 2001;139(5):636–42.

[104] Schibler A, von der Heiden A, Birrer R, et al. Prospective randomised treatment with recombinant human growth hormone in cystic fibrosis. Arch Dis Child 2003;88(12):1078–81.

[105] Moran A, Doherty L, Wang X, et al. Abnormal glucose metabolism in cystic fibrosis. J Pediatr 1998;133(1):10–7.

[106] Milla CE, Warwick WJ, Moran A. Trends in pulmonary function in cystic fibrosis (CF) patients correlate with the results of oral glucose tolerance test at baseline. Am J Respir Crit Care Med 2000; 162:891–5.

[107] Milla CE, Billings JL, Moran A. Diabetes is associated with dramatically decreased survival in women but not men with cystic fibrosis. Diabetes Care 2005;28:2141–4.

[108] Moran A, Hardin DS, Rodman DM, et al. Diagnosis, screening and management of cystic fibrosis related diabetes mellitus. A consensus conference report. Diabetes Res Clin Pract 1999;45:61–73.

[109] Lanng S, Thorsteinson B, Nerup J, et al. Diabetes mellitus in cystic fibrosis: effect of insulin therapy on lung function and infections. Acta Paediatr 1994;83:849–53.

[110] Diabetes therapy to improve BMI and lung function in CF. Available at: http://clinicaltrials.gov/show/ NCT00072904. Accessed March 25, 2007.

[111] Dobson L, Hattersley AT, Tiley S, et al. Clinical improvement in cystic fibrosis with early insulin treatment. Arch Dis Child 2002;87(5):430–1.

[112] Franzese A, Spagnuolo MI, Sepe A, et al. Can glargine reduce the number of lung infections in patients with cystic fibrosis related diabetes? Diabetes Care 2005;28:2333.

ELSEVIER
SAUNDERS

Clin Chest Med 28 (2007) 331–346

CLINICS
IN CHEST
MEDICINE

Inflammation and Anti-Inflammatory Therapies for Cystic Fibrosis

James F. Chmiel, MD, MPH[a,b,*], Michael W. Konstan, MD[a,b]

[a]*Division of Pediatric Pulmonology, Department of Pediatrics, Case Western Reserve University School of Medicine, 11100 Euclid Avenue, Cleveland, OH 44106, USA*
[b]*LeRoy Mathews Cystic Fibrosis Center, Rainbow Babies and Children's Hospital, 11100 Euclid Avenue, Cleveland, OH 44106, USA*

The majority of morbidity and mortality in cystic fibrosis (CF) results from progressive pulmonary disease that is characterized by a self-perpetuating cycle of airway obstruction, chronic bacterial infection, and excessive inflammation that results in bronchiectasis and death [1,2]. Relieving obstruction and controlling infection have been the cornerstones of therapy for decades. Recognition that inflammation is primarily responsible for the lung destruction in CF has prompted investigation into therapies directed toward attenuating the inflammatory response. This article provides an overview of the inflammatory response in the CF airway and the current understanding of anti-inflammatory therapies in CF.

Characteristics of the inflammatory response in the cystic fibrosis airway

To understand the approach to anti-inflammatory therapy for patients who have CF, it is necessary to review the inflammatory response in the CF airway. Patients who have CF have a predilection for infection with a limited spectrum of distinctive bacteria, such as *Staphylococcus aureus*, *Haemophilus influenzae*, *Pseudomonas aeruginosa*, *Burkholderia cepacia* complex organisms, *Stenotrophomonas maltophilia*, and *Achromobacter xylosoxidans*. Once challenged by viral or bacterial infection, massive numbers of neutrophils are recruited to the airway. Although inflammation is meant to contain infection, this fails in the CF airway, and the exaggerated inflammatory response is responsible for much of the pathology in the CF lung. The inflammatory response in CF begins early in life, becomes persistent, and is excessive relative to the burden of infection. Bronchoalveolar lavage fluid (BALF) from patients who have CF contains large concentrations of inflammatory mediators and massive amounts of neutrophils and neutrophil products [3–8]. This may not be surprising in adolescents and young adults, even those with mild disease, because most of these patients are chronically infected [7]; however, there is an impressive burden of inflammation even in infants who have CF [3,5,8–11]. BALF from infected infants who have CF contains greatly elevated concentrations of neutrophil chemoattractants, neutrophils, and neutrophil products compared with BALF from non-CF infants [3,10,11]. These inflammatory mediators are present, although at somewhat lower concentrations, in BALF from apparently uninfected infants who have CF [3]. The presence of inflammation in the absence of detectable pathogens might suggest that the inflammatory response in the CF lung operates independently of an infectious stimulus. These findings may also be explained by the failure to terminate the inflammatory response once the inciting stimulus has been eradicated and may represent an abnormal persistence of inflammation after clearance of early, transient infection [2]. Other studies suggest that the inflammatory response in CF is also excessive relative to the burden of infection [12,13].

This article was supported by NIH grant P30-DK27651 and by the U.S. Cystic Fibrosis Foundation.

* Corresponding author. 11100 Euclid Avenue, Cleveland, OH 44106.

E-mail address: james.chmiel@uhhospitals.org (J.F. Chmiel).

BALF from infants who have CF infected only with *H influenzae* contains more neutrophils and interleukin (IL)-8, a potent neutrophil chemoattractant, for any given burden of *H influenzae* than does BALF from infants who have underlying conditions other than CF who are infected with *H influenzae* [12,13]. Apoptosis seems to be delayed in neutrophils from patients who have CF [14,15], and this likely contributes further to the large number of neutrophils present in the CF airway. As they undergo necrosis, neutrophils release their damaging intracellular contents into the airway. Neutrophil DNA and actin increase the viscosity of CF sputum and impair mucociliary clearance. Neutrophils also release oxidants and proteases, including elastase. Excessive amounts of oxidants overwhelm the antioxidant defenses and contribute to lung injury. The huge excess of elastase similarly overwhelms the antiprotease screen in the airways and results in uninhibited proteolytic enzymatic activity. Elastase directly promotes structural damage by digesting elastin and other airway wall proteins; worsens airway obstruction by impairing ciliary beating, increasing mucus secretion, and increasing sodium reabsorption through activation of the epithelial sodium channel; promotes bacterial persistence by cleaving critical opsonins and receptors that are necessary for phagocytosis; and promotes the generation of neutrophil chemoattractants, particularly IL-8, leukotriene (LT)B_4, and the complement component C5a-like peptide [1,2]. Bacteria and their products also promote the generation of chemoattractants, which recruit more neutrophils into the airways, fueling the vicious cycle of inflammation that leads to lung destruction [2,16].

BALF from patients who have CF contains large concentrations of tumor necrosis factor–alpha (TNF-α), IL-1β, IL-6, IL-8, and granulocyte-macrophage colony-stimulating factor [4]. All of these proinflammatory cytokines have the common characteristic that their synthesis is promoted by transcription factor nuclear factor-kappa B (NF-κB), which is activated by cellular interaction with bacteria, bacterial products, and proinflammatory cytokines. Additional regulatory abnormalities may also occur that lead to excessive transcription of proinflammatory cytokine genes. Some studies have found that CF airways are relatively deficient in IL-10 and nitric oxide (NO) [17–20], both of which preserve the function of inhibitory protein-kappaB (IκB), the inhibitor of NF-κB. In situations where either or both

IL-10 and NO might be deficient, less IκB would be available to inhibit NF-κB, and proinflammatory mediator production would increase. Therefore, an imbalance between IκB and NF-κB would result in the prolonged and excessive production of the mediators responsible for the damaging inflammation. In addition, CF tissues seem to be deficient in peroxisome proliferator activating receptor (PPAR) [21]. When activated, PPAR forms a heterodimer with activated retinoid X receptor, which is able to modulate inflammation [22]. PPAR exerts its attenuating effects typically by inhibiting NF-κB activity via up-regulation of IκB [23] or by competition with NF-κB for helicases. CF airway epithelial cell lines seem to have less PPAR-γ activity than do non-CF airway epithelial cell lines [24]. Decreased PPAR expression leads to an imbalance between IκB and NF-κB that favors increased inflammation in CF. The proposed mechanisms are not mutually exclusive, and it is possible that a combination of these processes fuels the aggressive and damaging inflammatory cascade.

It seems that the most appropriate time to treat the excessive inflammatory response is relatively early in life, before the establishment of the vicious cycle of obstruction, infection, and inflammation and before the onset of structural damage to the airways. It is not known whether limiting inflammation in infancy promotes or retards the establishment of chronic infection. To some extent, the inflammatory response is likely to be protective early in the course of disease; however, published clinical trials suggest that anti-inflammatory therapy needs to begin early in the course of disease [25–27]. It seems plausible that as lung disease progresses, therapies such as the mechanical removal of secretions, antioxidants, and antiproteases, which limit the structural damage due to the inflammatory response, must accompany treatments aimed at reducing inflammation.

Therapies aimed at the inflammatory response in the cystic fibrosis airway

In addition to the regular use of antibiotics to treat the chronic bacterial infection in the CF airway, a direct attack on inflammation seems warranted because it is the major process leading to destruction of the lungs. There are several steps in the inflammatory process at which intervention may be targeted (Table 1). Because the overall

Table 1
Targets of anti-inflammatory therapies in CF

Target in inflammatory cascade	Therapies
Stimuli	
Bacteria/bacterial products	Antibiotics (macrolides [101–111])
Viruses	
Receptors	Etanercept, BIIL 284 BS [77], montelukast [78]
Intracellular signaling mechanisms	Corticosteroids [25,26,28–43], ibuprofen [27,32,44–52], IL-10 [53,54], interferon-γ [58], simvastatin [62–68], L-arginine [69–72], thiazolidinediones/pioglitazone [24,59,60,68], p38 mitogen-activated protein kinase inhibitors
Products	
Cytokines	Corticosteroids, ibuprofen, infliximab, IL-10, macrolides [112–117], N-acetyl cysteine [84,85], anti–IL-8
Eicosanoid modulators	Corticosteroids, BIIL 284 BS, ibuprofen, omega-3 fatty acids [79,80]
Leukocyte adhesion molecules	Anti–ICAM-1
Oxidants	N-acetyl cysteine, glutathione [86–89], β-carotene, vitamin C, vitamin E,
Proteases	α1-protease inhibitor [90–93], secretory leukoprotease inhibitor, monocyte/neutrophil elastase inhibitor [94], Depelstat [95–98]
DNA	Dornase-alfa [118–124]
Other	Hydroxychloroquine, methotrexate [125], cyclosporine-A [126]

inflammatory process can be viewed as a self-propagating cycle, significant efficacy at any step may result in a benefit to the patient who has CF. Because the neutrophil is the primary effector cell mediating the damaging inflammation in the CF airway, anti-inflammatory therapies must address, directly or indirectly, the neutrophil or its products. Therapies inhibiting neutrophil chemotaxis and the downstream consequences of neutrophil products are under investigation. Attention has focused primarily on the therapeutic potential of systemic and inhaled corticosteroids and ibuprofen; however, investigators recently have considered the anti-inflammatory capabilities of cytokines, intracellular signaling modulators, eicosanoid modulators, antioxidants, and antiproteases.

Corticosteroids

Corticosteroids possess several potent anti-inflammatory effects. They reduce the formation of mucus and edema; inhibit chemotaxis, adhesion, and activation of leukocytes; inhibit NF-κB activation; and interfere with the synthesis or actions of inflammatory mediators. In the past two decades, the use of systemic corticosteroids as a general anti-inflammatory therapy in CF has been considered based, in part, on the results of two 4-year, double-blind, placebo-controlled clinical trials [25,26].

In the first clinical trial of oral corticosteroids, children (1–12 years of age) who had CF with mild to moderate lung disease who received alternate-day prednisone (2 mg/kg) for 4 years, had better lung function, improved weight gain, and fewer hospital admissions and maintained constant immunoglobulin G concentrations with no apparent adverse effects during the study period [25]. This lack of adverse effects most likely relates to the small number of patients enrolled in the study (21 subjects in the treatment group and 24 subjects in the placebo group). A follow-up analysis 5 years after completion of the first trial reported that 14 of the 17 patients assigned to the steroid group who completed the trial developed growth retardation, two developed cataracts, and two developed glucose abnormalities [28]. In 1995, the results of a much larger multicenter trial were reported. Two alternate-day dosing regimens (2 mg/kg and 1 mg/kg) were compared with placebo over a 4-year period in 285 patients (6–14 years of age) who had CF with mild to moderate lung disease. Although beneficial effects on lung function were observed, particularly in patients infected with P aeruginosa, so were adverse effects, including glucose intolerance, growth impairment, and cataracts, even at the 1 mg/kg dose [26]. Follow-up 6 years after the completion of this trial demonstrated persistent deficits in growth after the therapy had been discontinued [29]. Subjects in the 1 mg/kg prednisone group also seemed to have an accelerated rate of decline in forced expiratory volume in 1 second (FEV_1) after discontinuation of the drug. In another trial, a shorter course of systemic corticosteroids was associated with increased forced vital capacity and FEV_1 and decreased serum IgG and cytokine concentrations [30], suggesting that short courses of steroids may be a useful adjunct to the treatment of exacerbations. The role of systemic steroids as a long-term maintenance therapy in CF seems to be limited; however, most studies of systemic corticosteroids have used relatively high doses (1–2 mg/kg every other day of prednisone). A Cochrane review of systemic steroids in CF concluded, "Oral corticosteroids at a prednisolone-equivalent dose of 1 mg/kg or 2 mg/kg alternate days appear to slow the progression of lung disease in CF, but benefit needs to be weighed against the occurrence of adverse events, especially development of cataracts and effect on linear growth. A risk benefit of low-dose alternate day corticosteroids would be important and the role of short-term use of oral corticosteroids should be more fully evaluated" [31]. Perhaps lower doses (0.1–0.25 mg/kg every other day) of systemic steroids might yield significant beneficial effects without the severe side effects documented in earlier studies. These studies might be difficult to undertake given the experience of the CF community with the previous corticosteroid studies.

Adverse effects associated with systemic corticosteroid administration have prompted investigations of inhaled corticosteroids. Because physicians are familiar with these drugs for the treatment of asthma, they have been widely prescribed as anti-inflammatory agents in CF [32,33]. The inhaled route might afford benefit with less risk than systemic administration, but systemic administration may be necessary to affect neutrophil migration. The clinical benefits of inhaled corticosteroids have been difficult to demonstrate in patients who have CF. None of the clinical trials of inhaled corticosteroids in CF have demonstrated convincing effects with respect to lung function or inflammatory markers in airway secretions [34–40]. These studies have been hampered by relatively small study populations and short observation periods. A Cochrane Review of inhaled corticosteroids in CF concluded that there is insufficient evidence to determine if they are beneficial or harmful [41]. In a large prospective, multicenter study, withdrawal of inhaled corticosteroids for 6 months was not associated with significant worsening of CF lung disease [42]. Patients in whom steroids were discontinued did

not have a change in lung function over time, an increased need for oral or intravenous antibiotics, or a shorter time to pulmonary exacerbation [42]. Although inhaled steroids may be of benefit in patients who have coexisting asthma, their use as a general anti-inflammatory agent in CF has not been substantiated. Potential long-term complications of inhaled corticosteroids, including adrenal suppression, growth failure, glucose intolerance, cataract formation, and decreased bone mineral density, have not been adequately evaluated in patients who have CF. Reports that inhaled corticosteroids may be associated with earlier acquisition of *P aeruginosa* are also concerning [43]. Because of this, caution should be heeded with respect to prescribing inhaled corticosteroids to young children who have CF. This may be the time when anti-inflammatory therapy would be most efficacious. Because no data exist that support the efficacy and safety of long-term inhaled corticosteroid for slowing the progression of lung disease in CF, additional trials with more patients, longer durations of therapy, and varying dosages are warranted.

Ibuprofen

Nonsteroidal anti-inflammatory drugs (NSAIDs) possess some of the same anti-inflammatory properties as corticosteroids but generally have fewer adverse effects, making them more suitable for long-term use. Ibuprofen has received the most attention because at high doses (those that achieve peak plasma concentration > 50 µg/ml) ibuprofen has specific activity against neutrophils, including inhibition of neutrophil migration, which has been demonstrated in an animal model of chronic pseudomonas endobronchial infection [44] and in patients who have CF [45]. Moreover, high concentrations of ibuprofen inhibit the activation of NF-κB and AP-1, two important proinflammatory transcription factors, probably by inhibiting several critical kinases, including IKKβ, ERK, p38 mitogen-activated protein kinase (MAPK), and cyclin-dependent kinases [46–48]. In addition, ibuprofen may exert some of its anti-inflammatory effect by activating PPAR-α and PPAR-γ [49]. At concentrations typically found in the serum of patients who have CF who are receiving high-dose ibuprofen, ibuprofen activated PPAR-γ in the CF airway epithelial cell lines, and this may account for some of its beneficial effects documented in CF [24]. Thus, ibuprofen should be considered as a broad-spectrum anti-inflammatory agent, much like corticosteroids.

The demonstration that oral administration of ibuprofen twice daily (in doses sufficient to interfere with neutrophil migration) to rats with endobronchial pseudomonas infection significantly decreased inflammation without increasing the lung burden of organisms [44] led to a 4-year, double-blind, placebo-controlled clinical trial of twice daily high-dose ibuprofen in 85 patients who had CF, 5 to 39 years of age, with mild lung disease [27]. Oral doses were individualized for each subject; the desired peak plasma concentration of 50 to 100 μg/ml was generally achieved with 20 to 30 mg/kg of ibuprofen. Compared with placebo, ibuprofen-treated patients had significantly less decline in pulmonary function measures, better preservation of body weight, fewer hospital admissions, and better Brasfield chest radiograph scores [27]. The effect was most pronounced in the youngest age group (5–13 years of age), in which the annual rate of decline in FEV_1 was reduced by 88% compared with the placebo group. There were no significant differences in adverse effects between the treatment groups (although the sample size was too small to detect even common effects), but two subjects could not tolerate long-term ibuprofen use because of increases in epistaxis in one and conjunctivitis in another. The incidence of gastrointestinal (GI) complications was lower in the ibuprofen group compared with placebo.

The results from this study were sufficiently compelling to recommend that high-dose ibuprofen therapy be considered for patients who have CF with mild lung disease, particularly younger patients. It is not known whether patients who have CF with more advanced lung disease would derive the same benefit from this therapy. Vigilant monitoring for adverse effects was recommended because relatively rare known side effects of ibuprofen would likely occur as more patients who have CF begin this therapy. Despite the knowledge that inflammation in the CF lung occurs early in the course of disease and is responsible for lung destruction and that the results of the ibuprofen trial suggest beneficial effects, this therapy has not been widely adopted. Fewer than 10% of patients who have CF per year were treated with ibuprofen between 1996 and 2000 [50]. Based on a survey of CF Care Centers in the United States, infrequent use of ibuprofen seems to be attributable to the complexity of obtaining a pharmacokinetic study to initiate therapy and concerns regarding safety [32]. With respect to the need for pharmacokinetic study to initiate therapy, establishing the appropriate dose in each patient seems to be necessary and is recommended to achieve the desired effect and to avoid risks associated with peak concentrations of ibuprofen that are too low or too high. Regarding safety, the factor most cited as a concern was GI hemorrhage, a known adverse effect of NSAIDs use. Based upon data from the U.S. Cystic Fibrosis Foundation National Registry, patients who had CF treated with ibuprofen in the United States between 1996 and 2000 had an increased risk of GI hemorrhage requiring hospitalization compared with those not treated with ibuprofen (relative risk, 2.12), but the overall incidence was less than 0.5% [50]. The excess risk of GI hemorrhage due to ibuprofen was 2.6/1000 treated patients, meaning that one patient had a GI hemorrhage that could be attributed to ibuprofen for every 384 patients receiving the drug. Thus, the benefits of this therapy seem to outweigh the associated risks. The incidence of GI hemorrhage might be reduced further by concomitant administration of antacids or proton pump inhibitors and by misoprostol (a PGE_1 analog). Renal failure associated with ibuprofen therapy has been the subject of a few case reports, but based upon U.S. CF Foundation Registry data, the incidence of renal failure is not increased among patients who have CF who are treated with ibuprofen [50].

The lack of additional data assessing the effectiveness of ibuprofen therapy for CF is another reason cited for infrequent use [32]. In 1999, a Cochrane Review concluded that there is evidence to suggest that NSAIDs may prevent pulmonary deterioration in subjects who have CF with mild disease, but further trials are required to confirm their beneficial effects on lung disease and nutritional status [51]. Since that time, additional data have accumulated. A 2-year, placebo-controlled, multicenter trial conducted in 145 patients who had CF in Canada demonstrated a beneficial effect of ibuprofen on lung function despite falling short of enrollment goals (L. Lands, personal communication, 2005). Ten-year follow-up data analysis of the patients who had CF enrolled in the original 4-year ibuprofen trial found that the beneficial effect of ibuprofen on lung function has persisted even though some patients in the ibuprofen arm discontinued the drug and some patients in the placebo arm initiated therapy at the end of the 4-year study period [50]. Seventeen years after the start of the 4-year trial, survival has been better in the patients randomized to ibuprofen (81%) compared with those randomized to placebo (70%). A more recent analysis of the CF Foundation Patient Registry focused on the benefit of long-term ibuprofen use on disease progression as measured by the rate of decline in FEV_1. For patients likely to benefit the most from this therapy (ie, children who have mild lung disease), those treated on average for 4 years had an annualized rate of decline in FEV_1 that was 33% less than those not treated with ibuprofen [52]. This is a substantial reduction in slope and represents slowing of the progression of lung disease. Thus, the benefits of high-dose ibuprofen therapy far outweigh the risks in young patients who have mild lung disease and should be considered a routine therapy for these patients.

Cytokines and anticytokines

Since the first clinical trial of corticosteroids for the treatment of CF pulmonary inflammation over 20 years ago, many new modulators of inflammation have been developed for the treatment of sepsis, rheumatoid arthritis, psoriasis, and inflammatory bowel disease. Because the inflammatory response in the CF lung shares many of the same features as some of these conditions, agents developed for treatment of other proinflammatory diseases may have efficacy in CF. Early studies consisted of evaluation of IL-1 receptor antagonist, anti–IL-8 antibody, and anti–ICAM-1 antibody. More recently, two TNF-α antagonists have been developed for the treatment of inflammatory bowel disease and rheumatoid arthritis. Etanercept (Enbrel), a soluble TNF receptor that can complex with TNF-α and prevent its interaction with native receptor, and infliximab (Remicade), a humanized monoclonal antibody against TNF-α, may be effective in the treatment of CF lung disease. Given the multitude of inflammatory pathways that are activated in CF and the redundancy inherent within cytokine networks, inhibition of any one mediator may not be sufficient to markedly limit the overall inflammatory response. Many investigators believe that the success of steroids and high-dose ibuprofen in limiting the CF inflammatory response is due to their broad spectrum of action.

Most cytokines are pleiomorphic, and although some demonstrate a preponderance of proinflammatory effects, others demonstrate a preponderance of anti-inflammatory effects. IL-10 possesses many anti-inflammatory properties. It inhibits the production of many proinflammatory cytokines; it stabilizes IκB, thereby limiting NF-κB activation and dampening the entire inflammatory response; it induces neutrophil apoptosis so that its absence probably contributes to the continued accumulation of neutrophils; and it decreases antigen presentation and T-cell stimulation, which may have important implications for the administration of viral gene therapy vectors. Because IL-10 terminates the inflammatory response, its absence might result in persistent inflammation even after a stimulus has been eradicated. The production of IL-10 is stimulated by TNF-α and lipopolysaccharide, which are abundant in the CF airway [4]. IL-10 is decreased, not increased, as one would predict. The effect of IL-10 on *P aeruginosa*–induced inflammation has been studied in animal models. IL-10 knockout mice have much worse endobronchial inflammation for the same inoculum of *P aeruginosa* compared with their wild-type littermates; conversely, administration of IL-10 to mice with chronic endobronchial pseudomonas infection is beneficial [53,54]. Thus, restoring IL-10 to the CF airway or administering it in pharmacologic quantities seems to be advantageous. A planned clinical trial of recombinant human IL-10 was stopped for reasons unrelated to CF, but this remains an interesting therapeutic option in CF.

One cytokine that has come to trial in CF is interferon (IFN)-γ. Because of the increase of the protein inhibitor of activated stat-1 in CF airway epithelial cells, the Jak-Stat signaling pathway is inefficient in CF, reducing mRNA production for IFN regulatory factor, nitric oxide synthase (NOS)-2, RANTES, and other Stat-1–dependent products [55–57]. The reduced production of NOS-2 leaves the cell producing less NO, which probably contributes to the inflammatory response by destabilizing IκB. These functions can be restored in cell models by the application of excess IFN-γ, although whether these levels can be achieved in vivo is unknown. A trial comparing inhaled IFN-γ (Actimmune) (500 and 1000 μg) to placebo demonstrated that although inhaled IFN-γ was in general well tolerated, it did not improve pulmonary function; alter sputum bacterial density; or affect sputum IL-8, neutrophils, elastase, myeloperoxidase, or DNA [58]. Patients randomized to receive 1000 μg but not 500 μg of inhaled IFN-γ had a statistically significant higher percentage of hospitalizations for pulmonary exacerbations than did patients randomized to receive placebo.

Modulators of intracellular signaling

Because the overproduction of cytokines in the CF airway likely contributes to the excessive inflammatory response in CF, it seems logical to alter the signaling pathways that account for the excess response. There is no consensus as to what these pathways are and how they may interact with the basic defect in CF. In vitro studies with selective modulators might clarify the various mechanisms; thus, if prudent choices are made, clinical trials may give insight into the mechanisms in vivo. High-dose ibuprofen and IL-10 inhibit NF-κB activation, thereby downregulating the inflammatory response at the transcriptional level. Other drugs that limit proinflammatory molecule transcription may be useful in the treatment of CF. Another mechanism of inhibiting NF-κB activity occurs via up-regulation of PPAR with the thiazolidinediones or glitazones [59,60]. The agonists troglitazone and ciglitazone activate PPAR in primary CF airway epithelial cells and CF epithelial cell lines, thus resulting in reduced production of IL-8, IL-6, and granulocyte-macrophage colony-stimulating factor in response to incubation with *P aeruginosa* [24]. A clinical trial of pioglitazone (Actos) is underway in patients who have CF. Other possibilities include inhibiting the MAPK pathways. The p40/p42 and p38 MAPK pathways are activated when bacteria interact with airway epithelial cells. Activation of the p38 MAPK pathway may prolong the half-life of cytokine mRNA molecules. This may have significance in CF because there seems to be sustained production of inflammatory cytokines even after a stimulus has been removed. Inhibiting the p38 MAPK pathway may help to terminate the inflammatory response. This may also inhibit the production of immunomodulatory cytokines such as IL-10.

Among the cell signaling pathways that are dysregulated in CF epithelial cells is the pathway that leads to the production of NO. Multiple studies have demonstrated decreased NO in exhaled air (eNO) from patients who have CF [19,20]. NO is a highly reactive signaling molecule with important antimicrobial and anti-inflammatory properties. The loss of NO production from the airways may contribute to bacterial infection

and overzealous inflammation in CF [55,61]. One potential cause of decreased eNO in CF is up-regulation of RhoGTPase, a cell signaling molecule that reduces the expression of NOS2 [62]. Up-regulation of the RhoGTPase pathway may also contribute to the overzealous inflammatory response by increasing production of IL-8. The RhoGTPase pathway can be inhibited by blocking 3-hydroxy-3-methylglutaryl-CoA reductase with the commercially available statins, such as simvastatin [62]. The statins have other anti-inflammatory effects, including the ability to inhibit neutrophil migration, decrease proinflammatory cytokine production, and increase transcriptional activation of PPAR [63–68]. A clinical trial of simvastatin in patients who have CF is underway.

L-Arginine, a substrate of NO synthases, is the precursor of NO. Arginase activity is increased in the blood and sputum of patients who have CF [69,70], and this may exacerbate the decreased eNO. In a rodent model of chronic *P aeruginosa* infection, L-arginine treatment was associated with reduced tissue damage, inhibited neutrophil recruitment, and reduced IL-1β [71]. In a small pilot study of CF, the administration of oral L-arginine was associated with increased eNO [72]. Whether L-arginine has the potential for use as an anti-inflammatory in CF remains to be studied in large prospective clinical trials.

Eicosanoid modulators

Eicosanoids are increased in the sputum and BALF from patients who have CF [7,73,74]. LTB$_4$, a potent neutrophil chemoattractant, is present in high concentrations in the CF airway [7]. Although it is difficult to determine the relative contribution of each chemoattractant present in the CF airway to the massive influx of neutrophils, once neutrophils are present, neutrophil-derived LTB$_4$ likely contributes to further neutrophil infiltration [75]. Neutrophil products such as elastase may also contribute to the chemotactic load by stimulating alveolar macrophages to release more LTB$_4$ [76]. Therefore, it seems logical that reducing LTB$_4$ production in the CF airway should have beneficial effects. BIIL 284 BS (Amelubant), a specific LTB$_4$ receptor antagonist, was recently studied in CF, but the study was terminated early due to a statistically significant increase in pulmonary-related serious adverse events in adults receiving BIIL 284 BS [77]. One possible explanation is that LTB$_4$ has some other previously unrecognized beneficial effect in CF, and its inhibition is detrimental. A more plausible explanation might be that the inhibitory effect of BIIL 284 BS on the LTB_4 pathway was too potent, resulting in impaired antimicrobial defenses and increasing the risk of an exacerbation. The results of this study demonstrate that care must be taken when selecting an anti-inflammatory agent for future clinical trials.

Although antagonists of the cysteinyl leukotriene receptor, such as montelukast (Singulair), may benefit patients who have CF with airway reactivity, it was previously thought that these agents were unlikely to affect the airway inflammatory response in CF because the cysteinyl leukotrienes (LTC_4, LTD_4, and LTE_4) are not important mediators of the neutrophil-dominant inflammation seen in CF. A pilot study has demonstrated that patients who received montelukast had decreases in sputum and serum concentrations of IL-8 and eosinophil cationic protein, decreased sputum myeloperoxidase, and increased serum and sputum levels of IL-10 in addition to an increase in FEV_1, peak expiratory flow, and forced expiratory flow at midexpiratory phase compared with patients who received placebo [78]. If verified in further studies, such effects would have important implications for patients who have CF. Another strategy to decrease LTB_4 in the CF airway is to redirect the metabolism of arachidonic acid from LTB_4 to the less potent chemoattractant LTB_5. This can be accomplished with fish oil preparations that contain omega-3 fatty acids, eicosapentaenoic acid, and docosahexanoic acid. These fatty acids also suppress IL-1β and TNF-α production. Oral supplementation of omega-3 fatty acids increases the incorporation of eicosapentaenoic acid into the neutrophil membrane and reduces the LTB_4/ LTB_5 ratio [79]. Although patients who have CF are capable of absorbing quantities of fish oil sufficient to incorporate omega-3 fatty acids into membrane phospholipids without adverse effects [80], the amount that would be needed on a daily basis is not tolerable. Altering the metabolic pathways of arachidonic acid might have beneficial effects in treating CF lung disease.

Antioxidants

Neutrophils release many toxic products, including oxygen radicals that contribute to local tissue damage and perpetuate inflammation via the release of neutrophil chemoattractants LTB_4 and IL-8. Elevated levels of oxidant products have been detected in the airways of CF mice [81] and of patients who have CF [82,83]. The oxidant–antioxidant imbalance likely contributes to the exaggerated and damaging inflammatory response seen in CF. Some of the biochemical abnormalities in CF can be reversed by supplementation with high-dose antioxidants, such as vitamins C and E and β-carotene. Further studies must be performed to demonstrate a beneficial effect on lung function. N-acetyl cysteine, initially developed as a mucolytic, is receiving renewed interest as an antioxidant and as an anti-inflammatory in CF. N-acetyl cysteine is a thiol compound that provides sulfhydryl groups and acts as a precursor of reduced glutathione and as a direct scavenger of reactive oxygen species [84]. In studies of CF, high-dose oral N-acetyl cysteine was associated with decreased sputum elastase, IL-8, and neutrophil burden [85]. The study was of short duration and was not powered to detect changes in pulmonary function. If N-acetyl cysteine reduces neutrophils and their products, then one would expect that the rate of pulmonary function decline would also be affected in the long term. Further large, randomized double-blind placebo controlled trials of N-acetyl cysteine in CF are warranted.

The oxidant–antioxidant imbalance may be directly exacerbated by abnormalities in cystic fibrosis transmembrane conductance regulator (CFTR). If glutathione is transported by CFTR [86], then abnormalities in CFTR would decrease the concentrations of this important antioxidant on epithelial surfaces, thus leaving the airway vulnerable to even ordinary levels of oxidative stress. Because decreased lung levels of glutathione, particularly reduced glutathione, have been demonstrated in CF mice [81] and in patients who have CF [87], it seems logical to augment the concentration of this active antioxidant in the CF lung. Glutathione levels in BALF can be significantly increased by treatment with aerosolized glutathione [88,89], and this treatment reduces superoxide production in response to phorbol myristyl acetate by inflammatory cells recovered from the BALF [88]. Inhaled glutathione has attracted attention in the lay press as a potential therapy in CF, but its therapeutic benefits and adverse effects have not been studied sufficiently in controlled clinical trials to warrant clinical use. Establishing an optimal formulation, route of delivery, dose, and dosing schedule of glutathione are required before long-term efficacy and safety studies can commence. Failure to do so may result in serious consequences for patients who elect to treat themselves with unapproved formulations.

Antiproteases

Early in life, neutrophils infiltrate the CF airway and release massive amounts of active proteases that overwhelm local antiprotease defenses, particularly alpha-1–protease inhibitor (α_1-PI) and secretory leukocyte protease inhibitor [8]. α_1-PI diffuses into the smaller airways and alveoli from the blood and is carried up the airway by the mucociliary escalator. Secretory leukocyte protease inhibitor is produced and secreted by airway mucosal cells and is the predominant protease inhibitor in the conducting airways. The concentration of α_1-PI in the BALF of patients who have CF is severalfold higher than in healthy subjects, but even in patients who have mild CF disease there is a several hundred– to several thousand–fold excess of elastase and other neutrophil proteases, which exceeds the capacity of the inhibitors [2,6,8]. The imbalance between the proteases and their inhibitors becomes worse during exacerbations and contributes to clinical deterioration. The challenge of inhibiting the enormous burden of active proteases in the CF airway is substantial. Because neutrophils reach the airway by migrating through the epithelium, much of the release of proteases occurs beneath the thick layer of mucus, which is difficult for inhibitors to penetrate. In model systems, this can be overcome by using the polymeric immunoglobulin receptor to deliver systemically administered α_1-antitrypsin to the luminal side of the airway epithelium [90]. The exogenous administration of antiproteases to supplement the increased but inadequate amount of endogenous antiproteases present in CF airways has been under investigation since 1990. In a preliminary study in 12 patients who had CF, aerosol delivery of plasma-derived α_1-antitrypsin (1.5–3 mg/kg twice daily for 1 week) was shown to effectively suppress active elastase in the airways [91]. A multicenter dose escalation clinical trial studying the efficacy and safety of plasma-derived α_1-antitrypsin administered by aerosol twice daily for 4 weeks also revealed a reduction in active elastase [92]. The use of this therapy is limited by expense, supply, and the inherent risks associated with administering a plasma-derived product. Nonetheless, enthusiasm for the investigation of

plasma-derived α_1-antitrypsin in treating CF has not waned; clinical trials are being considered. Because of the promising results from previous antiprotease studies, clinical investigations using recombinant human α_1-antitrypsin produced by transgenic sheep have been considered in CF. A phase II trial of transgenic α_1-antitrypsin in CF demonstrated modest results [93]. Subjects who received 125 or 250 mg of the study drug experienced a trend toward improvement in time to first pulmonary exacerbation and fewer total hospitalizations compared with subjects who received 62.5 mg of the study drug or placebo, but the results did not reach statistical significance [93]. Because this drug must be administered frequently and in large amounts, its development for use in CF has been slow. Aerosolization of recombinant secretory leukocyte protease inhibitor has also been studied. Further development of recombinant secretory leukocyte protease inhibitor has been stalled, likely due to the inability to produce sufficient quantities at a less than prohibitive cost. Another recombinant protein, monocyte/neutrophil elastase inhibitor, has been shown to protect rat lungs against injury from CF airway secretions [94] and is under development for a clinical trial in CF. Engineered protein inhibitor human neutrophil elastase (EPI-hNE4; Depelstat) is a highly specific and potent inhibitor of human neutrophil elastase and is also under clinical development for use in CF [95]. Preclinical studies demonstrated that EPI-hNE4 effectively inhibited the high levels of active neutrophil elastase present in sputum from children who had CF in vitro [96]. Depelstat also decreased neutrophil migration in cell culture and animal models without altering the clearance of *P aeruginosa* and prevented elastase activation of the epithelial sodium channel [96–98]. Phase II trials in CF are underway in Europe. Promising data demonstrate that antiprotease therapy has the potential to significantly affect inflammation in CF. To be effective, it may be necessary to inhibit all of the active elastase in the airways because even minute amounts interfere with opsonophagocytosis. Further investigation is required to determine the optimal agent and best route of administration.

Other therapies

Many therapies that are designed primarily for other purposes have some efficacy in interrupting the inflammatory response [99,100]. Therapies that prevent or control infection, particularly

P aeruginosa infection, are likely to reduce inflammation in the long term. A more aggressive use of antibiotics on a chronic basis might be effective in reducing the airway burden of bacteria, with the expectation that less inflammation would be present. Although the primary action of antibiotics is to neutralize bacteria, their therapeutic benefits may be enhanced by their anti-inflammatory properties. The use of macrolides in CF has garnered much recent interest. This stems from its use in diffuse panbronchiolitis, a disease that shares several features with CF. Treatment with erythromycin was associated with improved survival in patients who had diffuse panbronchiolitis [101]. A pilot study in lung transplant patients who had bronchiolitis obliterans found a beneficial effect of azithromycin (Zithromax) on lung function [102]. In three clinical trials in CF, azithromycin was found to increase lung function or to decrease the need for antibiotics for treatment of respiratory symptoms; no significant adverse effects were observed [103–105]. The results of these studies led the U.S. CF Foundation to conduct a 6-month, multicenter, placebo-controlled trial in 185 patients who had CF with mild to moderate lung disease and who had been infected with *P aeruginosa* for at least 1 year. Patients were randomized to receive thrice weekly placebo or azithromycin (250 mg for weight <40 kg, 500 mg for body weight ≥40 kg) [106]. Patients who received azithromycin demonstrated improvements in lung function, weight gain, and quality of life and a reduction in CF pulmonary exacerbations compared with patients who received placebo [106]. Azithromycin was found to be safe and well tolerated. Nausea, diarrhea, and wheezing were more common in the patients who received azithromycin [106]. The results of this trial have led the CF Foundation to recommend that chronic administration of azithromycin be considered in patients who have CF who are infected with *P aeruginosa*. Although macrolides have a beneficial effect on CF lung disease, their mechanism of action is less clear. In vitro and in vivo studies of macrolides have demonstrated bronchodilatory, anti-infective, and anti-inflammatory effects, depending on the model system. Typically, *P aeruginosa* is resistant to macrolide antibiotics, as determined by in vitro susceptibility testing. Conventional methods of antimicrobial susceptibility testing use low concentrations of actively dividing bacteria, whereas *P aeruginosa* organizes into a biofilm and likely exists in a stationary phase in the CF airway. The susceptibility of *P*

aeruginosa in the stationary phase to antibiotics differs from its susceptibility when in the growth phase. Azithromycin may be effective at killing *P aeruginosa* in the stationary phase. In vitro studies have demonstrated that azithromycin disrupts cell-to-cell communication (quorum sensing) between pseudomonads when organized into a biofilm, inhibits flagellin expression, and decreases adherence to tracheal epithelium [107–111]. Whether these effects occur in vivo is unknown. In addition to their antibacterial properties, macrolides seem to have significant anti-inflammatory properties. Erythromycin may inhibit neutrophil migration and elastase secretion. Macrolides also may reduce the production of proinflammatory mediators, including TNF-α, IL-1β, IL-8, and NO_2^- [112–117]. The ability of macrolides to down-regulate proinflammatory mediators may be due to inhibition of the transcription factors regulating the inflammatory pathways. Macrolides possess several properties that may affect various aspects of CF lung disease.

As neutrophils break down and disintegrate, they release their DNA. Large amounts of high-molecular-weight neutrophil DNA in the airway lumen increase the viscosity of CF sputum. The high viscosity and resistance to shearing effects of coughing further impair mucociliary clearance. Therefore, the most common lesion in CF is mucopurulent plugging of the airway. The highly anionic nature of the extracellular free DNA leads to many ionic interactions with other constituents in CF sputum. DNA also may bind aminoglycoside antibiotics and decrease their efficacy. Recombinant human DNase (dornase alfa; Pulmozyme) hydrolyzes DNA released from neutrophils, decreases the viscoelasticity of purulent secretions, and increases the ability of mucus to be cleared from the airway [118,119]. This aerosolized drug results in significant improvement in pulmonary function in patients who have CF and results in fewer pulmonary exacerbations in young patients who have CF with mild lung disease [120,121]. Analysis of the data from the Epidemiologic Survey of Cystic Fibrosis shows that administration of dornase alfa was associated with a slower rate of decline in FEV_1 after controlling for confounding variables [122]. Reducing the rate of decline in lung function is likely to affect survival to a much greater extent than increasing the FEV_1 transiently. Some of these effects may be due to a reduction in inflammatory mediators. In another clinical trial, treatment with dornase alfa was associated with decreased accumulation of IL-8, neutrophils, neutrophil elastase, and DNA in the BALF from patients who have CF over a 3-year period [123,124]. Thus, dornase alfa may be considered an anti-inflammatory therapy, although these effects are probably indirect.

In addition to antibiotics and classic anti-inflammatory therapeutics, other agents may be beneficial in treating CF pulmonary inflammation. Studies of the effects of hydroxychloroquine and low-dose methotrexate in CF [125] are underway. Although chemotherapeutics have been studied in refractory asthma, there have been few studies in CF. Low-dose cyclosporin A was found to decrease the need for systemic corticosteroids in four out of six pediatric patients who had CF in one case series [126]. Chest radiograph scores and height velocity also improved. These data suggest the need for further evaluation of chemotherapeutics in CF. Due to the toxicities of chemotherapeutics, studies in animal models are preferable before beginning large clinical trials. As with all treatments, the risks and potential benefits of the treatment must be balanced against the risks of the disease.

The use of ion transport regulators is also under investigation and may correct the airway surface fluid abnormality and improve clearance. Therapies that activate mutant CFTR might be expected to correct the airway surface fluid abnormality [1]. Gene replacement therapies also might have direct effects on decreasing inflammatory mediator production by epithelial cells in addition to decreasing the predilection for infection. A direct link between defective CFTR and the airway inflammatory response has not been proven. It is possible that correcting the basic defect might not fully obviate the host inflammatory response, especially in patients who have more severe lung disease. Although anti-inflammatory agents, antioxidants, and antiproteases might decrease the injurious products of inflammation, no neutralizing treatment is likely to equal the efficacy of physical removal of the damaging products. Airway clearance techniques, long a cornerstone of CF therapy, will continue to receive significant attention. Thus, nearly all therapies directed at any step in the pathophysiologic process directly or indirectly affect inflammation.

Summary

CF lung disease begins early in infancy for most patients and continues unabated throughout life. Inflammation is a key contributor to the progression of CF lung disease and is the primary cause of the chronic destructive changes that are responsible for the majority of morbidity and mortality in CF. Studies have demonstrated that anti-inflammatory therapies have a beneficial effect in CF. These therapies should be added to existing strategies aimed at decreasing the progression of CF lung disease and likely have to begin early in life before the onset of irreversible damage to the airway. To limit the persistent inflammatory response, these therapies have to be administered on a chronic basis. Although inhaled corticosteroids are the most frequently prescribed anti-inflammatory therapy in CF, their benefits, like their risks, have not been established. Ibuprofen is the best proven anti-inflammatory drug available, although its use in the CF community has not been widely adopted. Newer anti-inflammatory agents targeting intracellular signaling pathways and their products are under investigation and will likely come to clinical trial over the next few years. Progress has been slow, and, despite recent advances, more studies of anti-inflammatory agents are necessary to understand their mechanisms of action in the CF lung, to determine which agents would provide the most benefit to patients who have CF, and to determine which therapies should be initiated at what age and stage of lung disease [127]. A combination of anti-inflammatory medications or the development of agents that interfere with the signaling mechanisms responsible for promoting the transcription of proinflammatory mediators is necessary to significantly modify the inflammatory response and natural history of CF. Adding anti-inflammatory therapy to an already comprehensive program for treating the lungs may decrease morbidity and improve the quality of life for patients who have CF.

References

[1] Davis PB, Drumm M, Konstan MW. Cystic fibrosis: state of the art. Am J Respir Crit Care Med 1996; 154(5):1229–56.

[2] Chmiel JF, Konstan MW, Berger M. The role of inflammation in the pathophysiology of CF lung disease. Clin Rev Allergy Immunol 2002;23(1):5–27.

[3] Khan TZ, Wagener JS, Bost T, et al. Early pulmonary inflammation in infants with cystic fibrosis. Am J Respir Crit Care Med 1995;151(4):1075–82.

[4] Bonfield TL, Panuska JR, Konstan MW, et al. Inflammatory cytokines in cystic fibrosis lungs [Published erratum appears in Am J Respir Crit Care

Med 1996 Oct;154(4 Pt 1):1217]. Am J Respir Crit Care Med 1995;152(6 Pt 1):2111–8.

[5] Kirchner KK, Wagener JS, Khan TZ, et al. Increased DNA levels in bronchoalveolar lavage fluid obtained from infants with cystic fibrosis. Am J Respir Crit Care Med 1996;154(5):1426–9.

[6] Konstan MW, Hilliard KA, Norvell TM, et al. Bronchoalveolar lavage findings in cystic fibrosis patients with stable, clinically mild lung disease suggest ongoing infection and inflammation [published erratum appears in Am J Respir Crit Care Med 1995 Jan:151(1)260]. Am J Respir Crit Care Med 1994;150(2):448–54.

[7] Konstan MW, Walenga RW, Hilliard KA, et al. Leukotriene B4 is markedly elevated in the epithelial lining fluid of patients with cystic fibrosis. Am Rev Respir Dis 1993;148(4 Pt 1):896–901.

[8] Birrer P, McElvaney NG, Rudeberg A, et al. Protease-antiprotease imbalance in the lungs of children with cystic fibrosis. Am J Respir Crit Care Med 1994;150(1):207–13.

[9] Balough K, McCubbin M, Weinberger M, et al. The relationship between infection and inflammation in the early stages of lung disease from cystic fibrosis. Pediatr Pulmonol 1995;20(2): 63–70.

[10] Armstrong DS, Grimwood K, Carzino R, et al. Lower respiratory infection and inflammation in infants with newly diagnosed cystic fibrosis. BMJ 1995;310(6997):1571–2.

[11] Armstrong DS, Grimwood K, Carlin JB, et al. Lower airway inflammation in infants and young children with cystic fibrosis. Am J Respir Crit Care Med 1997;156(4 Pt 1):1197–204.

[12] Noah TL, Black HR, Cheng PW, et al. Nasal and bronchoalveolar lavage fluid cytokines in early cystic fibrosis. J Infect Dis 1997;175(3):638–47.

[13] Muhlebach MS, Stewart PW, Leigh MW, et al. Quantitation of inflammatory response to bacteria in young cystic fibrosis and control patients. Am J Respir Crit Care Med 1999;160(1):186–91.

[14] Tager AM, Wu J, Vermeulen MW. The effect of chloride concentration on human neutrophil functions: potential relevance to cystic fibrosis. Am J Respir Cell Mol Biol 1998;19(4):643–52.

[15] Watt AP, Courtney J, Moore J, et al. Neutrophil cell death, activation and bacterial infection in cystic fibrosis. Thorax 2005;60(8):659–64.

[16] Chmiel JF, Davis PB. State of the art: why do the lungs of patients with cystic fibrosis become infected and why can't they clear the infection? Respir Res 2003;4(1):8–21.

[17] Bonfield TL, Konstan MW, Berger M. Altered respiratory epithelial cell cytokine production in cystic fibrosis. J Allergy Clin Immunol 1999;104(1): 72–7.

[18] Bonfield TL, Konstan MW, Burfeind P, et al. Normal bronchial epithelial cells constitutively produce the anti-inflammatory cytokine interleukin-10,

which is downregulated in cystic fibrosis. Am J Respir Cell Mol Biol 1995;13(3):257–61.

[19] Balfour-Lynn IM, Laverty A, Dinwiddie R. Reduced upper airway nitric oxide in cystic fibrosis. Arch Dis Child 1996;75(4):319–22.

[20] Grasemann H, Michler E, Wallot M, et al. Decreased concentration of exhaled nitric oxide (NO) in patients with cystic fibrosis. Pediatr Pulmonol 1997;24(3):173–7.

[21] Ollero M, Junaidi O, Zaman MM, et al. Decreased expression of peroxisome proliferators activated receptor gamma in cftr -/- mice. J Cell Physiol 2004; 200(2):235–44.

[22] Green S. PPAR: a mediator of peroxisome proliferators action. Mutat Res 1995;333(1–2):101–9.

[23] Vanden Berghe W, Vermeulen L, Delerive P, et al. A paradigm for gene regulation: inflammation, NF-kappaB, and PPAR. Adv Exp Med Biol 2003;544: 181–96.

[24] Davis PB, Gupta S, Eastman J, et al. Inhibition of proinflammatory cytokine production by PPAR-gamma agonists in airway epithelial cells. Pediatr Pulmonol 2003;(Suppl 25):A246, 268–69.

[25] Auerbach HS, Williams M, Kirkpatrick JA, et al. Alternate-day prednisone reduces morbidity and improves pulmonary function in cystic fibrosis. Lancet 1985;2(8457):686–8.

[26] Eigen H, Rosenstein BJ, FitzSimmons S, et al. A multicenter study of alternate-day prednisone therapy in patients with cystic fibrosis. Cystic Fibrosis Foundation Prednisone Trial Group. J Pediatr 1995;126(4):515–23.

[27] Konstan MW, Byard PJ, Hoppel CL, et al. Effect of high-dose ibuprofen in patients with cystic fibrosis. N Engl J Med 1995;332(13) 848–844.

[28] Donati MA, Haver K, Gerson W, et al. Long-term alternate day prednisone therapy in cystic fibrosis. Pediatr Pulmonol 1990;5:A322, 277.

[29] Lai H-C, FitzSimmons SC, Allen DB, et al. Risk of persistent growth impairment after alternate-day prednisone treatment in children with cystic fibrosis. N Engl J Med 2000;342(12):851–9.

[30] Greally P, Hussain MJ, Vergani D, et al. Interleukin-1α, soluble interleukin-2 receptor, and IgG concentrations in cystic fibrosis treated with prednisolone. Arch Dis Child 1994;71(1):35–9.

[31] Cheng K, Ashby D, Smyth R. Oral steroids for cystic fibrosis. The Cochrane Database Syst Rev 1999; 4:CD000407.

[32] Oermann CM, Sockrider MM, Konstan MW. The use of anti-inflammatory medications in cystic fibrosis: trends, and physician attitudes. Chest 1999; 115(4):1053–8.

[33] Konstan MW, Butler SM, Schidlow DV, et al. Patterns of medical practice in cystic fibrosis. Part II: use of therapies. Pediatr Pulmonol 1999;28(4): 248–54.

[34] Schiotz PO, Jorgensen M, Flensborg EW, et al. Chronic *Pseudomonas aeruginosa* lung infection in

cystic fibrosis. A longitudinal study of immune complex activity and inflammatory response sputum sol-phase of cystic fibrosis patients with chronic *Pseudomonas aeruginosa* lung infections: influence of local steroid treatment. Acta Paediatr Scand 1983;72(2):283–7.

[35] van Haren EHJ, Lammers J-WJ, Festen J, et al. The effects of the inhaled corticosteroid budesonide on lung function and bronchial hyperresponsiveness in adult patients with cystic fibrosis. Respir Med 1995;89(3):209–14.

[36] Nikolaizik WH, Schoni MH. Pilot study to assess the effect of inhaled corticosteroids on lung function on patients with cystic fibrosis. J Pediatr 1996; 128(2):271–4.

[37] Balfour-Lynn IM, Klein NJ, Dinwiddie R. Randomised controlled trial of inhaled corticosteroids (fluticasone propionate) in cystic fibrosis. Arch Dis Child 1997;77(2):124–30.

[38] Bisgaard H, Pedersen SS, Nielsen KG, et al. Controlled trial of inhaled budesonide in patients with cystic fibrosis and chronic bronchopulmonary *Pseudomonas aeruginosa* infection. Am J Respir Crit Care Med 1997;156(4 pt 1):1190–6.

[39] Dauletbaev N, Viel K, Behr J, et al. Effects of short-term inhaled fluticasone on oxidative burst of sputum cells in cystic fibrosis patients. Eur Respir J 1999;14(5):1150–5.

[40] Wojtczak HA, Kerby GS, Wagener JS, et al. Beclomethasone diproprionate reduced airway inflammation without adrenal suppression in young children with cystic fibrosis: a pilot study. Pediatr Pulmonol 2001;32(4):293–302.

[41] Dezateux C, Walters S, Balfour-Lynn I. Inhaled corticosteroids for cystic fibrosis [Cochrane methodology review]. In: The Cochrane Library issue 4. Chichester (UK): John Wiley & Sons, Ltd.; 2003.

[42] Balfour-Lynn IM, Lees B, Hall P, et al. Multicenter randomized controlled trial of withdrawal of inhaled corticosteroids in cystic fibrosis. Am J Respir Crit Care Med 2006;173(12):1356–62.

[43] Schmidt J, Davidson AGF, Seear M, et al. Is the acquisition of pseudomonads in cystic fibrosis patients increased by use of inhaled corticosteroids? Unexpected results from a double blind placebo controlled study. Pediatr Pulmonol 1997;(Suppl 14): A318, 293–294.

[44] Konstan MW, Vargo KM, Davis PB. Ibuprofen attenuates the inflammatory response to Pseudomonas aeruginosa in a rat model of chronic pulmonary infection: implications for antiinflammatory therapy in cystic fibrosis. Am Rev Respir Dis 1990;141(1):186–92.

[45] Konstan MW, Krenicky JE, Finney MR, et al. Effect of ibuprofen on neutrophil migration *in vivo* in cystic fibrosis. J Pharmacol Exp Ther 2003;306(3): 1086–91.

[46] Scheuren N, Bang H, Munster T, et al. Modulation of transcription factor NF-kappaB by enantiomers of the nonsteroidal drug ibuprofen. Br J Pharmacol 1998;123(4):645–52.

[47] Tegeder I, Niederberger E, Israr E, et al. Inhibition of NF-κB and AP-1 activation by R- and S-flurbiprofen. FASEB J 2001;15(3):595–7.

[48] Tegeder I, Pfeilschifter, Geisslinger G. Cyclooxygenase-independent actions of cyclooxygenase inhibitors. FASEB J 2001;15(12):2057–72.

[49] Jaradat MS, Wongsud B, Phornchirasilp S, et al. Activation of peroxisome proliferators-activated receptor isoforms and inhibition of prostaglandin H(2) synthases by ibuprofen, naproxen, and indomethacin. Biochem Pharmacol 2001;62(12): 1587–95.

[50] Konstan MW, Schluchter MD, Storfer-Isser, et al. Use of ibuprofen for the treatment of airway inflammation in CF: an update. Pediatr Pulmonol 2002;(Suppl 24):164–5.

[51] Dezateux C, Crighton A. Oral non-steroidal anti-inflammatory drug therapy for cystic fibrosis [Cochrane methodology review]. In: The Cochrane Library issue 4. Chichester (UK): John Wiley & Sons, Ltd.; 2003.

[52] Schluchter MD, Konstan MW, Xue L, et al. Relationship between high-dose ibuprofen use and rate of decline in FEV_1 among young patients with mild lung disease in the CFF Registry. Pediatr Pulmonol 2004;(Suppl 27):A385, 322.

[53] Chmiel JF, Konstan MW, Saadane A, et al. Prolonged inflammatory response to acute pseudomonas challenge in IL-10 knockout mice. Am J Respir Crit Care Med 2002;165(8):1176–81.

[54] Chmiel JF, Konstan MW, Knesebeck JE, et al. IL-10 attenuates excessive inflammation in chronic pseudomonas infection in mice. Am J Respir Crit Care Med 1999;160(6):2040–7.

[55] Kelley TJ, Drumm ML. Inducible nitric oxide synthase expression is reduced in cystic fibrosis murine and human airway epithelial cells. J Clin Invest 1998;102(6):1200–7.

[56] Kelley TJ, Elmer HL. *In vivo* alterations of IFN regulatory factor-1 and PIAS1 protein levels in cystic fibrosis epithelium. J Clin Invest 2000;106(3): 403–10.

[57] Steagall WK, Elmer HL, Brady KG, et al. Cystic fibrosis transmembrane conductance regulator-dependent regulation of epithelial inducible nitric oxide synthase expression. Am J Respir Cell Mol Biol 2000;22(1):45–50.

[58] Moss RB, Mayer-Hamblett N, Wagener J, et al. Randomized, double-blind, placebo-controlled, dose-escalating study of aerosolized interferon gamma-1b in patients with mild to moderate cystic fibrosis lung disease. Pediatr Pulmonol 2005;39(3): 209–18.

[59] Zingarelli B, Sheehan M, Hake PW, et al. Peroxisome proliferator activator receptor-gamma ligands, 15-deoxy-Delta(12,14)-prostaglandin J2 and ciglitazone, reduce systemic inflammation in

polymicrobial sepsis by modulation of signal transduction pathways. J Immunol 2003;171(12): 6827–37.

[60] Ruan H, Pownall HJ, Lodish HF. Troglitazone antagonizes tumor necrosis factor-alpha-induced reprogramming of adipocyte gene expression by inhibiting the transcriptional regulatory functions of NF-kappaB. J Biol Chem 2003;278(30): 28181–92.

[61] Meng QH, Springall DR, Bishop AE, et al. Lack of inducible nitric oxide synthase in bronchial epithelium: a possible mechanism of susceptibility to infection in cystic fibrosis. J Pathol 1998;184(3): 323–31.

[62] Kraynack NC, Corey DA, Elmer HL, et al. Mechanisms of NOS2 regulation by Rho GTPase signaling in airway epithelial cells. Am J Physiol Lung Cell Mol Physiol 2002;283(3):L604–11.

[63] Dunzendorfer S, Rothbucher D, Schratzberger P, et al. Mevalonate-dependent inhibition of transendothelial migration and chemotaxis of human peripheral blood neutrophils by pravastatin. Circ Res 1997;81(6):963–9.

[64] Weber C, Erl W, Weber KS, et al. HMG-CoA reductase inhibitors decrease CD11b expression and CD11b-dependent adhesion of monocytes to endothelium and reduce increased adhesiveness of monocytes isolated from patients with hypercholesterolemia. J Am Coll Cardiol 1997;30(5):1212–7.

[65] Rezaie-Majd A, Maca T, Bucek RA, et al. Simvastatin reduces expression of cytokines interleukin-6, interleukin-8, and monocyte chemoattractant protein-1 in circulating monocytes from hypercholesterolemic patients. Arterioscler Thromb Vasc Biol 2002;22(7):1194–9.

[66] Martin G, Duez H, Blanquart C, et al. Statin-induced inhibition of the Rho-signaling pathway activates PPARalpha and induces HDL apoA-I. J Clin Invest 2001;107(11):1423–32.

[67] Zelvyte I, Dominaitiene R, Crisby M, et al. Modulation of inflammatory mediators and PPAR-gamma and NFkappaB expression by pravastatin in response to lipoproteins in human monocytes in vitro. Pharmacol Res 2002;45(2):147–54.

[68] Berger J, Moller DE. The mechanisms of action of PPARs. Annu Rev Med 2002;53:409–35.

[69] Grasemann H, Schwiertz R, Grasemann C, et al. Decreased systemic bioavailability of L-arginine in patients with cystic fibrosis. Respir Res 2006;7: 87–93.

[70] Grasemann H, Schwiertz R, Matthiesen S, et al. Increased arginase activity in cystic fibrosis airways. Am J Respir Crit Care Med 2005;172(12):1523–8.

[71] Hopkins N, Gunning Y, O'Croinin DF, et al. Anti-inflammatory effect of augmented nitric oxide production in chronic lung infection. J Pathol 2006; 209(2):198–205.

[72] Grasemann H, Grasemann C, Kurtz F, et al. Oral L-arginine supplementation in cystic fibrosis patients: a placebo-controlled study. Eur Respir J 2005;25(1):62–8.

[73] Cromwell O, Walport MJ, Morris HR, et al. Identification of leukotrienes D and B in sputum from cystic fibrosis patients. Lancet 1981;2(8239): 164–5.

[74] Sampson AP, Spencer DA, Green CP, et al. Leukotrienes in the sputum and urine of cystic fibrosis children. Br J Clin Pharmacol 1990;30(6):861–9.

[75] Ford-Hutchinson AW, Bray MA, Doig MV, et al. A potent chemokinetic and aggregating substance released from polymorphonuclear leukocytes. Nature 1980;286(5770):264–5.

[76] Hubbard RC, Fells G, Gadek J, et al. Neutrophil accumulation in the lung in alpha 1-antitrypsin deficiency: spontaneous release of leukotriene B4 by alveolar macrophages. J Clin Invest 1991;88(3): 891–7.

[77] Konstan MW, Doring G, Lands LC, et al. Results of a phase II clinical trial of BIIL 284 BS (a LTB_4 receptor antagonist) for the treatment of CF lung disease. Pediatr Pulmonol 2005;(Suppl 28):125–7.

[78] Stelmach I, Korzeniewska A, Stelmach W, et al. Effects of montelukast treatment on clinical and inflammatory variables in patients with cystic fibrosis. Ann Allergy Asthma Immunol 2005; 95(4):372–80.

[79] Panchaud A, Sauty A, Kernen Y, et al. Biological effects of a dietary omega-3 polyunsaturated fatty acids supplementation in cystic fibrosis patients: a randomized, crossover placebo-controlled trial. Clin Nutr 2006;25(3):418–27.

[80] Henderson WR Jr, Astley SJ, McCready MM, et al. Oral absorption of omega-3 fatty acids in patients with cystic fibrosis who have pancreatic insufficiency and in healthy control subjects. J Pediatr 1994;124(3):400–8.

[81] Velsor LW, van Heeckeren A, Day BJ. Antioxidant imbalance in the lungs of cystic fibrosis transmembrane conductance regulator protein mutant mice. Am J Physiol Lung Cell Mol Physiol 2001;281(1): L31–8.

[82] Jobsis Q, Raatgeep HC, Schellekens SL, et al. Hydrogen peroxide and nitric oxide in exhaled air of children with cystic fibrosis during antibiotic treatment. Eur Respir J 2000;16(1):95–100.

[83] Hull J, Vervaart P, Grimwood K, et al. Pulmonary oxidative stress response in young children with cystic fibrosis. Thorax 1997;52(6):557–60.

[84] Sadowska AM, Manuel-y-Kennoy B, De Backer WA. Antioxidant and anti-inflammatory efficacy of NAC in the treatment of COPD. Discordant in vitro and in vivo dose-effects: a review. Pulm Pharmacol Ther 2007;20(1):9–22.

[85] Tirouvanziam R, Conrad CK, Bottiglieri T, et al. High-dose oral N-acetylcysteine, a glutathione prodrug, modulates inflammation in cystic fibrosis. Proc Natl Acad Sci U S A 2006;103(12): 4628–33.

[86] Linsdell P, Hanrahan JW. Glutathione permeability of CFTR. Am J Physiol 1998;275(1 Pt 1): C323–6.

[87] Roum JH, Buhl R, McElvaney NG, et al. Systemic deficiency of glutathione in cystic fibrosis. J Appl Physiol 1993;75(6):2419–24.

[88] Roum JH, Borok Z, McElvaney NG, et al. Glutathione aerosol suppresses lung epithelial surface inflammatory cell-derived oxidants in cystic fibrosis. J Appl Physiol 1999;87(1):438–43.

[89] Griese M, Ramakers J, Krasselt A, et al. Improvement of alveolar glutathione and lung function but not oxidative state in cystic fibrosis. Am J Respir Crit Care Med 2004;169(7):822–8.

[90] Ferkol T, Cohn LA, Phillips TE, et al. Targeted delivery of antiprotease to the epithelial surface of human tracheal xenografts. Am J Respir Crit Care Med 2003;167(10):1374–9.

[91] McElvaney NG, Hubbard RC, Birrer P, et al. Aerosol alpha 1-antitrypsin treatment for cystic fibrosis. Lancet 1991;337(8738):392–4.

[92] Berger M, Konstan MW, Hilliard JB. Aerosolized prolastin (α_1-protease inhibitor) in CF. Pediatr Pulmonol 1995;20(6):421.

[93] Bilton D, Elborn S, Conway S, et al. Phase II trial to assess the clinical efficacy of transgenic alpha-1-antitrypsin (tg-hAAT) as an effective treatment of cystic fibrosis. Pediatr Pulmonol 1999;(Suppl 19): A289, 246.

[94] Rees DD, Rogers RA, Cooley J, et al. Recombinant human monocyte/neutrophil elastase inhibitor protects rat lungs against injury from cystic fibrosis airway secretions. Am J Respir Cell Mol Biol 1999;20(1):69–78.

[95] Grimbert D, Vecellio L, Delepine P, et al. Characteristics of EPI-hNE4 aerosol: a new elastase inhibitor for treatment of cystic fibrosis. J Aerosol Med 2003;16(2):121–9.

[96] Delacourt C, Herigault S, Delclaux C, et al. Protection against acute lung injury by intravenous or intratracheal pretreatment with EPI-HNE-4, a new potent neutrophil elastase inhibitor. Am J Respir Cell Mol Biol 2002;26(3):290–7.

[97] Honore S, Attalah HL, Azoulay E, et al. Beneficial effect of an inhibitor of leukocyte elastase (EPI-hNE-4) in presence of repeated lung injuries. Shock 2004;22(2):131–6.

[98] Harris M, Firsov D, Vuagniaux G, et al. A novel neutrophil elastase inhibitor prevents elastase activation and surface cleavage of the epithelial sodium channel expressed in Xenopus laevis oocytes. J Biol Chem 2007;282(1):58–64.

[99] Konstan MW. Evolving anti-inflammatory therapy in cystic fibrosis. In: Ramsey BW, Hodson ME, editors. New insights into cystic fibrosis. vol. 3 no. 2. New Jersey: Gardiner-Caldwell SynerMen; 1995. p. 7–11.

[100] Ramsey BW. Management of pulmonary disease in patients with cystic fibrosis [published erratum appears in N Engl J Med 1996 Oct;335(15):1167]. N Engl J Med 1996;335(3):179–88.

[101] Kudoh S, Azuma A, Yamamoto M, et al. Improvement of survival in patients with diffuse panbronchiolitis treated with low-dose erythromycin. Am J Respir Crit Care Med 1998;157(6 Pt 1):1829–32.

[102] Gerhardt SG, McDyer JF, Girgis RE, et al. Maintenance azithromycin therapy for bronchiolitis obliterans syndrome: results of a pilot study. Am J Respir Crit Care Med 2003;168(1):121–5.

[103] Jaffe A, Francis J, Rosenthal M, et al. Long-term azithromycin may improve lung function in children with cystic fibrosis. Lancet 1998;351(9100): 420.

[104] Wolter J, Seeney S, Bell S, et al. Effect of long term treatment with azithromycin on disease parameters in cystic fibrosis: a randomised trial. Thorax 2002; 57(3):212–6.

[105] Equi A, Balfour-Lynn IM, Bush A, et al. Long term azithromycin in children with cystic fibrosis: a randomised, placebo-controlled crossover trial. Lancet 2002;360(9338):978–84.

[106] Saiman L, Marshall BC, Mayer-Hamblett N, et al. Azithromycin in patients with cystic fibrosis chronically infected with Pseudomonas aeruginosa: a randomized controlled trial. JAMA 2003;290(13): 1749–56.

[107] Tateda K, Comte R, Pechere JC, et al. Azithromycin inhibits quorum sensing in Pseudomonas aeruginosa. Antimicrob Agents Chemother 2001;45(6): 1930–3.

[108] Nagino K, Kobayashi H. Influence of macrolides on mucoid alginate biosynthetic enzyme from Pseudomonas aeruginosa. Clin Microbiol Infect 1997; 3(4):432–9.

[109] Ichimiya T, Takeoka K, Hiramatsu K, et al. The influence of azithromycin on the biofilm formation of Pseudomonas aeruginosa in vitro. Chemotherapy 1996;42(3):186–91.

[110] Yamasaki T, Ichimiya T, Hirai K, et al. Effect of antimicrobial agents on the piliation of Pseudomonas aeruginosa and adherence to mouse tracheal epithelium. J Chemother 1997;9(1):32–7.

[111] Molinari G, Guzman CA, Pesce A, et al. Inhibition of Pseudomonas aeruginosa virulence factors by subinhibitory concentrations of azithromycin and other macrolide antibiotics. J Antimicrob Chemother 1993;31(5):681–8.

[112] Culic O, Erakovic V, Cepelak I, et al. Azithromycin modulates neutrophil function and circulating inflammatory mediators in healthy human subjects. Eur J Pharmacol 2002;450(3):277–89.

[113] Suzuki H, Shimomura A, Ikeda K, et al. Inhibitory effect of macrolides on interleukin-8 secretion from cultured human nasal epithelial cells. Laryngoscope 1997;107(12 Pt 1):1661–6.

[114] Suzuki H, Asada Y, Ikeda K, et al. Inhibitory effect of erythromycin on interleukin-8 secretion from exudative cells in the nasal discharge of patients with

chronic sinusitis. Laryngoscope 1999;109(3): 407–10.

[115] Ianaro A, Ialenti A, Maffia P, et al. Anti-inflammatory activity of macrolide antibiotics. J Pharmacol Exp Ther 2000;292(1):156–63.

[116] Feldman C, Anderson R, Theron AJ, et al. Roxithromycin, clarithromycin, and azithromycin attenuate the injurious effects of bioactive phospholipids on human respiratory epithelium *in vitro*. Inflammation 1997;21(6):655–65.

[117] Rubin BK, Tamaoki J. Macrolide antibiotics as biological response modifiers. Curr Opin Investig Drugs 2000;1(2):169–72.

[118] Shak S, Capon DJ, Hellmiss R, et al. Recombinant human DNase I reduces the viscosity of cystic fibrosis sputum. Proc Natl Acad Sci U S A 1990; 87(23):9188–92.

[119] Shah PL, Scott SF, Knight RA, et al. *In vivo* effects of recombinant human DNase I on sputum in patients with cystic fibrosis. Thorax 1996;51(2):119–25.

[120] Fuchs HJ, Borowitz DS, Christiansen DH, et al. Effect of aerosolized recombinant human DNase on exacerbations of respiratory symptoms and on pulmonary function in patients with cystic fibrosis. The Pulmozyme Study Group. N Engl J Med 1994; 331(10):637–42.

[121] Quan JM, Tiddens HA, Sy JP, et al. A two-year randomized, placebo-controlled trial of dornase alfa in young patients with cystic fibrosis with mild lung abnormalities. J Pediatr 2001;139(6):813–20.

[122] Konstan MW, Wagener JS, Pasta DJ, et al. Pulmozyme (dornase alfa) use is associated with a slower rate of lung function decline in patients with cystic fibrosis. Pediatr Pulmonol 2006;(Suppl 29):A370, 337.

[123] Paul K, Rietschel E, Ballmann M, et al. Effect of treatment with dornase alpha on airway inflammation in patients with cystic fibrosis. Am J Respir Crit Care Med 2004;169(9):719–25.

[124] Ratjen F, Paul K, van Koningsbruggen S, et al. DNA concentrations in BAL fluid of cystic fibrosis patients with early lung disease: influence of treatment with dornase alpha. Pediatr Pulmonol 2005; 39(1):1–4.

[125] Ballmann M, Junge S, von der Hardt H. Low-dose methotrexate for advanced pulmonary disease in patients with cystic fibrosis. Respir Med 2003; 97(5):498–500.

[126] Bhal GK, Maguire SA, Bowler IM. Use of cyclosporin A as a steroid sparing agent in cystic fibrosis. Arch Dis Child 2001;84(1):89.

[127] Konstan MW, Davis PB. Pharmacological approaches for the discovery and development of new anti-inflammatory agents for the treatment of cystic fibrosis. Adv Drug Deliv Rev 2002;54(11): 1409–23.

ELSEVIER
SAUNDERS

Clin Chest Med 28 (2007) 347–360

CLINICS
IN CHEST
MEDICINE

Macrolides in Cystic Fibrosis

John R. McArdle, MD[a,b,*], Jaideep S. Talwalkar, MD[a,c,d]

[a]Adult Cystic Fibrosis Program, Yale University School of Medicine, New Haven, CT 06520, USA
[b]Section of Pulmonary and Critical Care Medicine, Yale University School of Medicine, 333 Cedar Street,
P.O. Box 208057, New Haven, CT 06520, USA
[c]Department of Internal Medicine, Yale University School of Medicine, 333 Cedar Street, New Haven, CT 06520, USA
[d]Department of Pediatrics, Yale University School of Medicine, 333 Cedar Street, New Haven, CT 06520, USA

Cystic fibrosis (CF) is an autosomal recessive disorder affecting 1 in 3200 live births among Caucasians in the United States [1]. Once almost universally fatal in childhood, CF is still associated with premature mortality despite significant progress in the management of the many facets of this disease. Alterations in epithelial cell ion transport related to a defect in the cystic fibrosis transmembrane regulator (CFTR) result in increased sputum viscosity, leading to stasis of secretions and recurrent respiratory infection [2,3]. Multiple pathogens have been identified in the CF airways. *Pseudomonas aeruginosa* colonizes the majority of patients and it has been associated with an accelerated loss of lung function [4]. The assumption of a mucoid phenotype with biofilm formation impairs the effectiveness of phagocytes and antibiotics against *P aeruginosa* [5,6]. The host inflammatory response, which may be overabundant in this patient population, in conjunction with bacterial infection leads to tissue damage, bronchiectasis, and progressive respiratory insufficiency, with respiratory failure being the most common cause of death [3].

Inflammation in the CF airways is pronounced and may precede bacterial colonization of the lower airways [7]. Neutrophilic inflammation predominates in most patients, with increased levels of a number of proinflammatory cytokines found in the airways of patients who have CF, including tumor necrosis factor (TNF)-α and interleukin (IL)-1β, IL-8, and IL-6 [8]. Multiple neutrophil products lead to tissue damage and contribute to the chronic lung disease experienced by these patients.

Diffuse panbronchiolitis (DPB), a disease most common in Japan, shares several similarities with CF. Although it occurs most commonly in adults, DPB, like CF, is associated with chronic sinusitis, lower respiratory tract infections, and bronchiectasis, which can lead to respiratory failure and death, with 10-year survival rates as low as 12.4%. Patients suffering from this disease have a predilection to develop *P aeruginosa* infection with mucoid phenotype, as do patients who have CF. Macrolide antibiotic administration, namely the long-term use of erythromycin (EM), has resulted in a marked decrease in mortality, with marked reductions in mortality with long-term EM use [9,10].

Macrolides bind reversibly to the 50S subunit of bacterial ribosomes and thus interfere with translation of messenger RNA (mRNA) (Fig. 1) [8]. This inhibition of protein synthesis generally results in bacteriostatic effects, although macrolides can be bacteriocidal at higher concentrations. The predominant differences in the macrolides are related to the lactone rings, with 14-, 15-, and 16-member rings resulting in different pharmacokinetic and pharmacodynamic properties. Clarithromycin (CM) and EM are macrolides with 14-member lactone rings, whereas the lactone ring of azithromycin (AZM) contains 15 members (Fig. 2). AZM has a longer half-life with slower cellular efflux compared with EM

* Corresponding author. Section of Pulmonary and Critical Care Medicine, Yale University School of Medicine, 333 Cedar Street, P.O. Box 208057, New Haven, CT 06520.
E-mail address: john.mcardle@yale.edu (J.R. McArdle).

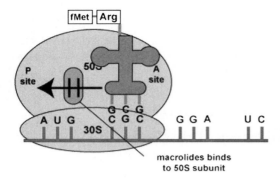

Fig. 1. Mechanism of action of macrolide antibiotics. Macrolide antibiotics bind to the 50S ribosomal subunit, preventing protein synthesis through inhibition of transfer RNA activity. (*Courtesy of* Gary E. Kaiser, PhD, Baltimore, MD.)

and CM, which can result in higher intracellular levels on prolonged administration [8]. Despite the results noted in patients who have DPB, macrolide concentrations that are achievable in human tissues are well below the minimum inhibitory concentrations (MICs) for *P aeruginosa*, and this class of antibiotic is not considered effective in the treatment of acute infections caused by this organism [11].

The improved outcome in DPB with macrolide therapy and the recognition of a number of anti-inflammatory and immunomodulatory effects of macrolides (discussed further below) have raised interest in a possible role for this class of

antibiotic in the treatment of patients who have CF. This article discusses the data supporting the use of macrolides, particularly AZM, in patients who have CF, possible mechanisms underlying its effects, and concerns engendered by the long-term use of these agents.

Clinical studies evaluating macrolide therapy in cystic fibrosis

In recent years, a number of clinical trials have been conducted to investigate the role of chronic macrolide therapy in patients who have CF (Table 1). The majority of these trials evaluated the use of AZM in patients who have CF who were chronically colonized with *P aeruginosa*. There is a significant amount of variability in study design, dosage, and outcome measures among these trials. The salient features of the larger trials are discussed individually.

Jaffe and colleagues [12] published the first experience with long-term AZM use. This trial was an open-label study in seven children who had end-stage lung disease or chronic airflow obstruction that was unresponsive to conventional therapy. All patients were culture positive for *P aeruginosa*. Variables followed included forced expiratory volume in 1 second (FEV_1), forced vital capacity (FVC), forced expiratory flow 25%–75%, peak expiratory flow rate, height, weight, and oxygen saturation. Patients were treated for at least 3 months with once-daily dosing for

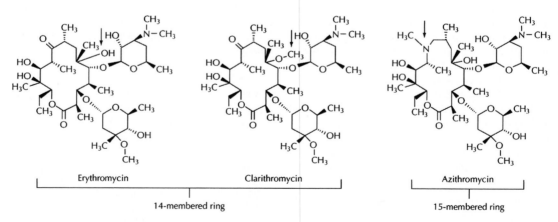

Fig. 2. Structure of common macrolide antibiotics. The difference between erythromycin and clarithromycin is the addition of a methoxy group at position 6 of the lactone ring (*arrow*). The addition of a nitrogen atom into the lactone ring creates the 15-membered azalide antibiotic, azithromycin (*arrow*). (*From* Nguyen T, Louis SG, Beringer PM, et al. Potential role of macrolide antibiotics in the management of cystic fibrosis lung disease. Curr Opin Pulm Med 2002;8: 521–9; with permission.)

a median treatment duration of 7 months. Significant differences were noted in FEV_1 and FVC, which increased by 11.0% and 11.3%, respectively, compared with pretreatment values. None of the other variables reached statistical significance.

Equi and colleagues [13] evaluated the impact of AZM on children 8 to 18 years of age. Their study was a randomized, double-blind, placebo-controlled, crossover design. Forty-one children who had CF were randomized to AZM or placebo for 6 months, followed by a 2-month washout period before they were crossed over to the alternative treatment arm. Patients randomized to the AZM arm received 250 mg daily if they weighed 40 kg or less or 500 mg daily if they weighed more than 40 kg. The primary outcome measure was the relative difference in FEV_1 between AZM and placebo treatment. Secondary outcomes included exercise testing, exacerbation rates, antibiotic use, quality of life (QOL), sputum microbiology, sputum IL-8, and elastase levels.

FEV_1 and FVC were consistently higher during the period of AZM therapy compared with placebo in both groups (placebo/AZM and AZM/placebo). Overall, 28 of 41 patients experienced improved lung function while on AZM. The median relative difference in FEV_1 of 5.4% significantly favored AZM therapy. FVC and forced expiratory flow 25%–75% also improved with AZM therapy relative to placebo. Likewise, there were significantly fewer antibiotic courses administered while patients were on AZM therapy. No significant differences were noted in the frequency of positive sputum cultures, bacterial density, sputum IL-8, elastase, exercise tolerance, or QOL. Therapy was well tolerated, with no evidence of ototoxicity on audiometry testing [13].

The first prospective, double-blind, placebo-controlled study on the use of AZM in adult patients who had CF was conducted by Wolter and colleagues [14]. Sixty patients who were clinically stable at the time of enrollment (defined as no change in symptoms or medications and no intravenous antibiotics or hospitalizations for 2 weeks before enrollment) were given AZM 250 mg once daily or placebo for 3 months. At baseline, mucoid and nonmucoid strains of *P aeruginosa* were cultured from 83.3% and 66.6% of patients, respectively. Outcome measures in this study included lung function, weight, and QOL using the Chronic Respiratory Disease Questionnaire. The investigators also performed serial bacteriologic investigation and measurement of serum inflammatory markers (C-reactive protein and erythrocyte sedimentation rate). The number of acute exacerbations of disease was recorded.

Patients randomized to AZM in this study maintained FEV_1 and FVC compared with baseline, whereas those randomized to placebo demonstrated declines in FEV_1 and FVC of 3.62% and 5.73%, respectively, relative to the AZM-treated group. There were also significant declines in the number of courses of intravenous antibiotic therapy and the number of days on intravenous antibiotics. The placebo group was composed of more men than the AZM group (67% versus 30%). Given that men who have CF generally have a slower rate of decline in lung function compared with women who have CF, these results are perhaps more impressive. C-reactive protein levels declined over time in the AZM group but not in the placebo group. Chronic Respiratory Disease Questionnaire scores improved in the AZM group relative to the placebo group. There was no difference in body mass index between the two treatment groups. There was no difference in bacteria isolated or colony counts among the two groups, nor was there a change from baseline, suggesting that the benefits achieved could not be explained solely by an antibacterial effect [14].

The largest double-blind, randomized, placebo-controlled trial assessing the use of AZM in patients who have CF was a multicenter trial conducted in the United States by the Macrolide Study Group [15]. A total of 185 patients 6 years of age and over with FEV_1 at least 30% predicted who had been infected with *P aeruginosa* for at least 1 year were randomized to AZM or placebo for 168 days with dosage based on body weight (250 mg three times weekly for patients who weighed less than 40 kg and 500 mg three times weekly for patients who weighed 40 kg or more). The primary outcome measure was change in FEV_1 from day 0 to completion of therapy. Weight gain and pulmonary exacerbations were secondary outcomes, and IL-8 and elastase levels in sputum and microbiologic evaluation were performed. Clinical evaluation of study participants included symptoms, physical examination, assessments of liver function, creatinine and hematology, and QOL evaluation by the Cystic Fibrosis Quality of Life Questionnaire. Audiology testing was conducted at 11 of the 23 centers.

Results of the United States study were similar to those published previously with regard to FEV_1 data, with the AZM group demonstrating a 4.4% improvement in mean FEV_1 percent predicted

Table 1
Published clinical trials on long-term macrolide use in cystic fibrosis

Authors	Study design/number of subjects	Drug/dosage/duration	Pseudomonas colonization on entry	Results
Jaffe et al [12] 1998	Open label/seven children	AZM/not specified; median duration 0.6 yr	All colonized with *P aeruginosa*	Median %FEV$_1$ increased 11.0%, median %FVC by 11.3%
Equi et al [13] 2002	Randomized, double-blind, placebo-controlled, crossover trial/41 children	AZM/250 mg daily (weight ≤40 kg) or 500 mg daily (weight >40 kg); 6 mo each arm	51% colonized with *P aeruginosa*	Median %FEV$_1$ increased 5.4% No change FVC Decreased antibiotic use while on AZM No change sputum elastase, IL-8
Wolter et al [14] 2002	Randomized, double-blind, placebo-controlled trial/60 adults	AZM/250 mg daily for 3 mo	83.3% colonized with mucoid *P aeruginosa*	Mean %FEV$_1$ 3.62% higher in AZM group Mean %FVC 5.73% higher in AZM group Decrease in intravenous antibiotic use Decrease CRP level Improved QOL score No change ESR or BMI
Saiman et al [15] 2003	Randomized, double-blind, placebo-controlled trial/185 patients age 6 yr and over	AZM/250 mg three times weekly (weight <40 kg) or 500 mg three times weekly (weight ≥40 kg) for 6 mo	All colonized with *P aeruginosa*	Mean difference %FEV$_1$ 6.2% Mean difference in %FVC 5.0% No difference in audiometry AZM group gained 0.7 kg more weight Hazard ratio for exacerbation 0.65, decreased hospitalization No difference in total QOL No difference in IL-8 or elastase
Clement et al [16] 2005	Randomized, double-blind, placebo-controlled trial/82 patients age 6 yr and over	AZM/250 mg three times weekly (weight <40 kg) or 500 mg three times weekly (weight ≥40 kg) for 12 mo	23% colonized with *P aeruginosa*	No difference in FEV$_1$/FVC ratio; decreased exacerbation and number of courses of additional antibiotics
Hansen et al [16] 2005	Observational cohort study/45 adults	AZM/250 mg daily; 1 yr treatment	90% colonized with *P aeruginosa*	Improved slope of FEV$_1$ and FVC decline Decreased percentage of patient colonized with *P aeruginosa* (90%–81%) improved weight and BMI

(continued on next page)

Table 1 (*continued*)

Authors	Study design/number of subjects	Drug/dosage/duration	Pseudomonas colonization on entry	Results
Pirzada et al [19] 2003	Retrospective study/20 patients	AZM/250 mg daily; median treatment 0.9 yr	All colonized with *P aeruginosa*	Mean %FEV$_1$ increased 8.9% Mean %FVC increased 11.6% BMI increased 1.1%; decreased pulmonary exacerbations requiring intravenous antibiotics by 48.3% compared with pretreatment period
Ordoñez et al [20] 2001	Prospective, single-blind study/10 adults	CM 500 mg BID; 6 wk treatment after 3 wk placebo	All colonized with *P aeruginosa*	No change in FEV$_1$/ FVC ratio; no change in sputum neutrophils, IL-8, elastase, TNF-α, or myeloperoxidase
Pukhalsky et al [21] 2004	Open-label, prospective study/27 children	CM 250 mg every other day for 1 yr	48% colonized with *P aeruginosa*	Improved FEV$_1$ and FVC (amount not quantified) Decreased sputum TNF-α, IL-8, IFN-γ and IL-4 No change in sputum elastase or protein level Increased peripheral blood lymphocyte response to PHA

Abbreviations: AZM, azithromycin; BMI, body mass index; CRP, C-reactive protein; CM, clarithromycin; ESR, erythrocyte sedimentation rate; %FEV$_1$, percent predicted forced expiratory volume in 1 s; %FVC, percent predicted forced vital capacity; IFN-γ, interferon-γ; IL-4, interleukin-4; IL-8, interleukin-8; PHA, phytohemagglutinin; QOL, quality of life; TNF-α, tumor necrosis factor–α.

compared with baseline and the placebo group demonstrating a 1.8% decline for a 6.2% treatment effect. FVC demonstrated a 5.0% treatment effect favoring AZM [15]. There were also significant decreases in the number of exacerbations in the AZM group (relative risk [RR], 0.65) and in the number of patients hospitalized (RR, 0.46). Weight gain favored the AZM group, with mean weight gain of 0.7 kg more in the AZM group. Overall QOL was unchanged, although the component of the CF QOL questionnaire dealing with physical functioning was significantly improved in patients treated with AZM. There was a trend toward decreased density of *P aeruginosa* in the AZM group compared with placebo, but this did not reach statistical significance. There

was no difference in audiology testing between the two groups, but the AZM group was significantly more likely to experience nausea, diarrhea, and wheezing (with differences of 17%, 15%, and 13% between AZM and placebo groups, respectively) [15].

A follow-up publication on the same group of patients stratified outcomes based on a number of patient and treatment variables, such as baseline FEV$_1$, concomitant therapies (eg, aerosolized tobramycin and rhDNAse), genotype, and the correlation of FEV$_1$ response and exacerbation rates [16]. Among patients randomized to AZM therapy, there was heterogeneity in FEV$_1$ response, with 26% of patients experiencing an increase of 10% or more and 10% of patients experiencing a decrease of 10% or more. When stratified based on FEV_1 response, those with an increase in FEV_1 of 5% or more had a similar decrease in the number of exacerbations compared with patients with less than 5% FEV_1 improvement (RR, 0.70 versus 0.61 compared with placebo). This suggests that at least some of the clinical benefit exists regardless of FEV_1 response. Patients who were not treated with inhaled tobramycin on study enrollment had higher FEV_1 at baseline than those on inhaled tobramycin and had a larger improvement in FEV_1 on AZM therapy. FEV_1 improvements were similar in patients regardless of baseline rhDNAse use and were not significantly different in patients who had an FEV_1 less than 60% predicted as compared with those who had an FEV_1 at least 60% predicted on study entry. Patients who were homozygous for $\Delta F508$ experienced greater FEV_1 benefit than those who were heterozygous for this mutation [16].

The data for exacerbation rates did not move in lockstep with data for FEV_1. Exacerbation rates declined more in patients who had FEV_1 values less than 60% at baseline compared with those who had FEV_1 values 60% or greater, (RR, 0.42 for the former group versus 0.82 for the latter). Decreases in exacerbations were slightly greater for tobramycin users compared with nonusers despite FEV_1 responses that favored nonusers. Patients treated with rhDNAse had a greater reduction in the risk for exacerbation compared with nonusers. These data suggest that the benefits of AZM persist in the face of a variety of other commonly used therapies and in patients who have different degrees of pulmonary function impairments [16].

Longer-term studies of AZM use have been published in recent years to assess the durability of treatment effect and safety with long-term administration. Clement and colleagues [17] published the results of a 1-year randomized, double-blind, placebo-controlled, multicenter trial of AZM in 82 patients 6 years of age and older who had FEV_1 at least 40% predicted. Only 19 of the 82 patients were infected with *P aeruginosa*. Dosage of AZM was three times weekly, 250 mg for those weighing more than 40 kg and 500 mg for those 40 kg or more. Patients treated with AZM did not have a significant difference in FEV_1 at 1 year compared with placebo-treated patients, but they had significant decreases in the number of pulmonary exacerbations and additional courses of oral antibiotics and prolongation of the time elapsed to the first exacerbation. These

results were similar in patients with or without *P aeruginosa* infection. This longer-term use of AZM was not met with an increased risk of adverse events and did not result in significant differences in body mass index and organisms isolated on sputum culture. Although an FEV_1 benefit was not noted in this trial, the data on exacerbation frequency were in line with data seen in other trials [17].

Two open-label, retrospective studies have evaluated longer-term AZM administration in patients who had chronic *P aeruginosa* infection. Hansen and colleagues [18] published results of an observational cohort study comparing clinical parameters in the 12 months before initiation of AZM therapy (250 mg daily). They demonstrated increased weight by a median of 0.8 kg, an improvement in the slope of FEV_1 decline, and a decrease in the number of sputum cultures growing *P aeruginosa* from 90% in the year before AZM therapy to 81% during treatment. Pirzada and colleagues [19] evaluated the effect of AZM (250 mg daily) on 20 patients who had progressive lung disease, defined as a decline in FEV_1 greater than 10% in the year before therapy initiation despite optimal conventional therapy. After a median of 0.9 years, they demonstrated improvement in mean FEV_1 from 50.2% predicted before therapy to 59.1% on treatment, with mean FVC increasing from 64.5% predicted to 76.1% predicted. Pulmonary exacerbations requiring intravenous antibiotics decreased by 48.3% on AZM therapy, and patients gained 3.9 kg on average. One patient discontinued therapy due to abdominal pain. A comparison group of 20 patients who had stable lung function over the year before therapy matched for age and sex did not demonstrate FEV_1 improvements over the same period and had lesser increases in body weight [19]. These studies provide additional data that the benefits of AZM therapy persist over longer treatment periods without significant toxicity.

Clarithromycin has been evaluated to a much lesser degree as long-term therapy in patients who have CF. Ordoñez and colleagues [20] performed a single-blind, prospective study on 10 adults who had CF and *P aeruginosa* infection. Patients were excluded if their FEV_1 was less than 30% predicted, if they had a change in medication or pulmonary exacerbation within the prior 4 weeks, if they had recent hemoptysis, or if they were colonized with atypical mycobacteria or *Burkholderia cepacia*. Patients were treated with placebo for 3 weeks followed by CM for 6 weeks at a dose of 500 mg twice daily. Outcome measures included pulmonary function, lung inflammation (neutrophil numbers), and sputum levels of TNF-α, IL-8, myeloperoxidase, and elastase. There was no difference in FEV$_1$, FVC, sputum neutrophils, or any of the sputum cytokine levels with clarithromycin therapy. The investigators also noted poor reproducibility for TNF-α measurements in sputum [20].

An open-label study by Pukhalsky and colleagues [21] examined the effects of a lower dose of CM (250 mg every other day) in 27 patients who had CF with a mean age of 12 years over a period of 1 year. Thirteen of the 27 patients were colonized with mucoid *P aeruginosa*. Significant increases in FEV$_1$ and FVC were noted compared with baseline, and there were significant declines in sputum IL-8 and TNF-α levels and in interferon-γ and IL-4 levels in sputum and blood. The ratio between interferon-γ and IL-4 increased significantly with treatment [21], suggesting a shift toward a TH-1 immune response, which has been suggested in animal models to be associated with a better outcome in the setting of chronic *Pseudomonas* infection [22]. The investigators noted that therapy with CM was associated with an increase in the response of peripheral blood lymphocytes to phytohemagglutinin, suggesting that activity of these cells was not being suppressed by CM [21].

A potential drawback to chronic macrolide use is the development of resistance to this class of agents on prolonged exposure. Phaff and colleagues [23] examined the frequency of macrolide resistance in *Staphylococcus aureus* and *Haemophilus influenzae* isolates from patients who had CF between 1999 and 2004, a period that saw an increase in AZM use to one third of the CF patient population. EM resistance among *S aureus* isolates increased from 6.9% to 53.8% over this period, and CM resistance among *H influenzae* increased from 3.7% to 37.5%. Patients receiving AZM therapy were less likely to have either of these agents present on culture than patients not receiving AZM. Prunier and colleagues [24] noted a high frequency of resistant *S aureus* isolates, with 53% of isolates resistant to macrolides. The mechanism of resistance most frequently involved the acquisition of a gene for an efflux pump or mutations in domain V of the 23S ribosomal RNA [24]. This region contains the peptidyl transferase region where proteins are synthesized.

In summary, AZM therapy is associated with a modest improvement in FEV$_1$ compared with placebo in a number of trials, with minimal toxicity and improvements in the rates of exacerbation and antibiotic use. A small amount of longer-term data suggests continued efficacy without substantial toxicity. Results on the use of CM are mixed, with divergent results in two studies with different doses, patient populations, and treatment durations. The long-term use of macrolides raises the concern for the selection of resistant bacteria, and there is evidence that *S aureus* and *H influenzae* strains are increasingly resistant to macrolide therapy in centers where AZM is used frequently.

Potential mechanisms underlying macrolide activity in cystic fibrosis

A number of theories have been proffered to explain the beneficial effects of macrolide therapy in patients who have CF. These theories can be roughly divided into two major categories: (1) the impact of macrolides on the offending pathogen, with *P aeruginosa* being the best studied, and (2) the impact on host defenses and inflammatory mechanisms (Table 2).

The impact of macrolides on P aeruginosa

P aeruginosa uses a number of different strategies to allow persistence in patients who have CF. Among these is the formation of an alginate biofilm, which allows the bacteria protection from antimicrobials and phagocytes [5]. Organisms exist within the biofilm in a stationary (as opposed to exponential) growth pattern, which can alter their sensitivity to cell-cycle–dependent antibiotics. *P aeruginosa* colonies also use quorum-sensing mechanisms, which allow the members of a colony to act as a group with regard to the expression of pathogenicity factors [25]. Macrolide therapy, especially AZM, has been found to interfere with a number of these features in a way that might benefit the host.

Delayed bactericidal effect

Macrolides do not exhibit antipseudomonal activity on conventional antimicrobial sensitivity testing. Tateda and colleagues [26] demonstrated, however, that extension of the incubation period for EM, AZM, and CM results in diminished viability of the organism, with evidence of bactericidal effects against PAO1, a laboratory strain of *P aeruginosa*, and 13 of 14 clinical specimens consisting of mucoid and nonmucoid phenotypes. In these experiments, protein synthesis by the organisms was diminished in a time-dependent fashion and seemed to correlate with antimicrobial effect. The concentrations of antibiotic were 1/128 MIC

Table 2
Proposed mechanisms of action for macrolide antibiotics in cystic fibrosis

Mechanisms	In vitro evidence
Antimicrobial activity	
P aeruginosa	
Cidal for stationary phase	↓MIC stationary phase compared with log phase
Alter structural proteins	↓Flagellin expression
Alter alginate expression	Inhibit production via inhibition of enzyme in biosynthetic pathway
Inhibit cell-to-cell signaling	Inhibition of quorum sensing by ↓ production of HSL signaling molecules
Alter exoproduct expression	↓Protease expression
Anti-inflammatory activity	
Inhibition of proinflammatory cytokines	Inhibition of NF-κB activation
	↓IL-8, IL-6, TNFα, ICAM-1 gene synthesis
Neutrophils	↓Chemotaxis, ↓oxidative burst, ↑intracellular cAMP, accelerate proapoptotic effect
Monocytes	↓IL-1β, IL-6, and TNFα, ↓MIP
Lymphocytes	↓Proliferation, ↑proliferation
Bronchial epithelial cells	↓IL-6, ↓IL-8, ↓ICAM-1
Sputum rheology	↓Goblet cell or epithelial mucin production in response to LPS
Interact with P-glycoproteins	Impair activity of multidrug transporters, may enhance intracellular concentrations of chemotherapeutic agents

Abbreviations: HSL, homoserine lactone; ICAM-1, intracellular adhesion molecule; LPS, lipopolysaccharide; MIC, minimum inhibitory concentration; MIP, macrophage inflammatory protein; TNF, tumor necrosis factor; ↑ increased; ↓ decreased.

Adapted from Saiman L. The use of macrolide antibiotics in patients with cystic fibrosis. Curr Opin Pulm Med 2004;10:515–23; with permission.

for AZM and CM and 1/64 MIC for EM, all of which are clinically achievable. AZM was noted to accumulate intracellularly between 12 and 36 hours of exposure, perhaps contributing to the delayed bactericidal effect [26]. Imamura and colleagues [27] evaluated PAO1 viability on exposure to AZM. They found that isolates were insensitive to AZM when in the exponential growth phase, but organisms in the stationary growth phase, such as those found in biofilms, displayed sensitivity to AZM. Furthermore, this sensitivity was inhibited by exposure to Ca^{2+} or Mg^{2+}. The effect of these ions on sensitivity suggests that the mechanism of AZM is at the level of the bacterial outer membrane because the lipopolysaccharides in the outer membrane are stabilized by binding to divalent cations. 1-N-phenylnaphthylamine assay demonstrated interaction of AZM with the outer membrane, increasing its permeability, which would be expected with the proposed mechanism of action [27].

CM and AZM have been demonstrated to provide synergy against pathogens isolated from patients who have CF, enhancing the effect of more traditional antimicrobials, such as tobramycin for *P aeruginosa* and trimethoprim-sulfamethoxazole and ceftazidime for *Stenotrophomonas maltophilia*, *B cepacia*, and *Achromobacter*

xylosoxidans [28]. These results are of interest because patients who have CF are commonly treated with combinations of AZM and inhaled tobramycin, and this synergy may provide additional therapeutic effects.

Interference with quorum sensing

Quorum sensing is a mechanism used by *P aeruginosa* and other bacteria to coordinate the activity of individual organisms to benefit the colony. Individual organisms are capable of producing autoinducer substances; in the case of *P aeruginosa*, the homoserine lactones (HSLs) 3-O C_{12}-HSL and C_4-HSL [29]. These autoinducers can leave the cell and, when present in sufficient concentrations, activate transcription regulators that turn on gene transcription for select pathogenicity factors, such as elastase and rhamnolipid. 3-O C_{12}-HSL can incite a host inflammatory response, stimulating IL-8 production, which leads to increased neutrophilic inflammation. 3-O C_{12}-HSL also leads to increased production of MUC5AC, a core mucin protein, suggesting that autoinducers may alter the properties of secretions. Signaling by this autoinducer seems to use extracellular signal–regulated kinase (ERK) ½ and I-kappa-B [30].

On exposure to AZM (2 mg/L), there is a marked decrease in HSL production by 70% to 90%. Experimental replacement of the deficient autoinducers improves but does not normalize the expression of transcription activator genes under the control of HSLs, suggesting that AZM interferes with signaling via another mechanism [29], such as the ERK $\frac{1}{2}$ pathways. Nalca and colleagues [31] demonstrated extensive inhibition of quorum sensing signaling by AZM with impaired virulence factor production, oxidative stress response, and motility. Interference with quorum sensing, as demonstrated by AZM, could yield organisms less capable of inducing tissue damage and increase the effectiveness of phagocytes and antibiotics at clearing infections.

Adherence and motility

The oropharyngeal barrier provides a line of defense against lower respiratory colonization. Patients who have CF have higher than normal adherence of *P aeruginosa* to the buccal mucosa, which may be a precursor to lung infection. Baumann and colleagues [32] demonstrated that the use of long-term, low-dose AZM diminished the adherence of *P aeruginosa* by 70% to near normal levels in 11 children who had CF, eight of whom were infected with mucoid strains.

Yamasaki and colleagues [33] likewise demonstrated decreased *Pseudomonas* adherence to acid injured murine tracheal epithelium in the presence of EM. This diminished adherence was associated with a significant decrease in pili expression. In addition to cellular adherence, *P aeruginosa* adheres to salivary and airway mucins by using flagella and nonpilus adhesins on the outer membrane of the organism. Carfartan and colleagues [34] reported their experiments with PAO1 and 13 pseudomonas strains isolated from patients who had CF to assess the adherence to purified bronchial mucins in the presence or absence of AZM. Adherence of *P aeruginosa* to mucins was present in all strains tested and was inhibited by 2 to 4 mg/L of AZM in four of five mucoid strains and six of eight nonmucoid strains. The inhibition of adherence seemed to be dose dependent, with 47.5% inhibition with 2 mg/L concentration and 56% with 4 mg/L concentration, with mucoid strains generally requiring the higher (but clinically achievable) concentration [34].

Flagella are expressed by *P aeruginosa* to facilitate motility, thereby allowing the organism to establish itself in a suitable environment. Flagella also allow congregation of organisms to facilitate

biofilm formation to elude host defenses. AZM, CM, and EM at sub-MIC concentrations decrease the expression of flagellin, with AZM and EM also inhibiting flagellin expression for several hours after antibiotic removal [35,36]. Colonies exposed to AZM demonstrate markedly decreased motility due to absence of flagella on the majority of organisms [37,38]. Flagellin is a potent stimulator of inflammation, and decreased expression may lead to attenuation of the inflammatory response on exposure to *Pseudomonas*.

Expression of pathogenicity factors

Prolonged exposure to AZM results in significant inhibition of protein synthesis by *P aeruginosa*. A variety of exoproducts are produced in decreased amounts in the presence of macrolide antibiotics, with AZM demonstrating enhanced effect compared with EM and CM. Virulence factors that are inhibited by AZM in vitro include elastase, protease, leucocidin, lecithinase, DNase, gelatinase, exotoxin A, phospholipase C, and pyocyanin [37,39–41]. Results on isolates from CF patients are more variable because exoproduct expression is less robust during periods of low growth, as is seen in many CF isolates [39]. Nonetheless, the tissue damage and inflammation that results from exotoxin expression could potentially be ameliorated by macrolide, particularly AZM, therapy.

Biofilm

Alginate biofilms produced by *P aeruginosa* allow protection to the organisms against dehydration, phagocytes, and antimicrobial agents. Alginate is immunostimulatory and induces a continuous antigen–antibody reaction at the airway surface [10]. Macrolide therapy has been shown to affect biofilm formation through a variety of mechanisms. AZM has been demonstrated to inhibit alginate production from mucoid *Pseudomonas* at low concentrations [42]. Impairment in bacterial motility also inhibits the effectiveness of biofilm formation [43]. In addition, in *P aeruginosa* colonies that produce biofilms, the response of neutrophils is reduced relative to the response to planktonic bacteria. Treatment with macrolides, including EM, AZM, CM, and roxithromycin, significantly increases chemiluminescence response in biofilms exposed to neutrophils, with AZM demonstrating the most pronounced effect [44]. When neutrophils were pretreated with macrolides before exposure to the biofilm, this chemiluminescence pattern was not seen, suggesting that the result is related to a macrolide effect on the biofilm rather than an effect on the neutrophils [44]. These experiments suggest a potential role for AZM or other macrolides in diminishing the protective effects of established biofilms and inhibiting the production of alginate necessary for new biofilm formation.

Effect of macrolides on host defenses

A number of alterations in airway physiology and inflammatory response have been ascribed to macrolide therapy. Whether some of these effects relate to alterations in host–pathogen interactions or are a direct result of this class of antibiotics on neutrophils and other effector cells is unclear. The possibility that macrolides alter the properties of sputum or ion transport is an area of active investigation. The pharmacokinetics of macrolides, most notably AZM, demonstrate intracellular accumulation in mononuclear cells with levels of 15.4 mg/L noted in a study of long-term use by Beringer and colleagues [45]. Another study of daily AZM (500 mg) in patients who had CF demonstrated accumulation in neutrophils and sputum at levels higher than those found in blood, with sputum concentrations remaining detectable for 10 days after cessation of administration. Levels in neutrophils 24 hours after administration were 2100 times that in the plasma [46]. Baumann and colleagues [47] noted an accumulation of AZM in sputum by two orders of magnitude when dosed at 250 mg daily. This accumulation in sputum and inflammatory cells suggests a possible impact of this agent on host properties.

Sputum composition and rheology

Tenacious, viscous sputum accumulates over time in the airways of patients who have CF, contributing to the pathogenesis of this disease by impairing mucociliary clearance. A number of investigators have assessed the impact of macrolides on the characteristics of sputum. $3\text{-}O\text{-}C_{12}\,HSL$ seems to stimulate increased production of the mucin protein MUC5AC, an effect that is inhibited by AZM administration [30]. CM and EM have also been noted to reduce MUC5AC mRNA expression in vitro [48]. Baumann and colleagues [47] demonstrated a dose-dependent reduction in sputum viscosity in patients who had CF at doses of 250 mg twice weekly or once daily. Similar findings on sputum consistency in patients without CF were noted in a study of 33 patients who had non-CF bronchiectasis after 4 months of AZM therapy [49]. Tamaoki and colleagues [50] demonstrated improvement in sputum elasticity, solid composition,

and volume without altering bacterial density after 8 weeks of low-dose CM in 31 patients who had conditions associated with increase sputum production.

Not every study has confirmed this effect on rheology. Shibuya and colleagues [51] found no difference in the transportability of CF or non-CF sputum even with high-dose EM exposure. This experiment was performed on already formed, expectorated sputum, suggesting that EM does not have an effect on sputum that has already been produced.

Ion transport. CFTR is a member of the ATP-binding cassette family of proteins and serves as a transporter of chloride ions [3]. Multidrug-resistance–associated protein (MRP) is another member of this family and serves as an efflux pump to transport compounds out of cells. Macrolides have been demonstrated to up-regulate MRP production, suggesting a possible role in the restoration of ion transport abnormalities [52]. Pradal and colleagues [53] treated seven patients who had CF with abnormal nasal potential difference (NPD) with AZM (500 mg once daily for 4 weeks). At the end of treatment, they demonstrated increased MRP mRNA production by nasal epithelial cells and improved NPD chloride response, which correlated with the degree of MRP mRNA induction.

There have been conflicting reports. Barker and colleagues [54] tested the effect of macrolides (CM and AZM) on NPD in CFTR knockout and $\Delta F508$ homozygote mice. Eighteen patients who had CF involved in a crossover study of long-term CM use also had NPD measured. There were no differences in the NPD in normal or CF mice or in the human CF patients treated with CM.

Impact on inflammatory cells. AZM accumulates in neutrophils over time [45,46], and a number of effects on neutrophil function in the face of AZM therapy have been observed. Aoshiba and colleagues [55] demonstrated acceleration of neutrophil apoptosis in a dose-dependent fashion on exposure to EM, with an increase in intracellular cAMP seemingly accelerating the onset of apoptosis. Neutrophil chemoattraction and migration have been demonstrated to be altered in in vivo and in vitro models [56–58]. Production of IL-8, a potent neutrophil chemoattractant, is reduced in neutrophils, airway epithelial cells, and macrophages in the presence of macrolide therapy [59–62]. Tsai and colleagues [57] demonstrated decreased cellular infiltration into mouse lungs exposed to *Pseudomonas* beads, correlating with decreased TNF-α levels. Human and mouse neutrophils exposed to AZM demonstrate decreased chemotaxis to chemokine-dependent and -independent chemoattractants associated with impairments in ERK 1 and ERK 2 activation.

Decreased IL-8 levels and neutrophilia in BAL fluid have been associated with macrolide therapy in patients who have DPB [63,64]. Patients who have undergone lung transplantation who experienced chronic rejection due to bronchiolitis obliterans syndrome have demonstrated improvement in FEV_1 with long-term AZM therapy [65]. The effects of AZM are heterogeneous in bronchiolitis obliterans syndrome, with predictors of response including BAL neutrophilia, elevated BAL IL-8 levels, and earlier initiation of AZM, suggesting that the benefits of therapy may be related to effects on neutrophilic inflammation [66]. The production of adhesion molecules, such as intracellular adhesion molecule–1, β2 integrins by bronchial epithelial cells, and neutrophils, is inhibited on exposure to macrolides, suggesting that chemoattractant and adhesion molecules participate in altered neutrophil migration on macrolide exposure [60].

Cytokine and chemokine production in a number of cell lines are affected by macrolide therapy. Bronchial epithelial cells stimulated with IL-1 produce lower amounts of IL-6 and IL-8 in the presence of macrolides. Production of IL-6, IL-8, IL-10, and TNF-α is reduced in whole blood in the presence of EM on stimulation with *P aeruginosa* or *Streptococcus pneumoniae* [10]. A possible mechanism for the inhibition of cytokine production involves inhibition of nuclear factor kappa B (NF-κB) or apoprotein-1 (AP-1), which serve as transcription factors regulating a variety of proinflammatory cytokines. EM inhibits NF-κB transcriptional activity for IL-8 in T cells [67], and CM inhibits the activation of NF-κB and AP-1 by TNF, staphylococcal enterotoxin A, and lipopolysaccharide in mononuclear cells and airway epithelial cells [68,69].

The results of human studies with AZM and CM in CF have not consistently revealed significant alterations in sputum inflammatory markers, making the significance of the in vitro and ex vivo findings uncertain [13,15,20].

Summary

Macrolide therapy, predominantly azithromycin, in patients who have CF has been demonstrated in multiple trials to improve lung function and decrease the frequency of infectious exacerbations. Toxicity is limited over periods of follow-up as long as 1 year, with nausea and diarrhea being the most common side effects, but concerns over the possibility of hepatotoxicity and ototoxicity with longer-term use remain. The mechanisms of macrolide effect on CF are not well understood, but a variety of effects on pathogenic bacteria and host inflammatory responses have been observed. The expression of *P aeruginosa* pathogenicity factors, motility, and protein synthesis seem to be altered on extended exposure to macrolides. Neutrophil recruitment and expression of superoxides and elastase may be altered by macrolide therapy, but these effects have yet to be confirmed in the airways of patients who have CF.

References

[1] Hamosh A, FitzSimmons SC, Macek M Jr, et al. Comparison of the clinical manifestations of cystic fibrosis in black and white patients. J Pediatr 1998; 132(2):255–9.

[2] Ramsey BW. Management of pulmonary disease in patients with cystic fibrosis. N Engl J Med 1996; 335(3):179–88.

[3] Gibson RL, Burns JL, Ramsey BW. Pathophysiology and management of pulmonary infections in cystic fibrosis. Am J Respir Crit Care Med 2003; 168(8):918–51.

[4] Kerem E, Corey M, Gold R, et al. Pulmonary function and clinical course in patients with cystic fibrosis after pulmonary colonization with Pseudomonas aeruginosa. J Pediatr 1990;116(5):714–9.

[5] Donlan RM. Role of biofilms in antimicrobial resistance. ASAIO J 2000;46(6):S47–52.

[6] Hentzer M, Teitzel GM, Balzer GJ, et al. Alginate overproduction affects Pseudomonas aeruginosa biofilm structure and function. J Bacteriol 2001; 183(18):5395–401.

[7] Khan TZ, Wagener JS, Bost T, et al. Early pulmonary inflammation in infants with cystic fibrosis. Am J Respir Crit Care Med 1995; 151(4):1075–82.

[8] Nguyen T, Louie SG, Beringer PM, et al. Potential role of macrolide antibiotics in the management of cystic fibrosis lung disease. Curr Opin Pulm Med 2002;8(6):521–8.

[9] Nagai H, Shishido H, Yoneda R, et al. Long-term low-dose administration of erythromycin to patients with diffuse panbronchiolitis. Respiration 1991; 58(3–4):145–9.

[10] Schultz MJ. Macrolide activities beyond their antimicrobial effects: macrolides in diffuse

panbronchiolitis and cystic fibrosis. J Antimicrob Chemother 2004;54(1):21–8.

[11] Southern KW, Barker PM. Azithromycin for cystic fibrosis. Eur Respir J 2004;24(5):834–8.

[12] Jaffe A, Francis J, Rosenthal M, et al. Long-term azithromycin may improve lung function in children with cystic fibrosis. Lancet 1998;351(9100):420.

[13] Equi A, Balfour-Lynn IM, Bush A, et al. Long term azithromycin in children with cystic fibrosis: a randomised, placebo-controlled crossover trial. Lancet 2002;360(9338):978–84.

[14] Wolter J, Seeney S, Bell S, et al. Effect of long term treatment with azithromycin on disease parameters in cystic fibrosis: a randomised trial. Thorax 2002; 57(3):212–6.

[15] Saiman L, Marshall BC, Mayer-Hamblett N, et al. Azithromycin in patients with cystic fibrosis chronically infected with Pseudomonas aeruginosa: a randomized controlled trial. JAMA 2003;290(13): 1749–56.

[16] Saiman L, Mayer-Hamblett N, Campbell P, et al. Heterogeneity of treatment response to azithromycin in patients with cystic fibrosis. Am J Respir Crit Care Med 2005;172(8):1008–12.

[17] Clement A, Tamalet A, Leroux E, et al. Long term effects of azithromycin in patients with cystic fibrosis: a double blind, placebo controlled trial. Thorax 2006;61(10):895–902.

[18] Hansen CR, Pressler T, Koch C, et al. Long-term azitromycin treatment of cystic fibrosis patients with chronic Pseudomonas aeruginosa infection; an observational cohort study. J Cyst Fibros 2005; 4(1):35–40.

[19] Pirzada OM, McGaw J, Taylor CJ, et al. Improved lung function and body mass index associated with long-term use of macrolide antibiotics. J Cyst Fibros 2003;2(2):69–71.

[20] Ordonez CL, Stulbarg M, Grundland H, et al. Effect of clarithromycin on airway obstruction and inflammatory markers in induced sputum in cystic fibrosis: a pilot study. Pediatr Pulmonol 2001;32(1):29–37.

[21] Pukhalsky AL, Shmarina GV, Kapranov NI, et al. Anti-inflammatory and immunomodulating effects of clarithromycin in patients with cystic fibrosis lung disease. Mediators Inflamm 2004;13(2):111–7.

[22] Johansen HK, Cryz SJ Jr, Hougen HP, et al. Vaccination promotes TH1-like inflammation and survival in chronic Pseudomonas aeruginosa pneumonia: a new prophylactic principle. Behring Inst Mitt 1997;(98):269–73.

[23] Phaff SJ, Tiddens HA, Verbrugh HA, et al. Macrolide resistance of Staphylococcus aureus and Haemophilus species associated with long-term azithromycin use in cystic fibrosis. J Antimicrob Chemother 2006;57(4):741–6.

[24] Prunier AL, Malbruny B, Laurans M, et al. High rate of macrolide resistance in Staphylococcus aureus strains from patients with cystic fibrosis reveals

high proportions of hypermutable strains. J Infect Dis 2003;187(11):1709–16.

[25] Van Delden C, Iglewski BH. Cell-to-cell signaling and Pseudomonas aeruginosa infections. Emerg Infect Dis 1998;4(4):551–60.

[26] Tateda K, Ishii Y, Matsumoto T, et al. Direct evidence for antipseudomonal activity of macrolides: exposure-dependent bactericidal activity and inhibition of protein synthesis by erythromycin, clarithromycin, and azithromycin. Antimicrob Agents Chemother 1996;40(10):2271–5.

[27] Imamura Y, Higashiyama Y, Tomono K, et al. Azithromycin exhibits bactericidal effects on Pseudomonas aeruginosa through interaction with the outer membrane. Antimicrob Agents Chemother 2005;49(4):1377–80.

[28] Saiman L, Chen Y, Gabriel PS, et al. Synergistic activities of macrolide antibiotics against Pseudomonas aeruginosa, Burkholderia cepacia, Stenotrophomonas maltophilia, and Alcaligenes xylosoxidans isolated from patients with cystic fibrosis. Antimicrob Agents Chemother 2002;46(4): 1105–7.

[29] Tateda K, Comte R, Pechere JC, et al. Azithromycin inhibits quorum sensing in Pseudomonas aeruginosa. Antimicrob Agents Chemother 2001;45(6): 1930–3.

[30] Imamura Y, Yanagihara K, Mizuta Y, et al. Azithromycin inhibits MUC5AC production induced by the Pseudomonas aeruginosa autoinducer N-(3-Oxododecanoyl) homoserine lactone in NCI-H292 cells. Antimicrob Agents Chemother 2004;48(9): 3457–61.

[31] Nalca Y, Jansch L, Bredenbruch F, et al. Quorum-sensing antagonistic activities of azithromycin in Pseudomonas aeruginosa PAO1: a global approach. Antimicrob Agents Chemother 2006;50(5):1680–8.

[32] Baumann U, Fischer JJ, Gudowius P, et al. Buccal adherence of Pseudomonas aeruginosa in patients with cystic fibrosis under long-term therapy with azithromycin. Infection 2001;29(1):7–11.

[33] Yamasaki T, Ichimiya T, Hirai K, et al. Effect of antimicrobial agents on the piliation of Pseudomonas aeruginosa and adherence to mouse tracheal epithelium. J Chemother 1997;9(1):32–7.

[34] Carfartan G, Gerardin P, Turck D, et al. Effect of subinhibitory concentrations of azithromycin on adherence of Pseudomonas aeruginosa to bronchial mucins collected from cystic fibrosis patients. J Antimicrob Chemother 2004;53(4):686–8.

[35] Kawamura-Sato K, Iinuma Y, Hasegawa T, et al. Effect of subinhibitory concentrations of macrolides on expression of flagellin in Pseudomonas aeruginosa and Proteus mirabilis. Antimicrob Agents Chemother 2000;44(10):2869–72.

[36] Kawamura-Sato K, Iinuma Y, Hasegawa T, et al. Postantibiotic suppression effect of macrolides on the expression of flagellin in Pseudomonas

aeruginosa and Proteus mirabilis. J Infect Chemother 2001;7(1):51–4.

[37] Molinari G, Guzman CA, Pesce A, et al. Inhibition of Pseudomonas aeruginosa virulence factors by subinhibitory concentrations of azithromycin and other macrolide antibiotics. J Antimicrob Chemother 1993;31(5):681–8.

[38] Molinari G, Paglia P, Schito GC. Inhibition of motility of Pseudomonas aeruginosa and Proteus mirabilis by subinhibitory concentrations of azithromycin. Eur J Clin Microbiol Infect Dis 1992;11(5): 469–71.

[39] Wagner T, Soong G, Sokol S, et al. Effects of azithromycin on clinical isolates of Pseudomonas aeruginosa from cystic fibrosis patients. Chest 2005; 128(2):912–9.

[40] Kita E, Sawaki M, Oku D, et al. Suppression of virulence factors of Pseudomonas aeruginosa by erythromycin. J Antimicrob Chemother 1991;27(3): 273–84.

[41] Mizukane R, Hirakata Y, Kaku M, et al. Comparative in vitro exoenzyme-suppressing activities of azithromycin and other macrolide antibiotics against Pseudomonas aeruginosa. Antimicrob Agents Chemother 1994;38(3):528–33.

[42] Ichimiya T, Takeoka K, Hiramatsu K, et al. The influence of azithromycin on the biofilm formation of Pseudomonas aeruginosa in vitro. Chemotherapy 1996;42(3):186–91.

[43] Saiman L. The use of macrolide antibiotics in patients with cystic fibrosis. Curr Opin Pulm Med 2004;10(6):515–23.

[44] Takeoka K, Ichimiya T, Yamasaki T, et al. The in vitro effect of macrolides on the interaction of human polymorphonuclear leukocytes with Pseudomonas aeruginosa in biofilm. Chemotherapy 1998; 44(3):190–7.

[45] Beringer P, Huynh KMT, Kriengkauykiat J, et al. Absolute bioavailability and intracellular pharmacokinetics of azithromycin in patients with cystic fibrosis. Antimicrob Agents Chemother 2005;49(12): 5013–7.

[46] Wilms EB, Touw DJ, Heijerman HGM. Pharmacokinetics of azithromycin in plasma, blood, polymorphonuclear neutrophils and sputum during long-term therapy in patients with cystic fibrosis. Ther Drug Monit 2006;28(2):219–25.

[47] Baumann U, King M, App EM, et al. Long term azithromycin therapy in cystic fibrosis patients: a study on drug levels and sputum properties. Can Respir J 2004;11(2):151–5.

[48] Shinkai M, Rubin BK. Macrolides and airway inflammation in children. Paediatr Respir Rev 2005; 6(3):227–35.

[49] Davies G, Wilson R. Prophylactic antibiotic treatment of bronchiectasis with azithromycin. Thorax 2004;59(6):540–1.

[50] Tamaoki J, Takeyama K, Tagaya E, et al. Effect of clarithromycin on sputum production and its rheological properties in chronic respiratory tract infections. Antimicrob Agents Chemother 1995;39(8): 1688–90.

[51] Shibuya Y, Wills PJ, Cole PJ. The effect of erythromycin on mucociliary transportability and rheology of cystic fibrosis and bronchiectasis sputum. Respiration 2001;68(6):615–9.

[52] Altschuler EL. Azithromycin, the multidrug-resistant protein, and cystic fibrosis. Lancet 1998; 351(9111):1286.

[53] Pradal U, Delmarco A, Morganti M, et al. Long-term azithromycin in cystic fibrosis: another possible mechanism of action? J Chemother 2005;17(4): 393–400.

[54] Barker PM, Gillie DJ, Schechter MS, et al. Effect of macrolides on in vivo ion transport across cystic fibrosis nasal epithelium. Am J Respir Crit Care Med 2005;171(8):868–71.

[55] Aoshiba K, Nagai A, Konno K. Erythromycin shortens neutrophil survival by accelerating apoptosis. Antimicrob Agents Chemother 1995;39(4): 872–7.

[56] Suzuki H, Asada Y, Ikeda K, et al. Inhibitory effect of erythromycin on interleukin-8 secretion from exudative cells in the nasal discharge of patients with chronic sinusitis. Laryngoscope 1999;109(3): 407–10.

[57] Tsai WC, Rodriguez ML, Young KS, et al. Azithromycin blocks neutrophil recruitment in Pseudomonas endobronchial infection. Am J Respir Crit Care Med 2004;170(12):1331–9.

[58] Shinkai M, Foster GH, Rubin BK. Macrolide antibiotics modulate ERK phosphorylation and IL-8 and GM-CSF production by human bronchial epithelial cells. Am J Physiol Lung Cell Mol Physiol 2006;290(1):L75–85.

[59] Fujii T, Kadota J, Morikawa T, et al. Inhibitory effect of erythromycin on interleukin 8 production by 1 alpha,25-dihydroxyvitamin D3-stimulated THP-1 cells. Antimicrob Agents Chemother 1996;40(6): 1548–51.

[60] Lin HC, Wang CH, Liu CY, et al. Erythromycin inhibits beta2-integrins (CD11b/CD18) expression, interleukin-8 release and intracellular oxidative metabolism in neutrophils. Respir Med 2000;94(7): 654–60.

[61] Oishi K, Sonoda F, Kobayashi S, et al. Role of interleukin-8 (IL-8) and an inhibitory effect of erythromycin on IL-8 release in the airways of patients with chronic airway diseases. Infect Immun 1994; 62(10):4145–52.

[62] Sunazuka T, Takizawa H, Desaki M, et al. Effects of erythromycin and its derivatives on interleukin-8 release by human bronchial epithelial cell line BEAS-2B cells. J Antibiot (Tokyo) 1999;52(1):71–4.

[63] Ogushi F, Tani K, Maniwa K, et al. Interleukin-8 in bronchoalveolar lavage fluid of patients with diffuse panbronchiolitis or idiopathic pulmonary fibrosis. J Med Invest 1997;44(1–2):53–8.

[64] Sakito O, Kadota J, Kohno S, et al. Interleukin 1 beta, tumor necrosis factor alpha, and interleukin 8 in bronchoalveolar lavage fluid of patients with diffuse panbronchiolitis: a potential mechanism of macrolide therapy. Respiration 1996;63(1):42–8.

[65] Gerhardt SG, McDyer JF, Girgis RE, et al. Maintenance azithromycin therapy for bronchiolitis obliterans syndrome: results of a pilot study. Am J Respir Crit Care Med 2003;168(1):121–5.

[66] Verleden GM, Vanaudenaerde BM, Dupont LJ, et al. Azithromycin reduces airway neutrophilia and interleukin-8 in patients with bronchiolitis obliterans syndrome. Am J Respir Crit Care Med 2006; 174(5):566–70.

[67] Aoki Y, Kao PN. Erythromycin inhibits transcriptional activation of NF-kappaB, but not NFAT, through calcineurin-independent signaling in T cells. Antimicrob Agents Chemother 1999;43(11):2678–84.

[68] Abe S, Nakamura H, Inoue S, et al. Interleukin-8 gene repression by clarithromycin is mediated by the activator protein-1 binding site in human bronchial epithelial cells. Am J Respir Cell Mol Biol 2000;22(1):51–60.

[69] Kikuchi T, Hagiwara K, Honda Y, et al. Clarithromycin suppresses lipopolysaccharide-induced interleukin-8 production by human monocytes through AP-1 and NF-kappa B transcription factors. J Antimicrob Chemother 2002;49(5):745–55.

ELSEVIER
SAUNDERS

Clin Chest Med 28 (2007) 361–379

CLINICS
IN CHEST
MEDICINE

Novel Therapies for the Treatment of Cystic Fibrosis: New Developments in Gene and Stem Cell Therapy

Viranuj Sueblinvong, MD, Benjamin T. Suratt, MD,
Daniel J. Weiss, MD, PhD*

*Division of Pulmonary and Critical Care Medicine, The University of Vermont and Fletcher Allen Health Care,
149 Beaumont Avenue, HSRF 231, Burlington, VT 05405, USA*

Cystic fibrosis (CF) was one of the first target diseases for lung gene therapy, and studies of lung gene transfer for CF have provided many important insights into the necessary components of successful gene therapy for lung diseases. Although initial demonstrations of successful gene transfer in cultured lung epithelial cells and in small animal models generated enthusiasm, further studies in primate models and in patients have been discouraging. In particular, despite a number of clinical trials, a viable therapeutic strategy has yet to emerge. This reflects a number of obstacles to successful, sustained, and repeatable gene transfer in the lung, some of which may be only be overcome with great difficulty. As such, research efforts have largely shifted focus from clinical studies to more fundamental studies that seek to delineate the cell and molecular biology of gene transfer to airway epithelium. More recently, studies evaluating the use of cell-based therapies using embryonic stem cells and adult stem cells cells for correction of defective CF airway epithelium have been vigorously pursued. Although these studies are in relative infancy, they may provide a viable therapeutic approach in future years.

This article summarizes the current status of gene- and cell-based therapies for CF lung disease. Included is a brief discussion of CF pathophysiology with reference to specific targets in the lung epithelium for gene transfer and a detailed discussion of the vectors that are potentially appropriate for gene transfer to lung, consideration of the physiologic and immunologic barriers to lung gene transfer, and a review of clinical gene transfer trials for CF. Finally, the recent studies evaluating cell-based therapies for CF and other lung diseases are critically reviewed.

Pathophysiology of cystic fibrosis and target cells for gene transfer

CF is an autosomal recessive disease caused by mutations in the gene encoding for the cystic fibrosis transmembrane conductance regulator (CFTR). In 1989, the gene was localized to chromosome 7 and found to consist of approximately 250,000 base pairs that encode an mRNA of 6.5 kb [1–3]. Over 1000 mutations have been identified, resulting in aberrant transcription, translation, cellular trafficking, or ion channel function [4].

Isolation of the CF gene led to the development of gene transfer vectors (constructs, such as replication-deficient viruses, that could function to deliver a normal copy of the CF gene) to replace the defective gene [5]. Because the pulmonary disease in CF, which is characterized by abnormal mucus secretion, chronic bacterial infection, and airway inflammation, is the major cause of morbidity and mortality, the lung was the first target organ for gene replacement. To have successful CFTR gene transfer, the biology of CFTR and its function and the necessary target cell(s) for gene therapy need to be understood. At the cellular level, CFTR is an apical membrane protein found in several types of lung epithelial cells that serves as a regulated chloride channel [6]. Through interactions between CFTR and the

---

* Corresponding author.
  E-mail address: dweiss@uvm.edu (D.J. Weiss).

amiloride-sensitive epithelial sodium channel (ENaC), absence of functional CFTR in CF epithelial cells results in sodium hyperabsorption and lack of cyclic adenosine monophosphate–mediated chloride secretion [7]. CFTR is important for other cellular functions, including posttranslational processing of high-molecular-weight glycoconjugates and cell surface receptors, pH regulation of intracellular organelles and airway surface liquid, regulation of membrane trafficking, secretion of mucus, and regulation of glutathione transport [8]. There are increasing data demonstrating that constitutive and stimulated release of soluble inflammatory mediators is increased from CF airway epithelial cells. This may reflect, in part, increased basal and stimulated cell signaling resulting from increased nuclear factor–κB activity, AMP-dependent kinase activity, or altered antioxidant homeostasis in cells with defective CFTR [9]. Although the mechanisms for many of these effects remain incompletely understood, they provide evidence of the complexity and multiple cellular effects that need to be considered with CFTR gene replacement.

At the organ level, CFTR in lung is localized primarily at the ciliated cells of the proximal airways and the ciliated cells of the submucosal glands, which are located primarily in the proximal airways. Whether CFTR is substantially expressed in other epithelial cell types remains unclear. Earlier studies suggesting expression in nonciliated airway epithelial cells of the airways and glands, including basal epithelial cells, have been contradicted by more recent studies demonstrating that, although CFTR mRNA may be found in these cells, levels of CFTR protein expression are low and of uncertain significance [10,11]. Moreover, although CFTR can be detected in type 2 alveolar epithelial cells, CFTR expression is generally highest in proximal as compared with distal airways and alveoli [10]. This suggests that targeting the ciliated cells, primarily in the submucosal glands, will have most effect on regulation of mucus and airway surface liquid and presumably ameliorate the most relevant pathophysiologic respiratory effects of defective CFTR. However, there is turnover of the differentiated ciliated epithelial cells, and targeting the underlying basal progenitor epithelial cells may be a more viable approach to provide for longer-lasting or even indefinite expression. Progress has been made toward identifying endogenous progenitor cells resident in proximal and distal airways, but no viable strategy for specifically targeting these cells with gene transfer vectors has been identified.

Targeting defective CFTR alone may not fully correct airways disease. This is exemplified by the development of the ENaC over-expressing mouse [12]. Unlike the CFTR knockout or delta F transgenic mice, which do not develop substantial airways disease, increased airway sodium absorption in the airways of the ENaC mice resulted in airway surface liquid volume depletion, increased mucus concentration, delayed mucus transport, and mucus adhesion to airway surfaces [12]. The mice also developed severe spontaneous lung disease, comparable to that in patients who have CF, including mucus obstruction, goblet cell metaplasia, neutrophilic inflammation, and poor bacterial clearance. This provides evidence of the important role of ENaC in the development of many of the clinical manifestations of CF lung disease. Whether replacing defective CFTR results in appropriate regulation of ENaC remains unclear. Further, because none of the vectors used or currently being used in human trials efficiently achieves gene transfer to submucosal glands, if normal CFTR and thus normal ENaC function in submucosal glands are necessary for normal airway clearance, current approaches are not likely to affect disease pathogenesis in the proximal airways. However, efficient gene transfer to surface epithelium in more distal airways could ameliorate distal airway disease and thereby affect the clinical course of the disease without necessarily achieving a "cure."

In vitro and preclinical gene transfer studies

A number of in vitro studies using several types of gene transfer vectors have demonstrated that delivery of a normal CF gene to cultured CF airway epithelial cells restores cyclic adenosine monophosphate–mediated chloride transport [10,13–15]. In these in vitro studies, only a relatively small percentage of the total cultured epithelial monolayer was required to express normal CFTR to restore normal chloride conductance. For example, expression of CFTR in as few as 6% to 10% of cultured CF airway epithelial cells restored normal chloride transport properties [16]. These early results suggest that even a relatively inefficient gene transfer process might be successful. Subsequent studies demonstrated that close to 100% of CF epithelial cells must be transduced with a normal copy of the CF gene to reduce the sodium hyperabsorption characteristic of CF [17]. These data indicate that if sodium hyperabsorption across surface epithelia plays a major role in the pathogenesis of CF lung disease, efficient in vivo gene delivery is required to restore normal airway function.

Preclinical in vitro studies in small animal models have added additional proof of the concept for clinical CF gene therapy. In an early study, the use of nonviral vectors in CF transgenic mice corrected defective CFTR-dependent chloride transport in tracheas [18]. Due to redundant chloride channels, the CF mouse models generally do not develop robust airways disease, and finding suitable endpoints in which to assess the amount of airway epithelium that needs to be corrected has been difficult. The most commonly used are bacterial clearance and inflammatory abnormalities, both of which can be corrected in CF mouse models to varying degrees by gene complementation or transduction with different vectors [19,20]. The correlation between numbers and types of epithelial cells expressing normal CFTR and the measured endpoints remains unclear. This is further complicated by the growing appreciation that CFTR expression in inflammatory cells such as macrophages, neutrophils, and lymphocytes may have a profound effect on lung inflammation and infection in CF [9,21,22]. It remains unclear as to which cells and how many of these cells must express normal CFTR in vivo to result in therapeutic effect.

Vectors for use in cystic fibrosis gene therapy

One of the most important aspects for successful gene transfer is the technique used to introduce the gene or DNA sequence into a target cell. A number of general approaches have been used, including physical methods to transiently disrupt cell surfaces, thus allowing gene entry into the cytoplasm and nucleus (electroporation, calcium phosphate precipitation), DNA packaging into recombinant viruses, and transfection with naked DNA or RNA sequences or DNA complexed to synthetic lipids (liposomes and lipoplexes) or synthetic polymers (polyplexes). With respect to gene transfer for CF lung disease, recombinant viral vectors and cationic liposomes have been most heavily investigated, but newer data are emerging with synthetic polymers and with condensed naked DNA. A hypothetical ideal vector for airway-based gene delivery for CF requires the characteristics listed in Box 1. The ideal vector would efficiently deliver the gene to the appropriate target cells without causing toxicity or inflammation. Whether the target cells

are differentiated ciliated epithelial cells or underlying basal progenitor cells would also influence the choice of vector and delivery approach. In the discussion of each vector that follows, toxicity and physical and immunologic barriers to effective transduction are considered. Adenoviruses are considered in most detail because many of the lessons learned from their use are applicable to other vectors.

Viral vectors

Adenovirus

Adenoviruses are trophic for respiratory epithelium and are able to transduce virtually all types of epithelial cells from trachea to alveoli. Although there are few direct comparative studies, gene transfer using recombinant adenovirus vectors (AdV) results in the highest level of airway and alveolar epithelial gene expression of any recombinant replication-defective viral vector. A number physical barriers and immunologic responses can impede effectiveness and clinical utility of AdV-mediated gene transfer, particularly to airway epithelium in CF. The receptors for adenovirus, the coxsackie-adenovirus receptor and the $\alpha_v\beta_3$ or $\alpha_v\beta_5$ integrins, are predominantly located on basolateral cell membranes of airway epithelial cells [23]. Tight junction complexes between airway epithelial cells and apical surface glycocalyx proteins can limit access of AdV to these receptors [24,25]. Theoretically, in the setting of acute and chronic lung injury where airway and alveolar epithelial cells may be damaged or sloughed and tight junctions disrupted,

---

Box 1. Hypothetical model vectors for use in CF gene therapy

Exhibits selective tropism for respiratory epithelium

Can target appropriate ciliated cells (surface and glands)

Does not provoke inflammatory or immune responses

Can survive in inflamed and chronically infected airways

Results in sustained gene expression without insertional mutagenesis or can be repeatedly readministered

Can be suitably manufactured in purified clinical-grade form

adenovirus vectors may have increased access to basolateral receptors. Support for this comes from studies demonstrating that experimental disruption of tight junctions with a variety of agents can increase adenoviral-mediated epithelial gene expression [13]. Increased mucins, edema, or inflammatory debris in airway and alveolar spaces of diseased lungs may impede access of vectors to the epithelial cells. For example, sputum from patients who have CF impeded AdV-mediated gene transfer in cultured sheep trachea [26]. Pre-existing antiadenovirus antibodies in sputum and bronchoalveolar lavage fluid (BALF) from some patients who have CF may contribute to this inhibitory effect, and removal of immunoglobulins from BALF has been demonstrated to improve adenovirus-vector mediated transduction [27,28]. Nitric oxide, a reactive metabolite generated during acute lung inflammation, has also been demonstrated to reduce AdV-mediated gene transfer in mouse lungs [29]. AdV-mediated gene expression in airway epithelium was decreased in animals with bronchopulmonary inflammation induced by prior inoculation with a clinically relevant pathogen, mucoid *Pseudomonas aeruginosa* [30]. Moreover, alveolar macrophages can phagocytose and inactivate a substantial proportion of AdV delivered to the airways of normal animals [31]. Whether this clearance is increased in injured lungs of patients who have CF has not been determined. The use of AdV is also limited by the duration of gene expression, which generally peaks at 3 to 4 days and then tapers off over a period of several weeks, thus necessitating repeated administrations for CF treatment.

The most pressing argument against the use of recombinant adenovirus vectors for CF gene therapy is that they provoke acute inflammatory and subsequent immunologic responses after airway delivery to normal lungs and to the lungs of patients who have CF [32]. Host responses are provoked by proteins on the adenovirus surface and by expression of adenoviral genes. Immunologic responses may also be due to expression of the desired protein, CFTR, which can theoretically be perceived as foreign by a recipient in whom the protein is not normally expressed, although in a murine CFTR knockout model, expression of human CFTR does not seem to elicit an immune response [33]. Readministration of adenovirus vectors is hampered by the development of neutralizing antiadenovirus antibodies that can significantly reduce efficiency of subsequent gene transfer to epithelial cells [32].

Despite these problems, significant progress continues to be made with respect to use of AdV in lung. Administration of AdV does not provoke additional inflammation in the lungs of mice with experimentally induced acute lung injury resulting from the administration of endotoxin or bleomycin or in the setting of ovalbumin-induced allergic airways inflammation [34,35]. These studies suggest that AdV may be less inflammatory when used in the acutely injured lung. Moreover, the use of helper virus-dependent, high-capacity adenovirus vectors containing no endogenous adenovirus coding sequences has proven to be less inflammatory in lung [36]. The use of a helper-dependent adenovirus vector also was found to decrease inflammation after bacterial infection in CFTR knockout mice [37]. Recent studies with helper-dependent AdV have demonstrated that they can be readministered to mice with minimal loss of transgene expression correlating with lower levels of antiadenoviral antibodies [38]. Similarly, modification of the adenovirus capsid by replacement of capsid proteins with other ligands that can interact with epithelial cell surface receptors or by coating of the capsid with polyethylene glycol ("pegylation") may decrease host inflammatory and immune responses [39]. Nonetheless, despite continued experimental interest and improvement in adenoviral vectors, they have fallen out of favor for clinical use in CF but are being investigated for use in gene therapy approaches to lung cancer.

Adeno-associated virus

Recombinant adeno-associated virus (AAV) vectors are trophic for respiratory epithelium and do not induce acute inflammatory responses in normal lung. A further characteristic of AAV-mediated gene transfer that is attractive for CF gene therapy is transgene expression for periods of months. Accordingly, AAV vectors have undergone substantial investigation for use in CF and in other diseases, such as hemophilia and several retinopathies [40]. Despite the lack of inflammatory responses to recombinant AAV vectors, physical barriers may impede the delivery of recombinant AAV vectors after airway administration. Bronchial secretions obtained from patients who have CF contain proteolytic activity that degrades AAV2 [41]. The presence of apical membrane glycoconjugates may also inhibit viral entry, although some data suggest that AAV particles may transcytose through barrier epithelium [42,43]. In addition, there are a number of AAV serotypes, human and from other sources including nonhuman primates and other species, that have been investigated and that have differences in their ability to transduce respiratory epithelium [44]. The most heavily studied has been human serotype 2 (AAV2), which preferentially binds to receptors, including heparan sulfate proteoglycan and coreceptors fibroblast growth factor receptor 1 and $\alpha_v\beta_5$ integrin receptor in the basolateral membranes [45,46]. Other serotypes, notably AAV5 and AAV6, bind to receptors located on the apical epithelial surface, such as 2,3-linked sialic acid moieties found on several glycoproteins, including the platelet-derived growth factor receptor [47,48]. They are more effective in transducing airway epithelial cells after airway administration. Unlike adenovirus, there also seem to be inefficiencies related to the processing of adeno-associated virus in the endocytic pathway because inhibition of ubiquitination or proteosome function significantly increases gene transfer efficiency to mouse airway with AAV2 [49,50]. Similarly, the phosphorylation of intracellular proteins can effect AAV vector–mediated expression [51]. AAV vectors are also limited by the size of cDNA that can be carried, and the size of the CFTR cDNA sequence (4.8 kb) is larger than that accommodated by AAV vectors [40]. This limitation has been overcome by several approaches, including the removal of unnecessary intronic sequences or the use of homologous in vivo recombination mediated by separate AAV vectors carrying different portions of the CFTR sequence [52]. Additionally, truncated CFTR can complement ion transport defects [53], suggesting that AAV vectors containing a smaller CFTR cDNA may be physiologically effective.

A further significant limitation to the effective use of AAV vectors for CF is that, despite relatively substantial levels of gene expression in mouse lung epithelium, only low-level gene expression has been demonstrated in airway epithelium of nonhuman primates and in patients. This includes low levels detected in recent clinical trials of AAV vectors in patients who have CF [54–57]. In part, this might be related to the presence of pre-exisiting neutralizing AAV antibodies, particularly in patients who have CF [58]. Thus, although recombinant AAV vectors remain promising for CF gene therapy, several issues remain with respect to the use of these vectors.

Other viral vectors

Several aspects of retrovirus- and lentivirus-mediated gene transfer make them potentially attractive vectors for use in CF. Because they are vectors that integrate into the host genome, gene expression is more likely to be sustained rather than transient. A number of other factors have rendered these vectors less useful for airway epithelial gene delivery. Alveolar macrophages phagocytose and inactivate airway-delivered retroviral vectors [59]. Cell-surface receptors used for retroviral and lentiviral cell entry are expressed at low levels in pulmonary epithelium, and the majority of receptors reside on the basolateral membrane of epithelial cells, making these cells more resistant to transduction with airway (apical) delivery of vectors [60]. Cell replication is required for retroviral infection and integration, and only low levels of transduction were observed in normal nonproliferating airway epithelium [61]. Higher levels of transduction were observed in cultures of proliferating airway epithelial cells and in wounded regenerating regions of trachea, suggesting that actively proliferating or remodeling airway epithelium is a preferential target [62]. However, the administration of retrovirus vector to lungs of mice with sulfur dioxide–induced acute lung injury resulted in gene expression in only a small percentage of tracheal epithelial cells [63]. In contrast, lentiviruses do not require cell division for entry and gene expression and have been pseudotyped with surface proteins that permit binding and entry to airway epithelium [64]. Nonetheless, levels of expression after airway administration of lentivirus vectors are low in animal models, and there is little information about the gene transfer efficiency of lentiviruses in injured lung [64]. As currently constructed, recombinant RNA viruses do not seem to be effective options for CF gene therapy. Moreover, enthusiasm for the use of integrating recombinant RNA vectors is low given the development of T-cell leukemia in two children after retrovirus-vector mediated therapy for severe combined immune deficiency [65].

Vectors based on other replication-incompetent viruses that have greater tropism for airway epithelial cells than adenovirus or AAV, such as Sendai virus, respiratory syncytial virus (RSV), and influenza virus, have been developed and have been reported to mediate efficient gene transfer to human airway epithelial cells and to airway in animal models [66–68]. Little is known about the immune response to these recombinant viruses, but the severe illness associated with some cases of RSV and influenza infections suggests that host inflammatory responses may be more significant for these vectors compared with adenovirus, AAV, or lentiviral vectors. Further, respiratory viruses, such as RSV and parainfluenza, are increasingly recognized as having a significant pathogenic effect in development of CF lung disease. As such, it seems unlikely that these vectors will find significant use.

Nonviral vectors

In general, nonviral vectors, including naked DNA, antisense oligonucleotides, RNAi, and complexes of DNA with cationic liposomes (lipoplexes) or cationic polymers (polyplexes), result in less efficient airway epithelial gene expression after airway or systemic administration to normal or to injured lung compared with viral vectors [69,70]. Transgene expression is also generally transient, and, although not well studied for all types, nonviral vectors are more likely to be degraded or inactivated in an inflammatory environment or impeded by increased mucins or surfactants found in injured lung [71,72]. Sputum from patients who have CF has been demonstrated to inhibit cationic liposome vector–mediated transfection of cultured cells and cultured sheep trachea [26]. Moreover, some nonviral vectors, particularly cationic liposomes, can provoke significant inflammatory and systemic responses when administered to the lung by airway or intravenous routes [73,74]. This results in part from immune stimulation by unmethylated CpG bacterial sequences in the plasmid DNA [75]. Recent cationic liposomal vectors have attempted to minimize the CpG sequences, but transduction and epithelial gene expression remains low [76]. Further, there have been promising results with condensed naked DNA in animal and clinical trials and with the continuing development of polyplex vectors, particularly those containing polyethylenimine [77]. As continuing significant improvements in nonviral vector technology occur, particularly in delivery, transduction effectiveness, and persistence of expression, these vectors may be more useful for clinical CF gene therapy.

Delivery of gene transfer vectors to lung epithelium

Delivering exogenous DNA or genes directly to the airways offers a unique and appealing opportunity for specifically targeting gene expression to airway and alveolar epithelium. A large body of literature and experience supports the feasibility of this approach. However, animal studies and the recent human studies (see below) have demonstrated that airway-directed gene delivery is not as simple as was originally anticipated [13,78]. The lung has evolved physical and immunologic barriers that can hinder effective transduction of epithelial cells (Fig. 1). Moreover, most studies of gene delivery techniques have been conducted in normal lungs. There is less available information regarding effective delivery techniques

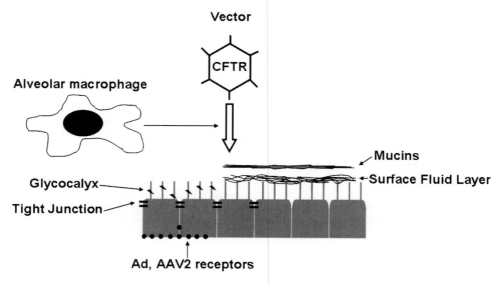

Fig. 1. Schematic of barriers to gene delivery in normal and injured lungs.

in acutely or chronically injured lungs, a more applicable setting for CF lung gene therapy. Much current work in gene therapy is directed toward overcoming the inflammatory and immune responses provoked by gene transfer vectors while maximizing vector delivery and subsequent gene expression. In this section, methods of administering gene transfer vectors to lung airways are reviewed. Physical and immunologic barriers are discussed, as are adjunct methods of delivery that can partly overcome some of these barriers.

General methods of airway gene delivery

Current techniques of delivering gene transfer vectors to airway epithelium include nasal deposition or instillation, direct instillation into the trachea or lower airways using a catheter or bronchoscope, and aerosolization and inhalation of vectors. Nasal deposition in obligate nasal breathers, such as rodents, can be effective in distributing vector throughout the lower airways. In humans, gene expression resulting from nasal deposition of vector is generally limited to nasal epithelia. Direct vector instillation into the trachea or lower airways in humans is achieved by bronchoscopic administration; this more often results in heterogenous deposition in limited portions of lung [78]. Multiple instillations are required to achieve more widespread vector distribution. Moreover, the resulting transgene expression is usually more evident in the epithelium of larger proximal airways. Catheter-directed instillation, particularly when using a bronchoscope, generally requires topical analgesia and sedation to be performed comfortably and safely. Techniques using spray devices inserted through the bronchoscope can improve vector distribution and deposition, particularly in distal airways [79].

Inhalation of aerosolized vector solutions can result in more diffuse transgene distribution throughout the lung and in increased distribution to distal airway and alveolar epithelium [80,81]. This approach is also easier to use clinically than direct intratracheal instillation. There are significant limitations to current aerosol techniques. Large amounts of vector are required because material is lost by deposition in the aerosolization equipment and on oro- or nasopharyngeal, laryngeal, or upper airway mucosa. Moreover, cationic liposomes may be disrupted during the aerosolization process [82]. Additionally, there is no standardized approach to nebulization of vector solutions and administration of the resulting

aerosol, and a number of different methods and nebulization devices have been described. A number of other factors, including droplet size and aerodynamic radius, density, hygroscopicity, and depth and rate of breathing influence where droplets are deposited. Administration of aerosolized vector solutions is inefficient, even with the most sophisticated devices and techniques. It is estimated that only 10% to 30% of aerosolized particles reach the lower airways [83]. This can be substantially rate limiting for clinical use of gene transfer vectors. Moreover, aerosols work best in normal lungs. Even lower amounts of vector delivery likely occur in injured and inflamed lungs.

Physical and immunologic barriers to airway-based vector delivery

Physical barriers that can impede vector access to lung epithelium include mucins and surfactants lining the airways and alveolar spaces. Mucociliary clearance and phagocytosis of vectors by airway and alveolar macrophages can decrease the amount of vector particles reaching the epithelium [13,78]. Further barriers for many vectors (viral and nonviral) include limited expression of receptors or relative binding sites on apical surfaces of lung epithelial cells and tight junction complexes that limit the access of apically applied vectors to these sites. The glycocalyx and other cell surface glycoconjugates may also decrease access to relevant receptors and binding sites [84].

Physical barriers may be increased in acute lung injury in which edema, increased mucin production, and inflammatory cellular debris can further impede the effective access of vectors to epithelial cells (Fig. 2). The inflammatory environment in an acutely injured lung may also hinder vector access and expression. Inflammatory cytokines, such as tumor necrosis factor-α and interferon-γ, nitric oxide–generated during acute lung injury, and other inflammatory substances present in diseased lungs, can decrease recombinant adenoviral-mediated expression [29]. Bronchial secretions and mucus from patients who have CF can interfere with adenovirus and cationic liposome-mediated transduction and contain proteolytic activity that can degrade AAV2 vectors [26–28]. Moreover, serum and BALF from normal patients and sputum from patients who have CF may contain antiadenovirus and anti-AAV antibodies that might also interfere with AdV-mediated transduction [27,58]. Physical and other barriers that can impede effective airway gene

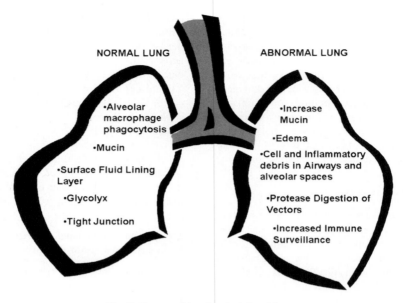

Fig. 2. Increased barriers in injured lung.

delivery have been mostly studied for AdV vectors. Many of the same barriers affecting AdV-mediated transduction of epithelial cells are applicable to other vectors, particularly nonviral vectors. For example, normal mucins can significantly impede cationic liposome-mediated transfection but have less effect on transduction mediated by AdV or synthetic polycationic vectors [26,85]. Similarly, surfactants can decrease cationic liposome-mediated transfection by disruption of the liposomes with subsequent decrease in gene transfer [71,72], whereas administration of AdV in surfactant can enhance gene expression [86].

There have been several attempts to develop methods to overcome some of these physical barriers. Modification of the transmembrane mucin MUC1, a major apical membrane glycoconjugate, by treatment with neuraminidase improved subsequent adenovirus-mediated gene transfer to cultured human airway epithelial cells [87]. Similarly, in cultured cells coated with sputum from patients who have CF, treatment with recombinant human DNAse but not mucolytic agents, including N-acetylcysteine, alginase, or lysine, improved AdV and cationic liposome-mediated gene transfer expression [72]. In a related study using sheep trachea in organ culture, removal of mucin resulted in a 25-fold increase in cationic liposome-mediated gene expression [26]. These studies illustrated the

role mucins may play in normal and injured lung but have not resulted in a clinically useful strategy for enhancing vector delivery.

The lung has a highly developed innate immune response to the introduction of foreign vector particles into the airways. For example, alveolar macrophages phagocytose and inactivate a large proportion of AdV and retrovirus vectors after intratracheal administration to normal lung [31,59]. Stimulation of inflammatory pathways and subsequent immune responses by the vector can limit the initial extent and duration of epithelial cell gene expression and can provoke undesirable clinical side effects. Pre-existing antibodies or the subsequent development of antibodies toward vectors, particularly virus vectors, can further limit readministration of these vectors [28,32,58]. Removal of immunoglobulins from CF BALF improved AAV5 vector–mediated epithelial transduction in a cell culture model [28]. Immune modulation has been used to enhance lung gene expression, predominantly inhibition of T-cell responses to administration of AdV [32,88,89]. Vector modifications, including use of helper-dependent adenovirus vectors, engineering vectors to target receptors located on apical epithelial surfaces (eg, the purinergic P2Y2 receptor), and coating vectors with polyethylene glycol to minimize inflammatory and immune responses are being actively investigated [39,90]. Whether these prove to be clinically safe and useful strategies, particularly in the setting of acute or chronic lung disease, has not been determined.

Adjunct methods for airway gene delivery

Several techniques have been demonstrated to augment expression after direct airway instillation of gene transfer vectors, particularly viral vectors, in cell culture and animal models [13,78]. Although the clinical applicability or feasibility of some of these approaches is unclear, methods using thixotropic solutions, surfactant, and perfluorochemical (PFC) liquid are based on clinical experience.

A number of agents have been demonstrated to alter cell surface barriers and enhance viral-mediated (and in some case nonviral-mediated) airway epithelial gene expression. Precipitating adenovirus, AAV2, or poly-L-lysine polyplex vectors with calcium phosphate results in a complex that exhibits increased nonspecific uptake on the apical surface of airway epithelial cells [91]. This approach abrogates the need to pass vectors through tight junctions to access basolateral receptors and enhances transgene expression in cultured lung epithelial cells and in mouse lung in vivo with no apparent toxicity. In contrast, EGTA, sodium caprate, and phospholipid detergents can disrupt tight junction protein complexes and increase vector access to basolateral receptors [92–94]. These potentially promising approaches have not been demonstrated to have efficacy in larger animal models or in injured lung, and it is not clear if they are clinically feasible.

Other more realistic clinical approaches include agents that can enhance vector dispersal or decrease clearance, including thixotropic solutions, surfactants, and PFC liquids. Thixotropic solutions, carboxymethyl cellulose, and other gels that become liquid with agitation have been used for intranasal delivery of nasal steroids. Delivery in a thixotropic solution increases the dwell time of the vector on the airway epithelium in part by impeding mucociliary clearance of vectors [95]. Delivering a CFTR-expressing adenovirus vector in a thixotropic solution enhanced the percentage of cells expressing an adenovirus transgene increase and the correction of chloride current defect in cultured human CF epithelial cells transduced compared with the same vector administered in phosphate-buffered saline [96]. Although the full range of thixotropic solution effect on enhanced gene expression is not understood and this

approach has not been tried in diseased lungs, the use of thixotropic solutions may become a valuable adjunct technique for lung gene delivery. Comparably, surfactant can be safely administered to the airways and has become a mainstay of treatment for respiratory failure in premature infants. Administering adenovirus vectors in surfactants increases total gene expression and enhances the distribution of expression [86]. Administering adenovirus vector in surfactant enhanced gene expression in rat lungs with experimentally induced pulmonary edema and lung injury [97]. This finding suggests that the use of surfactants during airway vector delivery may be effective in other forms of acute and chronic lung diseases, including CF. However, surfactants can impede gene expression mediated by naked DNA and by cationic liposomes and thus may not be applicable for all vectors. In parallel, PFC liquids have been safely used in clinical trials for acute lung injury in infants and adults. Although the use of PFC liquids is not a mainstay of treatment for acute lung injury, a considerable body of literature demonstrates that the use of PFC liquids enhances adenovirus- and AAV-mediated gene expression [13,78]. PFC liquids enhanced gene expression in models of acute and chronic lung injury [35,98]. The mechanisms of PFC effects include increased vector dispersal, inhibition of vector phagocytosis by macrophages, and transient opening of tight junctions [99]. Most recently, it has been demonstrated that the use of nebulized PFC enhances subsequent AdV-mediated gene expression in mice and in nonhuman primates [100]. This may be a more feasible clinical approach than intratracheal administration of PFC liquids.

Systemic administration of vectors for cystic fibrosis gene therapy

Intravenous administration has been used to deliver adenovirus and cationic liposome vectors to the lung. With this approach, the primary target is usually the pulmonary vascular endothelium rather than the airway and alveolar epithelium [101,102]. Nonetheless, although transgene activity has been described in airway and alveolar epithelial cells, expression is usually sparse and sporadic. Moreover, systemic administration of cationic liposomes and recombinant adenovirus vectors can provoke a significant inflammatory responses. Intravenous vector administration is more likely to be useful for diseases affecting the pulmonary vascular endothelium (eg, pulmonary hypertension) rather than for CF.

Human clinical trials

As of late 2006, a number of phase I and II gene transfer studies have been completed in patients who have CF. The vectors used have been recombinant adenovirus, recombinant AAV2, and cationic liposomes [54–57,74,103–106]. Most recently, condensed naked DNA has been evaluated [107]. Results from more recent studies are summarized in Table 1. Clinical effects, such as safety and lack of toxicity, are paramount, and most trials showed general safety of the vectors. Several of the trials conducted with recombinant adenovirus and with cationic liposome vectors included patients in whom local or systemic inflammatory responses developed. The other endpoints evaluated in the different trials were more variable. In many cases, small amounts of DNA transfer were observed in nasal, sinus, or bronchial brushings and biopsies. In fewer trials was mRNA detected, and only in several trials were relevant physiologic effects, such as correction of defective ion transport (predominantly in nasal mucosa after intranasal vector administration), observed.

These results are disappointing because despite a significant effort from many investigators, the trials have not revealed a successful strategy for CF gene therapy. Rather, they have highlighted the many problems that remain to be overcome. Particularly, with respect to vectors, despite more robust gene transfer than other vectors, recombinant adenoviruses have largely fallen out of favor because of significant problems with inflammatory and immune responses. Recombinant AAV and cationic liposome vectors are receiving continuing consideration, particularly because the biology of the different AAV serotypes is more completely appreciated, with continuing improvements to decrease inflammatory responses to cationic liposomal vectors. In recent randomized, double-blinded studies of repeated-dose, aerosolized AAV, there were no differences in adverse events, and there was confirmation of vector DNA transfer and a suggestion that the group receiving AAV had improvements in lung function and sputum inflammatory markers at 14 and 30 days but not at 60 or 90 days [56].

The trials to date have further evidenced one of the difficulties in gene therapy trials for CF lung disease—that of finding appropriate endpoints to measure in the absence of robust gene expression

[108]. Measurements of ion flux and potential differences are feasible in nasal epithelium but are technically challenging, and the procedure is well established only in a small number of centers. Because the nasal epithelium is a surrogate for gene transfer to the lower respiratory epithelium, a concerted effort is underway to develop better markers for lower airway gene expression. Measurements of ion flux and potential differences in the lower airways using bronchoscopic techniques have been reported for adults and children, but the technique is challenging and not well suited for trials with large numbers of patients. Other endpoints, such as improvement in lung function and decrease in inflammatory mediators, have been reported, most recently with the last AAV2 vector trials to be conducted [56,58]. Thus, in addition to efforts to improve gene transfer vectors, vector delivery, specific cell targeting, and persistence of gene expression and to decrease inflammatory and immune responses to vectors, a focused effort on improving the endpoints for measuring the success of physiologic gene transfer is being undertaken [108]. Few clinical trials for CF lung disease are in progress or planned for the near future.

Stem cells and cell-based therapies for cystic fibrosis lung disease

A developing potential therapeutic approach for CF and other lung diseases has been stimulated by recent reports demonstrating that several cell populations derived from adult bone marrow or from umbilical cord blood, including stromal-derived mesenchymal stem cells (MSCs), endothelial progenitor cells, and circulating fibrocytes, can localize to a variety of organs and acquire phenotypic and functional markers of mature organ-specific cells (Fig. 3) [109–112]. Whether the cells used in these studies were truly "stem" cells has not been rigorously demonstrated, and some of these studies are controversial [112–114]. Further, the fusion of marrow-derived cells with resident organ cells, rather than the phenotypic conversion of the marrow cells, has been demonstrated in several organs, notably in liver and skeletal muscle [115,116]. Nonetheless, even fusion of normal adult marrow–derived cells with diseased differentiated adult tissue might be a therapeutic approach. Additionally, embryonic stem cells can be induced in culture to develop markers of lung epithelium, and a human

Table 1
Representative recent clinical gene therapy trials for cystic fibrosis

Vector	Target site	Route	n	Summary	Reference
Compacted DNA nanoparticles	Nose/phase II multiple dose	Instillation	12	Safe; dose-dependent DNA in nasal scrapings at 2 wk; no mRNA expression; transient inflammation in some patients; partial to complete correction of ion transport in some patients	Konstan et al. (2004) [107]
AAV2	Lungs/phase II multiple dose	Aerosol	42	Safe; vector DNA in brushings; no mRNA expression; increase in FEV_1 at 14 and 30 d but not at 60, 90, or 150 d; decrease in sputum IL-8 at 14 d but not at 45 or 75 d; no change in sputum micro-organisms	Moss et al. (2004) [56]
AAV2	Nose/lungs/phase I multiple dose	Instillation or bronchoscope	25	Most patients had a local or systemic inflammatory response; variable DNA detected; mRNA and ion channel correction in a few patients	Flotte et al. (2003) [55]; Flotte et al. (2005) [57]
AAV2	Sinus/phase II single dose	Instillation	23	Safe; no change in sinusitis frequency or other end points	Wagner et al. (2002) [106]
Adenovirus	Nose/lungs/phase I single or multiple dose	Instillation or intrabronchial spray	34	Systemic response at high doses	Harvey et al. (2002) [105]
AAV2	Lung/phase I single dose	Aerosol	12	Safe; dose-dependent DNA in brushings; no detectable mRNA	Aitken et al. (2001) [54]
Adenovirus	Lung/phase I single dose	Aerosol	36	Systemic response to high doses; inefficient, transient gene expression	Joseph et al. (2001) [104]

(*continued on next page*)

Table 1 (*continued*)

Vector	Target site	Route	n	Summary	Reference
Cationic liposome	Lung/phase I single dose	Aerosol	8	Acute systemic responses; mRNA expression in 3 of 8	Ruiz et al. (2001) [74]
Cationic liposome	Nose/phase I-II single dose	Spray	11	Safe; no mRNA; no physiologic response	Noone et al. (2000) [146]
Cationic liposome	Nose/phase II multiple dose	Spray	10	Safe; evidence for mRNA and protein expression and physiologic effect	Hyde et al. (2000) [103]

embryonic stem cell line containing the ΔF508 CFTR mutation has been established [117–120]. Investigations using human embryonic stem cells are limited by scientific, ethical, and political considerations [121].

In lung, in vitro studies demonstrate that adult marrow–derived and cord blood–derived cells can be induced to express markers of airway or alveolar epithelial phenotype [112,114]. In some cases, the acquisition of functional phenotype in vitro has been demonstrated. For example, human marrow–derived MSCs cocultured with primary human airway epithelial cells express several airway epithelial markers, including cytokeratin, occludin, and CFTR [122]. MSCs obtained from the bone marrow of patients who have CF and transduced ex vivo to express wild-type CFTR partly correct defective CFTR-mediated chloride conductance when cocultured with primary airway epithelial cells obtained from patients who have CF [122]. Parallel in vivo studies in mouse models have suggested that bone marrow–derived cells can localize to lung and acquire phenotypic markers of airway and alveolar epithelium, vascular endothelium, and interstitial cells [112,114]. In humans, lung specimens from clinical

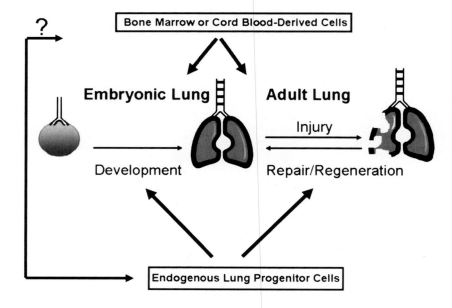

Fig. 3. Schematic of progenitor and stem cell participation in remodeling injured lung.

bone marrow transplant recipients demonstrate chimerism of epithelial and endothelial cells [123,124]. Similarly, lung specimens from lung transplant patients demonstrate chimerism of lung epithelium [125,126]. Many of these reports are based on sex-mismatched transplantation and in situ demonstration of Y chromosome–containing donor marrow–derived cells in recipient lungs by fluorescence in situ hybridization followed by immunohistochemical phenotyping of the donor-derived cells [127].

As analytical techniques have improved, despite earlier reports demonstrating substantial engraftment with donor-derived cells, more recent reports demonstrate that only small numbers of transplanted adult marrow–derived cells engraft in recipient lungs, particularly in airway or alveolar epithelium [112,128]. This includes only rare engraftment and CFTR expression in airway and intestinal epithelium after transplantation of adult marrow–derived cells containing wild-type CFTR to CFTR knockout mice [129,130]. Further, the mechanisms by which marrow-derived or cord blood–derived cells are recruited to lung and acquire airway or alveolar epithelial phenotype are poorly understood. Thus, although airway or alveolar epithelial engraftment by marrow-derived cells occurs, it is rare and has not been linked to potential therapeutic benefit.

Despite rare engraftment of airway or alveolar epithelium, there are an increasing number of studies demonstrating a functional role of adult marrow–derived cells in the mitigation of lung injury. This has been described in models of lung inflammation, emphysema, and fibrosis [131–133]. These effects have been observed with several cell populations, including MSCs. Systemic administration of MSCs immediately after intratracheal bleomycin administration decreased subsequent lung fibrosis and collagen accumulation [133]. Another population of marrow-derived cells, CD45+/CK+/CXCR4+ cells, contributed to airway epithelial re-epitheliazation in a tracheal allograft model [134]. Conversely, marrow-derived cells, including circulating fibrocytes, may contribute to the development of lung fibrosis [135–137]. The mechanisms for these effects are unknown but strongly suggest that marrow-derived cells can participate in lung injury and repair.

More recently, several reports have demonstrated that intratracheal, rather than systemic, administration of adult marrow–derived MSCs can mitigate lung injury. Intratracheal administration of MSCs 4 hours after intratracheal endotoxin administration decreased mortality, pulmonary edema, and BALF levels of the proinflammatory cytokines tumor necrosis factor–α and MIP-1β compared with endotoxin-only–treated mice [138]. There was little structural engraftment of airway or alveolar epithelium by the MSCs. Comparably systemic administration of MSCs to mice with bleomycin-injured lungs decreased levels of proinflammatory cytokines and levels of matrix metalloproteinase 2 and 9 in the lungs [133]. The mechanisms for these effects are unknown, but accumulating data suggest that MSCs may have significant immunomodulatory effects in the lung. Whether these cells can be used to modulate airways inflammation in CF or whether engraftment of marrow or cord blood–derived cells in airways epithelium can be used to correct defective CF airways epithelium are areas of active study but have not yielded viable therapeutic strategies.

Efforts to better identify and characterize resident progenitor cells and progenitor cell niches in the upper and lower airways and in alveoli may provide targets for sustained gene expression. Evidence in mice and humans suggests that there are regional niches of airway and submucosal gland progenitor cells with different phenotypic and functional characteristics [139–145]. Alveolar epithelium in patients who have CF contains primitive cuboidal cells that express primitive cell markers, including thyroid transcription factor and cytokeratin 7. This suggests that endogenous progenitor cell pathways in CF lungs may be altered, but this has not been extensively investigated. Progress toward identifying a specific pluripotential stem cell in the airway may allow for targeting with gene transfer vectors that provide sustained expression. Targeting of endogenous progenitor cells also requires methods to overcome the barriers to gene delivery.

Summary

Despite intense investigation and a number of clinical trials, a successful strategy for CF lung gene therapy remains elusive. Further developments in vector technology and in overcoming the barriers to cell targeting and sustained gene expression and improved understanding of inflammatory and immune responses are necessary. The use of embryonic or adult stem cells to remodel defective lung or to modulate inflammatory and immune reactions in lung is undergoing investigation and may provide future therapeutic approaches.

References

[1] Riordan JR, Rommens JM, Kerem BS, et al. Identification of the cystic fibrosis gene: cloning and characterization of complementary DNA. Science 1989;245:1066–73.

[2] Rommens JM, Iannuzzxi MC, Kerem BS, et al. Identification of the cystic fibrosis gene: chromosome walking and jumping. Science 1989;245:1059–65.

[3] Collins FS. Cystic fibrosis: molecular biology and therapeutic implications. Science 1992;256:774–9.

[4] Welsh MJ, Smith AE. Molecular mechanisms of CFTR chloride channel dysfunction in cystic fibrosis. Cell 1993;73:1251–4.

[5] Mulligan RC. The basic science of gene therapy. Science 1993;260:926–32.

[6] Rich DP, Anderson MP, Gregory RJ, et al. Expression of cystic fibrosis transmembrane conductance regulator corrects defective chloride channel regulation in cystic fibrosis airway epithelial cells. Nature 1990;347:358–63.

[7] Boucher RC. Airway epithelial fluid transport. Am Rev Respir Dis 1994;150:271–81, 581–93.

[8] Mehta A. CFTR: more than just a chloride channel. Pediatr Pulmonol 2005;39(4):292–8.

[9] Machen TE. Innate immune response in CF airway epithelia: hyperinflammatory? Am J Physiol Cell Physiology 2006;291(2):C218–30.

[10] Anson DS, Smith GJ, Parsons DW. Gene therapy for cystic fibrosis airway disease: is clinical success imminent? Curr Gene Ther 2006;6(2):161–79.

[11] Kreda SM, Mall M, Mengos A, et al. Characterization of wild-type and delta F508 cystic fibrosis transmembrane regulator in human respiratory epithelia. Mol Biol Cell 2005;16(5):2154–67.

[12] Mall M, Grubb BR, Harkema JR, et al. Increased airway epithelial Na+ absorption produces cystic fibrosis-like lung disease in mice. Nat Med 2004;10(5):487–93.

[13] Weiss DJ, Pilewski J. Current status of gene therapy for cystic fibrosis. Seminars in Pulmonary and Critical Care Medicine 2003;24:749–70.

[14] Griesenbach U, Geddes DM, Alton EW. Gene therapy progress and prospects: cystic fibrosis. Gene Ther 2006;13(14):1061–7.

[15] Rosenecker J, Huth S, Rudolph C. Gene therapy for cystic fibrosis lung disease: current status and future perspectives. Curr Opin Mol Ther 2006;8(5):439–45.

[16] Johnson LG, Olsen JC, Sarkadi B, et al. Efficiency of gene transfer for restoration of normal airway epithelial function in cystic fibrosis. Nat Genet 1992;2:21–5.

[17] Johnson LG, Boyles SE, Wilson J, et al. Normalization of raised sodium absorption and raised calcium-mediated chloride secretion by adenovirus-mediated expression of cystic fibrosis transmembrane conductance regulator in primary human cystic fibrosis airway epithelial cells. J Clin Invest 1995;95:1377–82.

[18] Hyde SC, Gill DR, Higgins CF, et al. Correction of the ion transport defect in cystic fibrosis transgenic mice by gene therapy. Nature 1993;362(6417):250–5.

[19] Ramalho AS, Beck S, Meyer M, et al. Five percent of normal cystic fibrosis transmembrane conductance regulator mRNA ameliorates the severity of pulmonary disease in cystic fibrosis. Am J Respir Cell Mol Biol 2002;27:619–27.

[20] Oceandy D, McMorran BJ, Smith SN, et al. Gene complementation of airway epithelium in the cystic fibrosis mouse is necessary and sufficient to correct the pathogen clearance and inflammatory abnormalities. Hum Mol Genet 2002;11:1059–67.

[21] Kostyk AG, Dahl KM, Wynes MW, et al. Regulation of macrophage chemokine expression by NaCl occurs independently of cystic fibrosis transmembrane conductance regulator. Am J Pathol 2006;169:12–20.

[22] Allard JB, Poynter ME, Marr KA, et al. Aspergillus fumigatus generates an enhanced Th2-biased immune response in mice with defective cystic fibrosis transmembrane conductance regulator. J Immunol 2006;177(8):5186–94.

[23] Walters RW, Grunst T, Bergelson JM, et al. Basolateral localization of fiber receptors limits adenovirus infection from the apical surface of airway epithelia. J Biol Chem 1999;274:10219–26.

[24] Wang G, Zabner J, Deering C, et al. Increasing epithelial junction permeability enhances gene transfer to mouse tracheal epithelium in vivo. Am J Respir Cell Mol Biol 2000;22:129–38.

[25] Pickles RJ, Fahrner JA, Petrella JM, et al. Retargeting the coxsackievirus and adenovirus receptor to the apical surface of polarized epithelial cells reveals the glycocalyx as a barrier to adenovirus-mediated gene transfer. J Virol 2000;74:6050–7.

[26] Kitson C, Angel B, Judd D, et al. The extra-and intercellular barriers to lipid and adenovirus-mediated pulmonary gene transfer to native sheep airway epithelium. Gene Therapy 1998;6:534–46.

[27] Perricone MA, Rees DD, Sacks CR, et al. Inhibitory effect of cystic fibrosis sputum on adenovirus-mediated gene transfer in cultured epithelial cells. Hum Gene Ther 2000;11:1997–2008.

[28] Rooney CP, Denning GM, Davis BP, et al. Bronchoalveolar fluid is not a major hindrance to virus-mediated gene therapy in cystic fibrosis. J Virol 2002;76(20):10437–43.

[29] Haddad IY, Sorscher EJ, Garver JI, et al. Modulation of adenovirus-mediated gene transfer by nitric oxide. Am J Respir Cell Mol Biol 1997;16:501–9.

[30] van Heeckeren A, Ferkol T, Tosi M. Effects of bronchopulmonary inflammation induced by Pseudomonas aeruginosa on adenovirus-mediated gene

transfer to airway epithelial cells in mice. Gene Therapy 1998;5:345–51.

[31] Worgall S, Leopold PL, Wolff G, et al. Role of alveolar macrophages in rapid elimination of adenovirus vectors administered to the epithelial surface of the respiratory tract. Hum Gene Ther 1997;8: 1675–84.

[32] Muruve DA. The innate immune response to adenovirus vectors. Hum Gene Ther 2004;15(12): 1157–66.

[33] Whitsett JA, Dey CR, Stripp BR, et al. Human cystic fibrosis transmembrane conductance regulator directed to respiratory epithelial cells of transgenic mice. Nat Genet 1992;2:13–20.

[34] Thorne PS, McCray PB, Howe TS, et al. Early-onset inflammatory responses in vivo to adenoviral vectors in the presence or absence of lipopolysaccharide-induced inflammation. Am J Respir Cell Mol Biol 1999;20:1155–64.

[35] Weiss DJ, Bonneau L, Liggitt D. Use of perflourochemical liquid allows earlier detection and use of less adenovirus vector for gene expression in normal lung and enhances gene expression in acutely injured lung. Mol Ther 2001;3(5 pt 1):734–45.

[36] Morsy MA, Gu MC, Motzel S, et al. An adenoviral vector deleted for all viral coding sequences results in enhanced safety and extended expression of a leptin transgene. Applied Biological Sciences 1998;95: 7866–71.

[37] Koehler DR, Sajjan U, Chow YH, et al. Protection of Cftr knockout mice from acute lung infection by a helper-dependent adenoviral vector expressing Cftr in airway epithelia. Proc Natl Acad Sci U S A 2003;100(26):15364–9.

[38] Koehler DR, Martin B, Corey M, et al. Readministration of helper-dependent adenovirus to mouse lung. Gene Therapy 2006;13(9):773–80.

[39] Croyle MA, Chirmule N, Zhang Y, et al. "Stealth" adenoviruses blunt cell-mediated and humoral immune responses against the virus and allow for significant gene expression upon readministration in the lung. J Virol 2001;75:4792–801.

[40] Flotte TR. Adeno-associated virus-based gene therapy for inherited disorders. Pediatr Res 2005;58(6): 1143–7.

[41] Virella-Lowell I, Poirier A, Chesnut KA, et al. Inhibition of recombinant adeno-associated virus (rAAV) transduction by bronchial secretions from cystic fibrosis patients. Gene Ther 2000;7: 1783–9.

[42] Duan D, Yue Y, Yan Z, et al. Polarity influences the efficiency of recombinant adenoassociated virus infection in differentiated airway epithelia. Hum Gene Ther 1998;9:2761–76.

[43] Bals R, Xiao W, Sang N, et al. Transduction of well-differentiated airway epithelium by recombinant adeno-associated virus is limited by vector entry. J Virol 1999;73:6085–8.

[44] Chao H, Liu Y, Rabinowitz J, et al. Several log increase in therapeutic transgene delivery by distinct adeno-associated viral serotype vectors. Mol Ther 2000;2:619–23.

[45] Summerford C, Samulski RJ. Membrane-associated heparan sulfate proteoglycan is a receptor for adeno-associated virus type 2 virions. J.Virol 1998;72:1438–45.

[46] Summerford C, Bartlett JS, Samulski RJ. Alpha-Vbeta5 integrin: a co-receptor for adeno-associated virus type 2 infection. Nat Med 1999;5:78–82.

[47] Walters R, Yi SM, Keshavjee S, et al. Binding of adeno-associated virus type 5 to 2,3-linked sialic acid is required for gene transfer. J Biol Chem 2001;276(23):20610–6.

[48] Halbert CL, Allen JM, Miller AD. Adeno-associated virus type 6 (AAV6) vectors mediate efficient transduction of airway epithelial cells in mouse lungs compared to that of AAV2 vectors. J Virol 2001;75:6615–24.

[49] Duan D, Yue Y, Yan Z, et al. Endosomal processing limits gene transfer to polarized airway epithelia by adeno-associated virus. J Clin Invest 2000;105: 1573–87.

[50] Yan Z, Zak R, Luxton GW, et al. Ubiquitination of both adeno-associated virus type 2 and 5 capsid proteins affects the transduction efficiency of recombinant vectors. J Virol 2002;76:2043–53.

[51] Sanlioglu S, Engelhardt JF. Cellular redox state alters recombinant adeno-associated virus transduction through tyrosine phosphatase pathways. Gene Ther 1991;6:1427–37.

[52] Halbert CL, Allen JM, Miller AD. Efficient mouse airway transduction following recombination between AAV vectors carrying parts of a larger gene. Nat Biotechnol 2002;20:697–701.

[53] Ostedgaard LS, Zabner J, Vermeer DW, et al. CFTR with a partially deleted R domain corrects the cystic fibrosis chloride transport defect in human airway epithelia in vitro and in mouse nasal mucosa in vivo. Proc Natl Acad Sci U S A 2002; 99:3093–8.

[54] Aitken ML, Moss RB, Waltz DA, et al. A phase 1 study of aerosolized administration of tgAAVCF to cystic fibrosis patients with mild lung disease. Hum Gene Ther 2001;12:1907–16.

[55] Flotte TR, Zeitlin PL, Reynolds TC, et al. Phase I trial of intranasal and endobronchial administration of a recombinant adeno-associated virus serotype 2 (rAAV2)-CFTR vector in adult cystic fibrosis patients: a two-part clinical study. Hum Gene Ther 2003;14(11):1079–88.

[56] Moss RB, Rodman D, Spencer LT, et al. Repeated adeno-associated virus serotype 2 aerosol-mediated cystic fibrosis transmembrane regulator gene transfer to the lungs of patients with cystic fibrosis: a multicenter, double-blind, placebo-controlled trial. Chest 2004;125(2):509–21.

[57] Flotte TR, Schwiebert EM, Zeitlin PL, et al. Correlation between DNA transfer and cystic fibrosis airway epithelial cell correction after recombinant adeno-associated virus serotype 2 gene therapy. Hum Gene Ther 2005;16(8):921–8.

[58] Halbert CL, Miller AD, McNamara S, et al. Prevalence of neutralizing antibodies against adeno-associated virus (AAV) types 2, 5, and 6 in cystic fibrosis and normal populations: Implications for gene therapy using AAV vectors. Hum Gene Ther 2006;17(4):440–7.

[59] McCray PB, Wang G, Kline JN, et al. Alveolar macrophages inhibit retrovirus-mediated gene transfer to airway epithelia. Hum Gene Ther 1997;8:1087–93.

[60] Wang G, Davidson BL, Melchert P, et al. Influence of cell polarity on retrovirus-mediated gene transfer to differentiated human airway epithelial epithelia. J Virol 1998;72:9818–26.

[61] Engelhardt JF, Yankaskas JR, Wilson JM. In vivo retroviral gene transfer into human bronchial epithelia of xenografts. J Clin Invest 1992;90: 2598–607.

[62] Halbert CL, Aitken ML, Miller AD. Retroviral vectors efficiently transduce basal and secretory airway epithelial cells in vitro resulting in persistent gene expression in organotypic culture. Hum Gene Ther 1996;7:1871–81.

[63] Johnson LG, Mewshaw JP, Ni H, et al. Effect of host modification and age on airway epithelial gene transfer mediated by a murine leukemia virus-derived vector. J Virol 1998;72:8861–72.

[64] Copreni E, Penzo M, Carrabino S, et al. Lentivirus-mediated gene transfer to the respiratory epithelium: a promising approach to gene therapy of cystic fibrosis. Gene Ther 2004;11(Suppl 1):S67–75.

[65] Hacein-Bey-Abina S, von Kalle C, Schmidt M, et al. A serious adverse event after successful gene therapy for X-linked severe combined immunodeficiency. N Engl J Med 2003;348:255–6.

[66] Slepushkin VA, Staber PD, Wang G, et al. Infection of human airway epithelia with H1N1, H2N2, and H3N2 influenza a virus strains. Mol Ther 2001;3:395–402.

[67] Zhang L, Peeples ME, Boucher RC, et al. Respiratory syncytial virus infection of human airway epithelial cells is polarized, specific to ciliated cells, and without obvious cytopathology. J Virol 2003;76: 5654–66.

[68] Ferrari S, Griesenbach U, Shiraki-Iida T, et al. A defective nontransmissible recombinant Sendai virus mediates efficient gene transfer to airway epithelium in vivo. Gene Ther 2004;11(22): 1659–64.

[69] Alton EW. United Kingdom Cystic Fibrosis Gene Therapy Consortium. Use of nonviral vectors for cystic fibrosis gene therapy. Proc Am Thorac Soc 2004;1(4):296–301.

[70] Simoes S, Filipe A, Faneca H, et al. Cationic liposomes for gene delivery. Expert Opin Drug Deliv 2005;2(2):237–54.

[71] Tsan MF, Tsan GL, White JE. Surfactant inhibits cationic liposome-mediated gene transfer. Hum Gene Ther 1997;8:817–25.

[72] Stern M, Caplen NJ, Browning JE, et al. The effect of mucolytic agents on gene transfer across a CF sputum barrier in vitro. Gene Therapy 1998;5:91–8.

[73] Scheule RK, St. George JA, Bagley RG, et al. Basis of pulmonary toxicity associated with cationic lipid-mediated gene transfer to the mammalian lung. Hum Gene Ther 1997;8:689–707.

[74] Ruiz FE, Clancy JP, Perricone MA, et al. A clinical inflammatory syndrome attributable to aerosolized lipid-DNA administration in cystic fibrosis. Hum GeneTher 2001;12:751–61.

[75] Yew NS, Wang KX, Przybylska M, et al. Contribution of plasmid DNA to inflammation in the lung after administration of cationic lipid:pDNA complexes. Hum Gene Ther 1999;10:223–34.

[76] Yew NS, Zhao H, Wu IH, et al. Reduced inflammatory response to plasmid DNA vectors by elimination and inhibition of immunostimulatory CpG motifs. Mol Ther 2000;1:255–62.

[77] Densmore CL. Polyethyleneimine-based gene therapy by inhalation. Expert Opin Biol Ther 2003;3(7): 1083–92.

[78] Weiss DJ. Delivery of gene transfer vectors to lung: obstacles and the role of adjunct techniques for airway administration. Mol Ther 2002;6:148–52.

[79] Cipolla DC, Gonda I, Shak S, et al. Coarse spray delivery to a localized region of the pulmonary airways for gene therapy. Hum Gene Ther 2000;11: 361–71.

[80] Sene C, Bout A, Imler JL, et al. Aerosol-mediated delivery of recombinant adenovirus to the airways of nonhuman primates. Hum Gene Ther 1995;6: 1587–93.

[81] Beck SE, Laube BL, Barberena CI, et al. Deposition and expression of aerosolized rAAV vectors in the lungs of Rhesus macaques. Mol Ther 2002; 6:546–54.

[82] Stern M, Sorgi F, Hughes C, et al. The effects of jet nebulisation on cationic liposome-mediated gene transfer in vitro. Gene Ther 1998;5:583–93.

[83] Muir DFC. Particle deposition. The lung: scientific foundations, 1839–1843. New York: Raven Press Ltd; 1991.

[84] Stonebraker JR, Wagner D, Lefensty RW, et al. Glycocalyx restricts adenoviral vector access to apical receptors expressed on respiratory epithelium in vitro and in vivo: role for tethered mucins as barriers to lumenal infection. J Virol 2004;78(24):13755–68.

[85] Ernst U, Ulrichskotter S, Schmalix WA, et al. Interaction of liposomal and polycationic transfection complexes with pulmonary surfactant. J Gene Med 1999;1:331–40.

[86] Jobe AH, Ueda T, Whitsett JA, et al. Surfactant enhances adenovirus-mediated gene expression in rabbit lungs. Gene Ther 1996;3:775–9.

[87] Arcasoy SM, Latoche J, Gondor M, et al. MUC1 and other sialoglycoconjugates inhibit adenovirus-mediated gene transfer. Am J Respir Cell Mol Biol 1997;17:422–35.

[88] Shean MK, Baskin G, Sullivan D, et al. Immunomodulation and adenoviral-mediated gene transfer to the lungs of non-human primates. Hum Gene Ther 2000;11:1047–55.

[89] Halbert CL, Standaert TA, Wilson CB, et al. Successful readministration of adeno-associated virus vectors to the mouse lung requires transient immunosuppression during the initial exposure. J Virol 1998;72:9795–805.

[90] Look DC, Brody SL. Engineering viral vectors to subvert the airway defense response. Am J Respir Cell Mol Biol 1999;20:1103–6.

[91] Fasbender A, Lee JH, Walters RW, et al. Incorporation of adenovirus in calcium phosphate precipitates enhances gene transfer to airway epithelia in vitro and in vivo. J Clin Invest 1998;102:184–93.

[92] Chu Q, St. George JA, Lukason M, et al. EGTA enhancement of adenovirus-mediated gene transfer to mouse tracheal epithelium in vivo. Hum Gene Ther 2001;12:455–67.

[93] Parsons DW, Grubb BR, Johnson LG, et al. Enhanced in vivo airway gene transfer via transient modification of host barrier properties with a surface-active agent. Hum Gene Ther 1998;9:2661–72.

[94] Coyne CB, Kelly MM, Boucher RC, et al. Enhanced epithelial gene transfer by modulation of tight junctions with sodium caprate. Am J Respir Cell Mol Biol 2000;23:602–9.

[95] Jiang C, Akita GY, Colledge WH, et al. Increased contact time improves adenovirus-mediated CFTR gene transfer to nasal epithelium of CF mice. Hum Gene Ther 1997;8:671–80.

[96] Seiler MP, Luner P, Moninger TO, et al. Thixotropic solutions enhance viral-mediated gene transfer to airway epithelia. Am J Respir Cell Mol Biol 2002;27:133–40.

[97] Factor P, Mendez M, Mutlu GM, et al. Acute hyperoxic lung injury does not impede adenoviral-mediated alveolar gene transfer. Am J Respir Crit Care Med 2002;165:521–6.

[98] Weiss DJ, Strandjord TP, Liggitt D, et al. Perflubron enhances adenoviral-mediated gene expression in lungs of transgenic mice with chronic alveolar filling. Hum Gene Ther 1999;10:2287–93.

[99] Weiss DJ, Beckett T, Bonneau L, et al. Transient increase in lung epithelial tight junction permeability: an additional mechanism for enhancement of lung transgene expression by perfluorochemical liquids. Mol Ther 2003;8:927–35.

[100] Weiss DJ, Bonneau L, Liggitt D. Inhalation of nebulized perflubron enhances adenovirus mediated gene expression in lung epithelium. Mol Ther 2003;5:S68.

[101] McLean JW, Fox EA, Baluk P, et al. Organ-specific endothelial cell uptake of cationic liposome-DNA complexes in mice. Am J Physiol Heart Circ. Physiol 1997;273:H387–404.

[102] Huard J, Lochmuller H, Acsadi G, et al. The route of administration is a major determinant of the transduction efficiency of rat tissues by adenoviral recombinants. Gene Ther 1995;2:107–15.

[103] Hyde SC, Southern KW, Gileadi U, et al. Repeat administration of DNA/liposomes to the nasal epithelium of patients with cystic fibrosis. Gene Ther 2000;7:1156–65.

[104] Joseph PM, O'Sullivan BP, Lapey A, et al. Aerosol and lobar administration of a recombinant adenovirus to individuals with cystic fibrosis: I. Methods, safety, and clinical implications. Hum Gene Ther 2001;12:1369–82.

[105] Harvey BG, Maroni J, O'Donoghue KA, et al. Safety of local delivery of low- and intermediate-dose adenovirus gene transfer vectors to individuals with a spectrum of morbid conditions. Hum Gene Ther 2002;13:15–63.

[106] Wagner JA, Nepomuceno IB, Messner AH, et al. A phase II, double-blind, randomized, placebo-controlled clinical trial of tgAAVCF used maxillary sinus delivery in patients with cystic fibrosis with antrostomies. Hum Gene Ther 2002;13:1349–59.

[107] Konstan MW, Davis PB, Wagener JS, et al. Compacted DNA nanoparticles administered to the nasal mucosa of cystic fibrosis subjects are safe and demonstrate partial to complete cystic fibrosis transmembrane regulator reconstitution. Hum Gene Ther 2004;(12):1255–69.

[108] Griesenbach U, Boyd AC. UK Cystic Fibrosis Gene Therapy Consortium. Pre-clinical and clinical endpoint assays for cystic fibrosis gene therapy. J Cyst Fibros 2005;4(2):89–100.

[109] Korbling M, Estrov Z. Adult stem cells for tissue repair: a new therapeutic concept? N Engl J Med 2003;349(6):570–82.

[110] Prockop DJ. Further proof of the plasticity of adult stem cells and their role in tissue repair. J Cell Biol 2003;160(6):807–9.

[111] Herzog EL, Chai L, Krause DS. Plasticity of marrow-derived stem cells. Blood 2003;102(10):3483–93.

[112] Weiss DJ, Berberich MA, Borok Z, et al. National Heart Lung Blood Institute/Cystic Fibrosis Foundation Workshop Report adult stem cells, lung biology, and lung disease. Proc Am Thorac Soc 2006;3:193–207.

[113] Wagers AJ, Christensen JL, Weissman IL. Cell fate determination from stem cells. Gene Ther 2002;9(10):606–12.

[114] Neuringer IP, Randell SH. Lung stem cell update: promise and controversy. Monaldi Arch Chest Dis 2006;65(1):47–51.

[115] Wang X, Willenbring H, Akkari Y, et al. Cell fusion is the principal source of bone-marrow-derived hepatocytes. Nature 2003;422:897–901.

[116] Camargo FD, Green R, Capetanaki Y, et al. Single hematopoietic stem cells generate skeletal muscle through myeloid intermediates. Nat Med 2003;9: 1520–7.

[117] Pickering SJ, Minger SL, Patel M, et al. Generation of a human embryonic stem cell line encoding the cystic fibrosis mutation deltaF508, using preimplantation genetic diagnosis. Reprod Biomed Online 2005;10(3):390–7.

[118] Denham M, Cole TJ, Mollard R. Embryonic stem cells form glandular structures and express surfactant protein C following culture with dissociated fetal respiratory tissue. Am J Physiol Lung Cell Mol Physiol 2006;290(6):L1210–5.

[119] Mateizel I, De Temmerman N, Ullmann U, et al. Derivation of human embryonic stem cell lines from embryos obtained after IVF and after PGD for monogenic disorders. Hum Reprod 2006; 21(2):503–11.

[120] Coraux C, Nawrocki-Raby B, Hinnrasky J, et al. Embryonic stem cells generate airway epithelial tissue. Am J Respir Cell Mol Biol 2005;32(2):87–92.

[121] Brown JK, Hogan BLM, Randell SH, Stripp B, Weiss DJ. Human Embryonic Stem Cell Research: an official ATS Research Policy Statement. Am J Respir Crit Care Med 2006;173:1–3.

[122] Wang G, Bunnell BA, Painter RG, et al. Adult stem cells from bone marrow stroma differentiate into airway epithelial cells: potential therapy for cystic fibrosis. Proc Natl Acad Sci U S A 2005;102(1):186–91.

[123] Suratt BT, Cool CD, Serls AE, et al. Human pulmonary chimerism after hematopoietic stem cell transplantation. Am J Respir Crit Care Med 2003; 168(3):318–22.

[124] Mattsson J, Jansson M, Wernerson A, et al. Lung epithelial cells and type II pneumocytes of donor origin after allogeneic hematopoietic stem cell transplantation. Transplantation 2004;78(1):154–7.

[125] Kleeberger W, Versmold A, Rothamel T, et al. Increased chimerism of bronchial and alveolar epithelium in human lung allografts undergoing chronic injury. Am J Pathol 2004;162(5):1487–94.

[126] Spencer H, Rampling D, Aurora P, et al. Transbronchial biopsies provide longitudinal evidence for epithelial chimerism in children following sex mismatched lung transplantation. Thorax 2005; 60(1):60–2.

[127] Trotman W, Beckett T, Goncz KK, et al. Dual Y chromosome painting and in situ cell-specific immunofluorescence staining in lung tissue: an improved method of identifying donor marrow cells in lung following bone marrow transplantation. Histochem Cell Biol 2004;121(1):73–9.

[128] Chang JC, Summer R, Sun X, et al. Evidence that bone marrow cells do not contribute to the alveolar epithelium. Am J Respir Cell Mol Biol 2005;33(4): 335–42.

[129] Loi R, Beckett T, Goncz KK, et al. Limited restoration of defective cystic fibrosis lung epithelium in vivo with adult marrow derived cells. Am J Resp Crit Care Med 2006;173:171–9.

[130] Bruscia EM, Price JE, Cheng EC, et al. Assessment of cystic fibrosis transmembrane conductance regulator (CFTR) activity in CFTR-null mice after bone marrow transplantation. Proc Natl Acad Sci U S A 2006;103(8):2965–70.

[131] Ishizawa K, Kubo H, Yamada M, et al. Bone marrow-derived cells contribute to lung regeneration after elastase-induced pulmonary emphysema. FEBS Lett 2004;556(1–3):249–52.

[132] Yamada M, Kubo H, Kobayashi S, et al. Bone marrow-derived progenitor cells are important for lung repair after lipopolysaccharide-induced lung injury. J Immunol 2004;172(2):1266–72.

[133] Ortiz LA, Gambelli F, McBride C, et al. Mesenchymal stem cell engraftment in lung is enhanced in response to bleomycin exposure and ameliorates its fibrotic effects. Proc Natl Acad Sci USA 2003; 100(14):8407–11.

[134] Gomperts BN, Belperio JA, Burdick MD, et al. Circulating progenitor cells traffic via CXCR4/ CXCL12 in response airway epithelial injury. J Immunol 2006;176:1916–27.

[135] Epperly MW, Guo H, Gretton JE, et al. Bone marrow origin of myofibroblasts in irradiation pulmonary fibrosis. Am J Respir Cell Mol Biol 2003; 29(2):213–24.

[136] Hashimoto N, Jin H, Liu T, et al. Bone marrow-derived progenitor cells in pulmonary fibrosis. J Clin Invest 2004;113(2):243–52.

[137] Schmidt M, Sun G, Stacey MA, et al. Identification of circulating fibrocytes as precursors of bronchial myofibroblasts in asthma. J Immunol 2003; 171(1):380–9.

[138] Gupta N, Su X, Serikov V, et al. Intrapulmonary administration of mesenchymal stem cells reduces LPS induced acute lung injury and mortality. Proc Am Thoracic Soc 2006;3:A25.

[139] Reynolds SD, Giangreco A, Power JH, et al. Neuroepithelial bodies of pulmonary airways serve as a reservoir of progenitor cells capable of epithelial regeneration. Am J Pathol 2000;156:269–78.

[140] Hong KU, Reynolds SD, Giangreco A, et al. Clara cell secretory protein-expressing cells of the airway neuroepithelial body microenvironment include a label-retaining subset and are critical for epithelial renewal after progenitor cell depletion. Am J Respir Cell Mol Biol 2001;24:671–81.

[141] Giangreco A, Reynolds SD, Stripp BR. Terminal bronchioles harbor a unique airway stem cell population that localizes to the bronchoalveolar duct junction. Am J Pathol 2002;161:173–82.

[142] Schoch KG, Lori A, Burns KA, et al. A subset of mouse tracheal epithelial basal cells generates large colonies in vitro. Am J Physiol Lung Cell Mol Physiol 2004;286(4):L631–42.

[143] Engelhardt JF, Schlossberg H, Yankaskas JR, et al. Progenitor cells of the adult human airway involved in submucosal gland development. Development 1995;121:2031–46.

[144] Zepeda ML, Chinoy MR, Wilson JM. Characterization of stem cells in human airway capable of reconstituting a fully differentiated bronchial epithelium. Somat Cell Mol Genet 1995;21:61–73.

[145] Hollande E, Cantet S, Ratovo G, et al. Growth of putative progenitors of type II pneumocytes in culture of human cystic fibrosis alveoli. Biol Cell 2004; 96(6):429–41.

[146] Noone PG, Hohneker KW, Zhou Z, et al. Safety and biological efficacy of a lipid-CFTR complex for gene transfer in nasal epithelium of adults patients with cystic fibrosis. Mol Ther 2000;1(1):105–14.

ELSEVIER
SAUNDERS

Clin Chest Med 28 (2007) 381–404

CLINICS
IN CHEST
MEDICINE

Infection Control Practice in Cystic Fibrosis Centers

Jonathan B. Zuckerman, MD[a,b,*], David B. Seder, MD[a,b]

[a]Department of Medicine, The University of Vermont College of Medicine, E-126 Given Building,
89 Beaumont Avenue, Burlington, VT 05405-0068, USA
[b]Division of Pulmonary and Critical Care, Maine Medical Center, 22 Bramhall Street, Portland, ME 04102, USA

A biological paradox prevails in most patients who have cystic fibrosis (CF). At the systemic level, host immunity seems to be robust, and no overt abnormality in cell-mediated or humoral immunity is implicated in the disease. However, increasing evidence points to local host defense abnormalities in patients who have CF that predispose the lungs to chronic infection by a specific spectrum of pathogenic organisms. The downstream mechanistic connections between the primary airway epithelial ion transport defects that define CF and the proclivity for lung infection have yet to be fully elucidated.

Despite these gaps in knowledge (which have been rapidly closing in recent years), much has been accomplished in the clinical arena. Over the past several decades, the median life expectancy of patients who have CF has improved from 25 years in 1985 to nearly 38 years in 2005 [1]. This improvement in longevity has been attributed to enhancements in nutritional treatment, coordination of care at accredited CF centers, and judicious use of antimicrobial therapy. Advancements in patient outcomes have come at some cost, however. Traditional principles of infectious disease mandate that the source of infection be identified, that the organism be recovered, that antimicrobial sensitivities of the organism delineated, and that an adequate duration of therapy be established to eradicate the infection. In CF, most studies support a less orthodox approach. By virtue of the fact that patients who have CF develop

chronic lower respiratory tract infection in which secretions typically contain on the order of 10^8 colony forming units per milliliter of pathogenic bacteria [2], permanent endpoints to antimicrobial therapy are not feasible. As a consequence, maturing patients who have CF, often having received multiple courses of "chronic suppressive" therapy, accumulate drug resistant bacteria over time.

Accruing medical evidence points to patient-to-patient (PTP) transmission as another mechanism by which patients develop deep-rooted infection. Acquisition of certain respiratory pathogens is often associated with more rapid decline in pulmonary function and with early mortality. In some circumstances, changes in respiratory tract flora may limit options for lung transplantation. Because of the broad personal implications of infection, the issues of chronic suppressive antimicrobial therapy and infection control are emotionally charged for patients and their families, provoking fears, protests, and a strong desire to participate in healthcare decisions.

In this article, we outline some of the major historical events that signaled the need to better understand mechanisms of infection in CF. We discuss general principles of infection control, focusing on issues of particular importance to patients who have CF. We describe the major pathogens associated with the CF airway, provide a review of findings from inpatient and outpatient studies of infection control, and provide an outline of future directions for investigation.

Major historical events in cystic fibrosis infection control

Since its early characterization and subsequent description, the *Burkholderia cepacia* complex

This work was supported by grant no. ZUCKER03A0 from the Cystic Fibrosis Foundation.

* Corresponding author. Division of Pulmonary and Critical Care, Maine Medical Center, 22 Bramhall Street, Portland, ME 04102.

E-mail address: zuckej@mmc.org (J.B. Zuckerman).

chestmed.theclinics.com

(BCC) has had a unique place in the psychology of the CF community. Widely present in many surroundings, it can be contracted de novo from an environmental source or through direct or indirect patient contact. The importance of these pathogens relates to the effect on life expectancy of patients who have CF, the frequency of severe infection, and the innate antimicrobial resistance of the organisms. PTP transmission has been clearly documented, but catastrophic outbreaks are rare. International spread of BCC has taken place over several decades, with recognition depending on careful analysis of stored sputum samples, centralized testing facilities and repositories, and the development of new genetic methodologies for species and strain identification. Here we present a review of some of the most dramatic examples of BCC spread, the recognition of which has prompted the introduction of effective and sometimes unpopular infection control practices at CF centers worldwide.

The "cepacia syndrome," a fatal condition characterized by rapidly progressive pulmonary decline and antibiotic-resistant systemic infection, was first described in 1984 [3]. In most patients, infection with BCC is not so evident. Given the slow progression of disease and the lack of sophisticated genetic testing then available, interpersonal transmission was difficult to demonstrate [4]. In 1986, investigators showed a decrease in the incidence of BCC after implementation of strict infection-control techniques [5], but PTP transmission was not proven until 1990. At that time, newly applied genetic testing verified the spread of BCC infection by "social contact" among children at a CF summer program in the United States [6]. Soon a vivid picture began to unfold as CF Centers from different continents reported PTP spread of BCC. The Summer Camp Study Group described the epidemic spread of BCC at three North American CF summer camps in 1990. Strict epidemiologic surveillance detected a 6.1% incidence of new BCC pulmonary infection among previously uninfected campers. Sputum specimens revealed an epidemic strain of genetically identical isolates, and exhaustive environmental water sampling failed to disclose a natural reservoir of the organism [7]. Interpersonal transmission of BCC was recognized contemporaneously in Europe. CF centers in Edinburgh and Manchester in the United Kingdom, noting a rise in the prevalence of BCC infection, analyzed the stored sputum specimens of 210 patients recovered between 1986 and

1992. Molecular testing revealed a particular genotype, subsequently designated electrophoretic type–12 (ET-12), that was highly transmissible and strongly associated with the cepacia syndrome [8]. The ET-12 strain was detected in Edinburgh in 1989, where an exercise class facilitated transmission between nine patients, and in Manchester in 1990, where seven cases were linked to a 1991 hospital Christmas party. Between 1990 and 1992, cross-infection between patients at the two centers was clearly documented [9]. Although the country of origin was not clearly established for ET-12, transmission between the European and North American continents occurred as campers from the United Kingdom who had a high prevalence of BCC carriage visited summer programs in Ontario [9]. A subsequent partial segregation policy, separating BCC-positive and BCC-negative patients, was instituted in Manchester in 1992, but it failed to contain the spread of the organism. This was followed by a strict segregation policy, under which the incidence of cases fell after 1994 [10].

In the wake of these discoveries, the fear of epidemic spread grew, and between 1993 and 1994, the CF summer camps were closed. There ensued an international effort to define, characterize, and better contain these pathogenic organisms. BCC-infected patients were segregated from uninfected peers, and the current molecular classification system was developed, along with national laboratories and specimen repositories. A major Mississippi outbreak involving multiple BCC strains and affecting CF and non-CF patients carried an overall mortality rate of almost 50%. This epidemic introduced the concept of BCC as a class of important respiratory pathogens with public health repercussions outside of the CF community [11] and raised the possibility that non-CF patients could be infected and serve as a reservoir for further spread. When an American company proposed to spray certain *Burkholderia* species from airplanes onto ginseng crops, opposition was galvanized by the CF foundation and resulted in an EPA scientific advisory panel recommendation against the commercial use of *Burkholderia* as a biopesticide (John LiPuma, personal communication, 2006). Cohorting of BCC-infected patients was reconsidered when the ET-12 strain replaced another *B cepacia* strain in five patients who had stable lung function, three of whom developed the cepacia syndrome. A fourth also suffered rapid clinical decline [12]. Transplant centers reported a high incidence of postsurgical mortality in patients harboring BCC [13,14], leading some to question whether BCC-infected patients should be offered lung transplantation [15]. Thereafter, many centers refused to list patients chronically infected with these organisms.

During this period, inpatient segregation policies were standardized and refined, and infected patients were asked to respect voluntary segregation outside of the hospital. In the outpatient environment, segregation by appointment times and room assignments was suggested [10], and patients were discouraged from associating in office waiting rooms. The previously tight social networks that had existed in the 1980s and early 1990s became fragmented. Hopes that more specific knowledge of the individual BCC pathogens would lead to a relaxation of segregation policies were abandoned when the putative genetic transmissibility markers BCESM and cblA (specific to ET-12) were shown to be insensitive [16,17], and case clusters were described in *Burkholderia* species other than *B cenocepacia* [18–21].

Perhaps the most unexpected BCC outbreak occurred despite the use of standard precautions and segregation policies at Children's Hospital Boston (CHB). Around 2001, the Cystic Fibrosis Foundation *Burkholderia cepacia* Research Laboratory and Repository recognized an abrupt increase in the prevalence of an unusual phenotype of *B multivorans* clustered at CHB. This was followed by the application of taxonomic methods and genetic "fingerprinting," which resulted in the description of Genomovar VI (subsequently designated *B dolosa*) and in the identification of the epidemic SLC6 strain [21,22]. As infection control measures at CHB were strengthened beyond those recommended by the CF Foundation, stored specimens at the repository dating back to 1992 were exhaustively reviewed, revealing that multiple specimens previously identified as atypical *B multivorans* were more accurately classified as *B dolosa*.

In Boston, intensive environmental testing of surfaces, water supplies, medical equipment, hospital rooms, physicians, and staff members did not reveal an environmental reservoir of infection. A chronologic examination of outpatient and inpatient visits suggested overlapping visits between previously infected patients and patients who had newly acquired infections within 6 to 12 months of the identification of the new infection. Given this finding, and despite the lack of an identified hospital-based reservoir, the outbreak triggered

a strengthening of the infection control program, including environmental surveillance measures, revised cleaning practices, intensified cohorting of patients infected with *B dolosa*, the strict institution of contact precautions, and partial segregation for all hospitalized patients who had CF, whether or not they were colonized with transmissible or virulent bacteria [23].

A case-control study showed that lung function measured by forced expiratory volume in 1 second declined more rapidly in patients who were infected with *B dolosa* than in a matched group of uninfected patients and a cohort infected with *B multivorans*. During an 18-month reference period, the relative risk of death associated with *B dolosa* infection was 10.8 compared with control group [23]. One patient died of fulminant cepacia syndrome in the absence of advanced structural lung disease (Figs. 1 and 2), and others experienced clinical decline well in advance of positive sputum cultures. Some patients expressed reluctance to attend appointments or to be hospitalized at CHB, but as tighter infection control practices were implemented, the incidence of new cases ceased. At the time of this writing, no new infections have been documented since January of 2005 (David Waltz, personal communication, 2006). Whether the decline in new cases was the result of the infection control measures instituted within CHB or of a heightened awareness among the clinic population of the dangers of interpatient contact in social settings away from the hospital is impossible to determine.

Several investigators have commented on the devastating psychologic effect of BCC infection

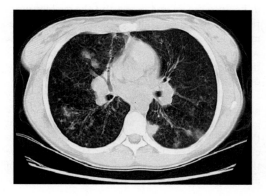

Fig. 1. Premorbid CT scan of the chest from a 19-year-old woman who has CF. The scan shows patchy peripheral opacities and diffuse but relatively mild bronchiectasis. Over 8 weeks in 2001, the patient experienced rapidly progressive and fatal *B dolosa* infection (*Courtesy of* David Waltz, MD, Boston, MA).

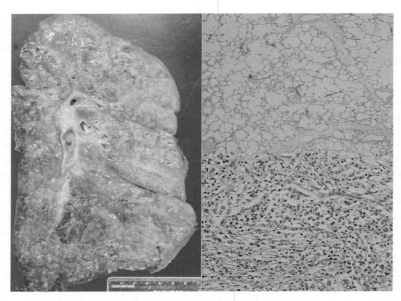

Fig. 2. Autopsy revealed acute and organizing bronchopneumonia involving 80% to 90% of the lung parenchyma. Blood and lung tissue cultures were positive for *B dolosa*. (*Courtesy of* David Waltz, MD, Boston, MA.)

on the CF community, noting an increased incidence of depression, social isolation, and loneliness in their patients since modern segregation practices began [24,25]. Most CF physicians agree that patient compliance with segregation practices is incomplete, and some complain that strict policies contribute to a "plague mentality" in the community and stigmatization of patients who are infected. Although all agree that BCC-infected patients should be treated with sensitivity and provided with social and emotional support, it is difficult to see an end in sight to the current practices of segregation and contact precautions. It remains impossible to know which patients will die with rapidly progressive lung and systemic infections or where virulent, transmissible, and multidrug-resistant strains will emerge.

These devastating accounts of the community effects of transmissible strains of BCC have galvanized CF centers worldwide and have set the stage for the development of current infection control practices. The following sections examine the broader evidence for PTP transmission of airway pathogens among patients who have CF.

Transmission of selected respiratory pathogens to patients who have cystic fibrosis

There is strong evidence that nosocomial PTP spread of infection may occur in CF and non-CF patients. However, many questions remain. For example, how pervasive is the problem of PTP spread in patients who have CF relative to rates of environmental acquisition? How much of an impact do innate features of an organism have on transmissibility? It has only been relatively recently that the CF community has had the tools and collective data to fully address such questions.

When reviewing the infection control literature, one should be aware of potential methodologic limitations of some of the early work in this area. Microbiologic techniques that attempt to define the relatedness of isolates by bacterial protein expression or antibiotic sensitivity profile are less reliable than more recently developed molecular approaches [26]. Pulsed-field gel electrophoresis (PFGE), a method by which bacterial genomic DNA is cleaved by low-frequency cutting endonucleases and then subjected to phoresis in a pulsatile electric field, has become the gold standard technique for obtaining molecular "fingerprints" of bacterial isolates, and criteria for grading relatedness of bacterial strains have been accepted [27].

A number of early attempts to confirm PTP transmission of *Pseudomonas aeruginosa* (PA) were hampered by the use of biochemical methods. A study at the Southhampton General Hospital in the United Kingdom highlighted this problem by incorporating newer genetic techniques into the protocol. A total of 496 morphotypes of PA were isolated from 69 patients over a 9-month period during outpatient visits. Antimicrobial sensitivity patterns were used to estimate cross-infection. Antibiogram similarities were shown to be coincidental by PFGE. In addition, serial isolates from individual patients were demonstrated to be genotypically indistinguishable despite differences in antibiotic sensitivity profiles [26], a finding corroborated by others [28–30]. Likewise, a group of investigators from the CF Center in Hannover, Germany studied the genetic fingerprints of 835 PA isolates using field-inversion gel electrophoresis, which was found to be more helpful than standard phenotypic testing to establish relatedness of isolates [31]. Further comparative descriptions of the methodology used for microbial characterization have been recently published [32,33].

The following sections examine biological characteristics of three important bacterial pathogens of the CF airway (PA, *Staphylococcus aureus* [SA], and BCC) and reviews of the evidence for PTP transmission and risk factors for acquisition of these pathogens. The summary tables that accompany these sections focus on studies after 1990 because many of the earlier studies were plagued by the technical limitations previously highlighted.

P aeruginosa

Organism characteristics and clinical impact
PA is an aerobic gram-negative bacillus that is found in many natural habitats, including water and soil. Niches have been identified in domestic and hospital settings. Approximately 77% of adult patients who have CF in the United States harbor PA (Fig. 3) [1]. A number of steps leading to chronic airway infection with this organism have been described. The process starts with acquisition, followed by attachment, persistent colonization, and chronic infection. In the acquisition phase, patients are typically asymptomatic. During the attachment phase, which may be mediated by characteristics of the organism and damage to the respiratory epithelium [34], an initial period of intermittent colonization seems to precede persistent infection [35]. At this stage, most patients note a minimal change in respiratory symptoms. Chronic infection is characterized by persistent recovery of PA from respiratory secretions for more than 6 months or the development of a specific antibody response to PA [34]. It is during the chronic infection phase that the mucoid phenotype typically develops [36], characterized by alginate biofilm formation. In the United States, 66% of adults harbor mucoid strains of PA, although the prevalence varies considerably by CF center (Fig. 4) [1]. PA growing in biofilms seems to adapt to an anaerobic environment and to become more fastidious due to alterations of the life cycle and resistance to antimicrobial agents [37]. The role of the exopolysaccharide alginate in this process has been reviewed extensively elsewhere [38,39].

Most patients who have CF become chronically infected with a single PA genotype [30,40], although in 20% to 30% of patients, transient

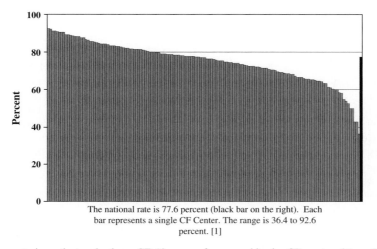

The national rate is 77.6 percent (black bar on the right). Each bar represents a single CF Center. The range is 36.4 to 92.6 percent. [1]

Fig. 3. PA infection rate in patients who have CF 18 years of age or older by CF center. (*From* 2005 Annual Data Report to the Center Directors. Cystic Fibrosis Patient Registry, Bethesda, MD; used with permission.)

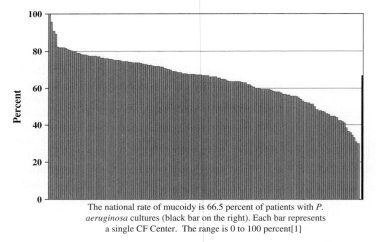

The national rate of mucoidy is 66.5 percent of patients with *P.
aeruginosa* cultures (black bar on the right). Each bar represents
a single CF Center. The range is 0 to 100 percent[1]

Fig. 4. Patients who have reported mucoid PA by CF center. (*From* 2005 Annual Data Report to the Center Directors.
Cystic Fibrosis Patient Registry, Bethesda, MD; used with permission.)

or permanent coinfection with more than one genotype occurs [33]. Chronic infection with PA
seems to be associated with worse pulmonary
function [41,42] and shorter life expectancy [43].
Patients who have multidrug resistant PA
(MDR-PA) undergo more rapid pulmonary decline and earlier listing for lung transplantation
than their noninfected peers [44]. At centers in
the United Kingdom, patients who have epidemic
strains of PA have been found to experience more
frequent pulmonary exacerbations [45] and accelerated loss of lung function [46].

Evidence of person-to-person transmission

The precise mode of acquisition of PA has
been a longstanding area of research interest.
Some groups have proposed that initial colonization of the CF airway usually comes from
environmental sources. At the CF Center in
Brussels, investigators examined the relatedness
of 166 PA isolates from 31 patients who had CF
using PFGE and found that the majority of
patients maintain the same or a related genotypic
strain over time [30]. Another study performed at
the Danish CF Center examined 310 strains of PA
from 240 patients who had CF and environmental
samples. Extensive environmental testing included
air sampling in patient care areas. Only 6 of 1000
environmental swabs (0.6%) demonstrated PA. A
total of 20 patient specimens with identical phage
and serotype were compared with the environmental specimens by PFGE and were found to
be distinct, supporting the notion that hygienic
precautions at the center were effective [47]. A

cross-sectional study was performed in the North
Staffordshire CF Clinic examining patients ranging from 1 to 54 years of age to assess the relatedness of PA isolates in the clinic population. From
1993 to 1998, environmental and patient-derived
PA isolates were collected, and patients were divided into six categories based on degree of contact. Members of the CF team also had throat
and nasal cultures for PA. Environmental swabs
were obtained from pediatric and adult clinics, inpatient wards, and a local school attended by
many of the patients. PA isolates were genotyped
by PFGE. In the original cross-sectional study,
only three matched PA genotypes were found in
paired patients who had little contact. Over the
next 5 years, PA isolates from patients and the
local environment were compared. Generally,
patients remained colonized with the same strain
and did not share the strain, refuting the concept
of segregation based on PA status [48]. A study at
the CF Center in Sao Paulo, Brazil used random
amplified polymorphic DNA typing to show
that cross infection was uncommon in the outpatient arena [49]. At the Royal Brompton Hospital
(London, England) Kerr and colleagues [50] sam-
pled stethoscopes and the hands of health care
workers on an inpatient CF unit and recovered
PA from only 1 of 76 samples. Laraya-Cuasay
and colleagues [51] studied 25 patients who had
CF at St. Christopher's Hospital (Philadelphia,
Pennsylvania) to see whether patients infected
with PA posed a risk to family members. Transmis-
sion/carriage of PA was found to be rare in healthy
family members (4/468 cultures). Based on such

evidence, some have argued that segregation of patients based on PA sputum culture results may lead to significantly increased expense, decreased clinic flexibility, and social stigmatization without corresponding gains in infection control [25].

In contrast, a growing number of reports suggest PTP spread of PA. Many of these studies are more recent and used sophisticated study designs and methodologies. At the CF Center in Hannover, Germany, molecular fingerprinting of PA isolates over a 4-year period led investigators to conclude that 12 of 40 patients acquired PA during time spent at recreation camps, clinics, or rehabilitation centers. After the institution of a hygienic precautions program, only one additional case developed in the next 2 years [52]. At the same center, the distribution and population dynamics of PA was evaluated in a contaminated hospital environment (ie, the inpatient CF ward). Multiple areas within the ward were checked, including water pipes, sinks, inhalers, toys, and cosmetics. Samples taken from multiple environmental sites showed that 45% of the rooms in the ward with PA-colonized patients and 30% of the outpatient clinics rooms were contaminated. They also found a high frequency of PA in sinks and water reservoirs. Hospital personnel and stethoscopes were not found to be contaminated [53]. At the Danish CF Center in Copenhagen, Denmark, investigators studied 22 patients who attended a 1-week winter camp. At the start of the trip, 5 of 22 patients did not harbor PA. After return, all 22 patients carried PA, and PFGE confirmed that these strains had been transmitted through social contact with other campers [54].

Groups in the United Kingdom and Australia have identified highly transmissible strains of PA, including the Liverpool epidemic strain (LES), the Manchester transmissible strain, the Midlands 1 strain, and the Melbourne strain. McCallum and colleagues [55] reported genotypically confirmed superinfection of four PA-positive patients who had a new strain of PA after contact with other infected patients who had CF on a hospital ward. In a report from the groups in Manchester and Edinburgh, airborne MDR-PA was detected in rooms on the inpatient ward during respiratory treatments [56]. Air sampling was performed 15 to 30 feet from the patient, which is beyond the 3-ft radius typically seen with droplet spread. The investigators point out that during their study, a PA-naive inpatient acquired the MDR strain. Six additional patients were identified, but no environmental source was found despite extensive

testing [56]. Another recent study of an inpatient ward points to possible airborne spread of the LES PA [57].

Circumstantial evidence further supports the concept of PTP transmission of PA. Scott and Pitt [58] examined the distribution of PA strains from 31 medical centers in England and Wales. A large data set comprising 1225 isolates demonstrated that although 72% of patients had unique PA genotypes, more than 20% across the network of centers carried similar genotypes, including the Manchester transmissible, LES, and Midland 1 forms, a clustering phenomenon suggestive of organism transmission [58]. Data collected at two CF centers in Wisconsin as part of a neonatal CF screening project showed that risk factors for early acquisition of PA included interspersed care of young patients who had CF with older patients who had CF and increased social contact between patients who had CF [59,60]. At the Danish CF Center, the point prevalence of chronic PA infection decreased from 65% in 1980 to 45% in 1995 after institution of patient segregation and early treatment for newly acquired PA [61,62]. Investigators in Australia showed that the prevalence of an epidemic strain of PA at the CF center decreased from 21% to 14% over 3 years after the institution of a segregation program [63]. At the center in Liverpool, a longitudinal study of PA isolates from sputum samples obtained during inpatient stays and outpatient visits used PFGE to evaluate the spread of MDR-PA through the local CF population. Four patients are described who acquired a MDR-PA after inpatient treatment, replacing their pre-existing strain of PA. No point source or environmental reservoir was identified in the hospital, suggesting cross-infection of patients through nosocomial social contact [55]. Jones and colleagues [64] found that during a 4-year, prospective study at the CF center in Manchester, England, standard infection control measures did not seem to limit the spread of an epidemic strain of PA, whereas a segregated cohort of patients remained free of infection. Table 1 summarizes findings of studies from 1990 to present that have examined PTP spread of PA in patients who have CF [65–70].

Identified risk factors for P aeruginosa *transmission*

Nosocomial transmission of PA has been well characterized in the non-CF population. Important lessons for health care workers can be learned

Table 1
Selected evidence for PTP spread of PA and SA in patients who have CF

Organism	Country	Year	No.	Setting	Comments
PA	Germany	1991, 1994, 1995	32–47	OP/IP	Indirect evidence of PTP spread and contamination of an inpatient ward [40,52,53]
	Belgium	1993	31	OP	No observed PTP spread [30]
	France	1993	21	OP/Home	Little evidence of PTP spread, except between twins [65]
	Denmark	1995	240	IP/OP	No nosocomial source of PA [47]
	Netherlands	1995	91	Camp	Little evidence of PTP spread at a summer camp [66]
	England	1996	120	OP	Evidence of frequent PTP spread through a pediatric CF program [67]
	USA	1997	123	OP	Increased risk of PA spread with mixed clinic care and increased social contact [59,60]
	Ireland	1998	50	OP/school	PTP spread suggested by shared clones within families and those attending the same school [68]
	Denmark	2000	22	Camp	Evidence of PTP spread at a camp [54]
	England	2001	72	OP	No observed spread [48]
	Brazil	2001	96	OP	No evidence of significant PTP spread [49]
	England	2001	4	IP	Evidence of superinfection with a new PA strain by PTP contact [55]
	England	2001	154	OP	Evidence of cross infection with MDR-PA [69]
	England	2002	NA	IP	Evidence of significant cross infection associated with hospitalization [173]
	Australia	2002	152	IP/OP	No spread from patients to health care workers [50]
	England	2004	849	OP	Epidemiologic evidence of PTP spread of transmissible genotypes [58]
	Australia/New Zealand	2005	325	OP	Reduced prevalence of an epidemic PA strain after segregation [63]
	England	2005	~250	OP	Four year prospective trial suggesting segregation prevents PTP spread [64]
SA	Germany	1993	53	Camp	Evidence of PTP spread of SA in patients who had CF attending a summer camp [99]
	Netherlands	1997	18	OP	Indirect evidence of PTP spread based on persistence of common types [101]
	Australia	1997	177	IP/OP	Evidence of nosocomial PTP spread but not with casual social contact [100]
	USA	2000	157	OP	Indirect evidence of PTP spread based on persistence of common types [70]
	Germany	2000	389	OP	Indirect evidence of PTP spread within families based on genotype [94]
	England	2005	45	OP/IP	Identification of risk factors for MRSA acquisition suggests nosocomial spread [102]

Abbreviations: IP, inpatient; OP, outpatient.

from a reported outbreak of PA in a neonatal intensive care unit at Columbia Presbyterian Medical Center. PA was found on 10 of 165 health care workers, where risk factors for colonization of the hands included artificial fingernails, nail wraps, and age [71]. CF sputum prolongs survival of PA (and BCC) on environmental surfaces [72] perhaps due to the presence of amino acid nutrients [73]. PA and BCC were transmissible by handshaking for 180 minutes when embedded in CF sputum versus 30 minutes when transported in normal saline [72]. It is therefore critical that good hand hygiene be practiced in the care of this patient population.

Despite the findings of Jones and colleagues [56] that PA may spread by droplet nuclei, most direct studies have demonstrated viable organisms only in larger droplets that tend to sediment to the floor within 3 feet of the patient [72,74]. A recent consensus document stresses the finding that PTP spread of PA is most likely via direct and indirect contact or by droplets rather than by aerosols [32].

The potential for PA transmission has been identified in a number of health care and environmental settings and is associated with various pieces of health equipment, including sinks and drains [53,72,75], hospital water supply [76], contaminated dental equipment [77], contaminated nebulizers [78–80], mist tents [81], whirlpools, and hot tubs [82].

S aureus

Organism characteristics and clinical impact

S aureus (SA) is a hardy, nonspore-forming bacterial species. Microscopically, these gram-positive spherical organisms typically arrange in clusters—hence the genus designation that derives from the Greek expression for "bunch of grapes." SA frequently resides in the nares or on the skin of patients who have CF or in nonaffected patients. A recent study estimates United States prevalence of SA nasal carriage to be 32% in the general population [83]. It is commonplace for individuals to

be repeatedly colonized with SA for stretches of time, punctuated by organism-free intervals. In the 1940s, it was recognized that many SA isolates produce a beta-lactamase (penicillinase) [84] that inactivates a range of antibiotics. This led to development of semisynthetic penicillinase-resistant compounds in the 1960s. Shortly thereafter, methicillin-resistant SA (MRSA) strains began to emerge in the hospital setting [85]. High-level resistance requires the presence of a gene, designated *mec*, that encodes an altered penicillin-binding protein (PBP 2a) [86,87]. In 1988, Boxerbaum and colleagues [88] predicted that MRSA would become a significant pediatric nosocomial pathogen despite the finding of only 3% prevalence in their clinic population at that time. In recent years, community strains of MRSA have become more common, and this has precipitated changes in the recommended empiric treatment strategies for out-of-hospital infections [89,90]. The prediction has also borne out in the CF community, where the estimated prevalence in the United States is almost 20% (Fig. 5) [1].

Other forms of antimicrobial resistance are being recognized. Phaff and colleagues [91] found that patients who had CF who were chronically treated with azithromycin over a 4-year study period had a high prevalence of macrolide resistant SA and *Haemophilus* sp. (54% and 37%, respectively) compared with nontreated control subjects. This finding has been confirmed elsewhere, although selective pressure for MRSA has not been observed with macrolides [92,93].

The clinical impact of SA and MRSA in patients who have CF remains incompletely

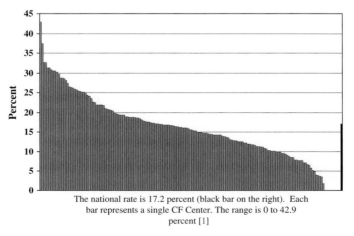

The national rate is 17.2 percent (black bar on the right). Each
bar represents a single CF Center. The range is 0 to 42.9
percent [1]

Fig. 5. MRSA infection rate by CF center. (*From* 2005 Annual Data Report to the Center Directors. Cystic Fibrosis Patient Registry, Bethesda, MD; used with permission.)

defined. Goerke and colleagues [94] assessed the epidemiology of SA in families with and without CF using PFGE. They found that the nasal prevalence of SA was higher in patients who had CF who were not prescribed antimicrobial medications compared with healthy control subjects and patients who had CF who were treated with antibiotics, suggesting that individuals who have CF may have a higher susceptibility to this organism [94]. Most patients seem to harbor the same genotype for at least 3 months [94,95]. Miall and colleagues [96] reported that MRSA infection in pediatric patients who have CF does not seem to significantly worsen respiratory function but may adversely affect growth, frequency of exacerbations, and x-ray scores. Infection with SA does not seem to shorten life expectancy. In fact, a recent study indicates that chronic SA infection predicts a mild survival benefit, possibly by delaying establishment of chronic gram-negative infection [97]. Small-colony variants of SA may be a particular problem in the patients who have CF, although data about appropriate detection and treatment strategies are only beginning to emerge. Small-colony variants may cause less tissue damage than typical Staphylococci but tend to be more fastidious [98]. These forms are associated with chronic infection and resistance to antibiotic therapy, and isolates are difficult to identify in the clinical microbiology lab due to very slow growth.

Evidence of person-to-person transmission

Although evidence of PTP transmission of SA (and MRSA) is well documented, particularly in the hospital setting, there are fewer such reports in the CF literature (Table 1). One group used PFGE to confirm the acquisition of new SA strains in four patients who had CF after a 4-week stay at a CF summer camp [99]. Givney and colleagues [100] investigated MRSA infection in a CF unit using phage-typing and PFGE analysis. Findings demonstrated transmission from the general hospital population to inpatients who had CF. There was one instance of possible transmission between two patients who had CF. Infection with this organism does not seem to occur frequently with simple social contact [100], but strain transmission may occur regularly within CF families [94,101].

Identified risk factors for acquisition

Patients who have CF seem to carry the same susceptibility to infection by SA through direct or indirect contact as unaffected individuals, particularly in the hospital setting [100]. Repeated

contact with health care facilities and broad-spectrum antibiotics, particularly ciprofloxacin and cephalosporins [102], increases the risk of exposure of patients who have CF to infection with MSSA and MRSA.

B cepacia *complex*

Organism characteristics and clinical impact

B cepacia was identified in the late 1940's at Cornell University [103], although it was originally assigned to the genus *Pseudomonas*. Members of the *B cepacia* complex (BCC) are motile, strictly aerobic, gram-negative bacilli that are widely present in soils and water. Initially described as the cause of "sour skin" onion rot, members of BCC have demonstrated commercial promise as biopesticides, acting as potent fungicides and nematocides. Selected species within the complex may be effective biodegradation agents, having the ability to break down toxic compounds found in pesticides and herbicides [104,105]. *Burkholderia* spp. have been identified in a number of ecologic niches and have been discovered in certain foods [106], commercial products [107,108], and landscaping preparations [109].

The BCC, now comprising 10 or more designated species differentiated by phenotypic and genotypic features, possesses a large and plastic genome that may increase the frequency of genetic mutations [105,110,111]. In humans, it has been described as a pathogen largely in individuals who have CF, where approximately 3% of patients carry these organisms (Fig. 6). BCC has also been reported to infect patients who have malignancy and chronic granulomatous disease [112]. Occasionally, immune-competent hosts are affected, and spread between CF and non-CF patients has been implicated in some reports [11,113]. These organisms seem to be capable of evading the host immune response by invading and surviving within alveolar macrophages and airway epithelial cells [114]. Antimicrobial resistance of BCC organisms may be mediated by a drug-effexor pump (bcrA); by the ability to create biofilms [115], siderophores, exopolysaccharides, and hemolysins; and by resistance to the protective effects of β-defensins and respiratory mucin [115–117]. For some strains, there are no effective antimicrobial therapies, and well publicized cases of progressive pneumonia, bacteremia, and death have lent urgency to the institution of effective infection control measures [3,9].

Before the application of genetic methodologies, speciation of BCC in the laboratory using

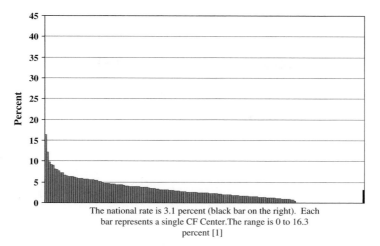

The national rate is 3.1 percent (black bar on the right). Each
bar represents a single CF Center. The range is 0 to 16.3
percent [1]

Fig. 6. *B cepacia* complex infection rate by CF center. (*From* 2005 Annual Data Report to the Center Directors. Cystic Fibrosis Patient Registry, Bethesda, MD; used with permission.)

phenotypic assays was difficult. Misidentification rates were as high as 36% [118]. The development of genetic techniques in the 1990s led to the ability to distinguish "genomovars" among phenotypically similar isolates and eventually led to the current classification scheme [113,119]. Genetic characterization and storage of BCC isolates is now routinely performed through specialized reference laboratories in many countries, including the United States, the United Kingdom, Italy, Belgium, and Canada. At least 10 species have been described [111], and an ever-increasing number of distinct strains within each species are being identified (Table 2). Although a variety of specialized techniques have been developed, full genetic characterization typically requires culture on antibiotic-impregnated agar plates, followed by phenotyping, polymerase chain reaction amplification, and restriction fragment length polymorphism analysis. Various genotyping methods may then be used to distinguish strains within a species.

Based on United States National Registry data from the mid 1990s, median survival of CF patients who harbor BCC seems to be almost a decade shorter than that of the CF population as a whole and approximately three decades shorter than that

Table 2
Burkholderia cepacia complex taxonomy and clinical features

Genomic species	Binomial designation	Distribution[a]	Comments
Genomovar I	*B cepacia*	3%	cblA homologs have been isolated
Genomovar II	*B multivorans*	39%	
Genomovar III	*B cenocepacia*	46%	ET12 lineage has been described in this species
Genomovar IV	*B stabilis*	<1%	
Genomovar V	*B vietnamiensis*	6%	
Genomovar VI	*B dolosa*	4%	Boston outbreak associated with high mortality
Genomovar VII	*B ambifaria*	<1%	
Genomovar VIII	*B anthina*	<1%	
Genomovar IX	*B pyrroncinia*	<1%	
Genomovar X	*B ubonensis*	Not identified as a CF pathogen	

Abbreviations: IP, inpatient; OP, outpatient.
[a] Distribution in United States isolates from the *B cepacia* repository [114].
Data from Reik R, Spilker T, Lipuma JJ. Distribution of *Burkholderia cepacia* complex species among isolates recovered from persons with or without cystic fibrosis. J Clin Microbiol 2005;43:2927.

of a cohort never infected with PA or BCC [120]. Infection with certain strains of *B cenocepacia* and *B dolosa* has been linked to an accelerated decline of lung function and increased mortality [23,121–123] and to an increased risk of poor outcome after lung transplantation [13,14,124]. Poor outcomes have been described with more "benign" species [125,126], so it is misleading to consider any species of *B cepacia* innocuous. It may be more predictive to recognize virulent or highly transmissible strains within any of the *Burkholderia* species than to single out one or two species as the "bad actors" [127].

Evidence of patient-to-patient transmission

When the relentlessly progressive and fatal cepacia syndrome was initially described in 1984, it was generally assumed that infection with *P cepacia* was a marker of underlying CF disease progression rather than being attributable to the organism itself. Affected patients were therefore allowed to socialize freely with their uninfected peers. In 1986, the successful use of infection control practices to limit the spread of disease was reported, thereby suggesting transmission from a common environmental source or through PTP contact [5]. The presence of environmental reservoirs was rapidly established [128–130], but rigorous demonstration of PTP BCC spread was not reported until 1990, when LiPuma and colleagues [131] used novel ribotyping methodologies to prove the "social" transmission of genetically identical *B cenocepacia* strains [6]. There is extensive evidence for PTP spread of BCC, and a summary of recent studies demonstrating transmission is found in Table 3 [132–138].

Identified risk factors for transmission

Within *B cenocepacia*, two putative genetic markers of transmissibility have been described: (1) BCESM, which contains elements homologous to negative transcriptional regulatory genes [139], and (2) cblA, which encodes a giant cable pilus that facilitates cellular adhesion [140]. In one study, BCESM and cblA were sensitive (94% and 59%, respectively) and specific (75% and 100%, respectively) for *B cenocepacia* transmissibility among patients [141]. Although *B cenocepacia* has in recent years been the most prevalent species infecting patients who have CF in the United States, Canada, and the United Kingdom [113], certain epidemic *B cenocepacia* strains, such as the PDHC strain common in the mid-Atlantic United States, lack BCESM and cblA. Although

the majority of outbreaks in the United States, Canada, and the United Kingdom are related to *B cenocepacia* (Genomovar III), smaller outbreaks have occurred in patients infected with *B multivorans* and *B dolosa* [21]. Thus, although certain high-risk strains have been identified, advances in the ability to distinguish between *Burkholderia* spp. and strains have not allowed for consistent prediction of virulence or transmissibility, and ongoing inpatient and outpatient segregation of all BCC-infected patients is recommended, irrespective of species [32].

Known risk factors for the transmission of BCC include certain patient behaviors, such as close or intimate social contacts [7], handshaking, or prolonged time shared within close quarters (eg, on car rides or in hospital rooms). Acquisition of BCC has been reported after hospitalization on a ward known to house other patients who have BCC [23,130] and after exposure to certain nosocomial reservoirs, such as colonized nebulizers or spirometry equipment [142,143], bronchodilator solutions [108,144, 145], or tube feeding dye [146]. These risk factors have been cataloged in recent excellent reviews [32,147]. The message from a series of reports worldwide is clear: If the spread of BCC is to be contained, then laboratories, health care teams, hospital organizations, and patients must work cooperatively to ensure the safety of the community.

Other organisms

A range of organisms have been identified as pathogens in the CF airway, although they are of less epidemiologic importance than PA, methicillin sensitive *Staphylococcus aureus* (MSSA)/MRSA, and BCC. PTP transmissibility of these organisms (aside from the viral pathogens) seems to be low and is not as well understood as with the other species. Infection of patients who have CF with these organisms has been reviewed elsewhere [32,147,148] and is summarized in Table 4 [149–151]. Viral infections deserve special mention because it is believed that these organisms may frequently initiate pulmonary exacerbations [152].

General infection control recommendations

A set of general guidelines for infection control has been promulgated by the Healthcare Infection Control Practices Advisory Committee, an organization formed in 1991 by the Centers for Disease Control and Prevention to check nosocomial infections. A key mandate of this group was

Table 3
Evidence for PTP spread of BCC in patients who have CF (studies since 1990)

Site	Year	No.	Location	Comments/references
USA	1990	16	CFF interns	Focused on single case of proven transmission by "social contact" between two individuals [6]
UK	1993	—	OP/camp	Transmission of identical isolates [9]
UK	1993	17	OP/IP	Epidemiology and genetic testing to evaluate BCC outbreak at a single center [132]
USA, Canada	1994	181	Camp	Transmission of identical isolates [7]
UK, Canada	1994	83[b]	IP/OP	Demonstrated geographic clusters of BCC by electrophoretic type (ET), identified "ET-12" strain [8]
USA	1994	18	IP	Epidemiologic study showed concurrent hospitalization/rooming a strong RF for development of BCC
UK, Canada	1995	[c]	IP/OP	Genetic typing of Canadian and UK clusters for comparison [133]
[a]	1996	298	IP/OP	Genetic epidemiology used to identify strain clusters in distinct geographical locations [134]
France	1997	71	IP/OP	French BCC isolates analyzed, cluster of distinct strain suggests PTP transmission [135]
USA	1998	268	IP	23 CF and 245 non-CF patients over 5 yrs at one hospital, multiple strains involved [11]
Australia	1999	6	IP	B gladiola among six inpatients shown to be BCC ET-12 on genetic analysis of isolates [136]
USA	2001	69	IP/OP	Isolates over 20 yr suggest BCESM- and cblA-negative epidemic cenocepacia strain
Canada	2002	447	Mixed	Clusters of genetically identical strains strongly suggest transmissibility [137]
USA	2003	360	Mixed	Identified identical cenocepacia, multivorans, and dolosa strains in 29 cities [21]
Europe	2004	131	Mixed	Epidemic clusters compared with genetic transmissibility markers. [141]
Italy	2005	225	Mixed	Geographic clusters of genetically identical strains found in national epidemiologic survey [138]
USA	2006	36	IP/OP	B dolosa outbreak epidemiology, unique strain cluster suggests PTP spread despite precautions [23]

[a] Canadian laboratory processed specimens from patients in Canada, USA, UK, Australia, and France.

[b] 83 specimens, unknown number of patients.

[c] 28 specimens, uncertain number of patients.

to develop practical protocols for isolation precautions in the hospital setting. Hand hygiene guidelines were developed in collaboration with the Society for Healthcare Epidemiology of America, the Association of Professionals in Infection Control and Epidemiology, and the Infectious Disease Society of America. These general recommendations apply to individuals who have CF, particularly in the inpatient environment, and can be accessed at www.cdc.gov/ncidod/dhqp/guidelines.html. This material has been summarized for CF health care workers (HCWs) in a recent review [147].

There are two tiers of precautions recommended for patients in the health care setting. "Standard precautions" are intended for all inpatients regardless of their microbiologic diagnosis, whereas "transmission-based precautions" apply only to patients harboring epidemiologically important pathogens that may be spread to others in the absence of special preventative measures.

Standard precautions

This approach incorporates the major features of protocols developed in the 1980s, such as "universal precautions" (designed to reduce the transmission of blood-borne organisms after the start of the HIV epidemic) and "body substance isolation" (designed to reduce the transmission of pathogens from moist body substances). The basic tenet of standard precautions is that all blood, body fluids (secretions and excretions other than sweat, regardless of whether or not they contain

Table 4
Other selected respiratory pathogens in patients who have CF

Organism	Comments
Haemophilus influenza	Often recovered in childhood. Course may be variable. Overall prevalence is 17% [1]. Acquisition may be from the environment or via PTP spread [32].
Stenotrophomonas maltophilia	Most frequently recovered in adults who have advanced lung disease. Overall prevalence is 12% [1]. Environmental acquisition seems to be more common than PTP outside the hospital setting [32].
Achromobacter xylosoxidans	Most frequently recovered in adults who have advanced lung disease. Overall prevalence is 4% [147]. Environmental acquisition seems to be more common than PTP outside the hospital setting [32].
Mycobacterium tuberculosis	Uncommon in the CF population. Primary mode of acquisition is PTP.
Nontuberculous mycobacteria (eg, *M avium* complex, *M abscessus, M gordonae*)	Recognized with increased frequency (all patients on chronic macrolide therapy should be monitored for mycobacterial species). Prevalence is about 13% in adult patients in the United States [149]. Environmental acquisition is the rule.
Respiratory viruses (eg, influenza, rhinovirus, adenovirus, respiratory syncytial virus, parainfluenza, metapneumovirus)	Patients who have CF do not seem to be more susceptible to viral infection [150], although these infections seem to be associated with pulmonary exacerbations and lung function decline over time [151,152].
Fungi (eg, *Aspergillus* spp.)	Environmental acquisition is the rule. Colonization is common, particularly in adults. True infection is rare except in the post–lung transplant population. Allergic bronchopulmonary aspergillosis is reported in 5% of patients 18 yr of age or older [1].

visible blood), nonintact skin, and mucous membranes may harbor potentially transmissible pathogens regardless of the clinical status of the patient or HCW. The central practices of standard precautions include:

> *Hand hygiene* before and after all patient contacts; after handling blood, body fluids, secretions, and excretions (except sweat); and after removing gloves. Hand washing should include the use of a non-antimicrobial soap for routine cleaning and an antimicrobial or waterless antiseptic agent for specific circumstances (see contact precautions). Each method seems to be equally effective, although when hands are physically soiled, soap and water should be used [153].
>
> *Gloves* should be worn when contacting blood, body fluids, secretions, excretions from mucous membranes, nonintact skin, and potentially contaminated equipment.
>
> *Other protective gear*, including a mask, a face shield, an eye shield, and a gown should be worn during procedures that are likely to generate splashes or sprays of blood, body fluids, secretions, and excretions.

Additional recommendations for proper maintenance and handling of patient-care equipment, linen, room and ward environments, and sharp instruments are outlined in the Healthcare Infection Control Practices Advisory Committee document [154]. These Category IB recommendations (strongly recommended for implementation and supported by certain experimental, clinical, or epidemiologic studies and a strong theoretical rationale) are designed to reduce the risk of transmitting micro-organisms in hospitals from recognized and unrecognized sources of infection.

Transmission-based precautions

There are three types of precautions in this category: airborne precautions, droplet precautions, and contact precautions. These divisions are based on the rationale that certain patients harbor organisms that have a propensity to spread by specific routes. The overall strategy holds that targeted organism- and host-specific approaches may be more effective for thwarting in-hospital spread of infection in these circumstances. Two additional modes of spread—common vehicle transmission (whereby infection is spread through contaminated items such as food, water, medications, devices, or equipment) and vector-borne transmission (via intermediate hosts such as flies, rats, and mosquitoes)—are encountered infrequently in hospitals within developed countries and are not discussed further here.

Subcategories of transmission-based precautions may be combined for diseases that have multiple routes of spread. Whether used alone or in combination, they are to be used as an adjunct to standard precautions [154]. Patients who have CF have a propensity to harbor MDR organisms during hospitalization, even if such organisms have not been previously identified on outpatient cultures. This issue should be considered when crafting infection control guidelines for inpatient care at individual CF centers.

Contact precautions: This set of rules is designed to minimize direct or indirect contact with epidemiologically important microorganisms. In addition to standard precautions, basic components of this set include:
  Private room.
  Gloves worn when entering the room. Remove gloves before leaving the room and wash hands immediately with antimicrobial soap or waterless antiseptic agent.
  Gown worn when entering the room, if contact with the patient or with potentially contaminated surfaces is anticipated. Remove gown before leaving the room.
  Patient transport from the room for essential purposes only. Precautions should be maintained during transport to minimize contamination of other equipment or environmental surfaces.
  Dedicate noncritical equipment to a single patient. Common equipment should be cleaned and disinfected appropriately.

Droplet precautions: These rules should be used in addition to standard precautions when the patient is known to have or is suspected of having organisms that can be transmitted by large-particle droplets (>5 μm in diameter; see www.cdc.gov/ncidod/dhqp/guidelines.html for listing) generated during activities such as coughing, sneezing, and talking. Basic components of this guideline set include:
  Private room.
  Mask worn when working within 3 feet of the patient. It may be most practical to put on the mask upon entry to the patient room.
  Mask worn by the patient during transport.

This category is often a source of confusion for HCWs. Although patients who have CF

generate large numbers of contaminated droplets during airway clearance and breathing treatments, the organisms being expelled are typically not epidemiologically important pathogens to HCWs or immunocompetent patients who do not have CF (a complete listing of organisms for which droplet precautions are recommended can be found at www.cdc.gov/ncidod/dhqp/guidelines.html). Therefore, contact precautions are appropriate for care provided in the patient room. Appropriate measures should be taken outside the patient room to minimize contamination of environmental surfaces on the ward, particularly if patients who have CF receive care on a designated unit.

Airborne precautions: In addition to standard precautions, airborne precautions should be used if a patient is known to be infected with organisms that can be shed in droplet nuclei (median diameter <5 μm), which can remain suspended in the air for prolonged periods and dispersed by air currents (see www.cdc.gov/ncidod/dhqp/guidelines.html). Basic components of this set include:
  Patient should be placed in a room with monitored negative pressure in relation to surrounding areas. There should be at least six air exchanges per hour in the room, and discharged air should be directed or filtered so as not to contaminate other areas of the hospital.
  Appropriate respiratory protection using a National Institute for Occupational Safety and Health-approved mask system worn by all HCWs entering the patient room.
  Patient transport should be minimized, and the patient must wear a mask if transportation is necessary for essential testing.

There have been reports of apparent contamination of inpatient rooms with respirable particles containing CF pathogens [56,155]. This has not been a consistent finding and has not been shown to pose a significant risk to HCWs or patients who do not have CF. Therefore, current recommendations from the most recent consensus document for CF infection control do not call for implementation of airborne precautions in most circumstances [32]. A complete listing of organisms for which airborne precautions are recommended can be found at www.cdc.gov/ncidod/dhqp/guidelines.html.

Selected infection control issues for patients who have cystic fibrosis

A number of infection control matters are of special concern to patients who have CF, their families, and CF care teams. In some instances, there is little evidence on which to base firm recommendations, although a recently published, comprehensive consensus document provides a generous set of guidelines that can inform discussions and local planning [32]. The following topics are frequent sources of questions.

Nebulizer and airway clearance device care

Nebulizers and airway clearance devices can become contaminated with respiratory pathogens [79], so it is critical that patients and HCWs master proper cleaning and maintenance of this equipment. Thoroughly cleaned devices have been shown to retain good performance over time [156].

Two steps should be taken to properly prepare respiratory equipment: cleaning and disinfection. Cleaning involves the physical removal of bulky contaminants. Dried and caked materials should be thoroughly cleaned from surfaces of the device with soap and water because disinfection is impaired by films or crusts of organic substances. Disinfection involves sufficient killing of pathogenic organisms to render a hygienic surface. Any of a number of acceptable methods [157] may be used to disinfect reusable items (after reviewing the manufacturers' recommendations):

Boil items in water for 5 minutes.
Immerse items in a 1:50 dilution of household bleach (5.25%–6.15% sodium hypochlorite) for 3 minutes, 70% to 90% ethyl or rubbing (isopropyl) alcohol for 5 minutes [158], or 3% hydrogen peroxide for 30 minutes.
Microwave items for 5 minutes [159,160]
Wash items in a dishwasher with a cycle that maintains 70°C or higher for at least 30 minutes [147,161].

Vinegar (acetic acid) should not be used to clean respiratory equipment because it has been shown to be unreliable for cleaning surfaces contaminated with Staphylococcal spp. and Escherichia coli [157]. All equipment should be air dried after cleaning. Unit dose medications are recommended for use in nebulizers to decrease the risk of contamination [142,144]. Patients are not to share respiratory equipment, even if they reside in the same household.

C difficile carriage and infection

In recent years, C difficile infections in the general public have increased in frequency, severity, and resistance to treatment [162]. Patients who have CF have a higher rate of asymptomatic carriage of C difficile than the population at large [163,164]. This is likely a result of repeated exposure to antibiotic therapy and hospital environments. Furthermore, patients who have CF with C difficile infection may experience atypical symptoms (eg, abdominal discomfort without diarrhea, which may mimic distal intestinal obstruction syndrome) and may present with an unusual radiographic pattern [165]. Therefore, a high index of suspicion should be maintained for this condition, and appropriate contact precautions should be instituted when the diagnosis is made or entertained.

Outpatient infection control and patient segregation

Individuals who have CF may harbor MDR or transmissible respiratory pathogens that can contaminate outpatient facilities. This has become a significant concern because epidemics have been reported at a number of CF centers worldwide. A recent study indicates that shedding of respiratory pathogens into the local environment occurs in more than 10% of outpatient encounters, regardless of whether the patient presents with acute pulmonary symptoms or for routine surveillance care [166]. To minimize direct and indirect patient contact, waiting room time should be minimized. Patients who are in the office concurrently should observe the "3-foot rule," which means to maintain an arm's distance of separation to minimize the risk of cross-infection by droplet spread. The 3-foot rule is recommended for all social situations where patients who have CF may congregate [32].

It is generally accepted that patients harboring BCC or MRSA should be stringently separated from other patients who have CF in the outpatient setting. One popular approach is to have patients who are infected with these organisms scheduled into the final clinic slots to minimize interaction with other patients. The issue of whether segregation of patients who have MDR or epidemic strains of PA is preferable to the rigorous application of accepted infection control measures is debated [25]. Some CF centers have chosen to segregate patients based on PA status and for other pathogenic species. Although this policy has not taken hold worldwide—particularly in the United States—the strategy has been embraced at some locations where epidemic strains have been identified. A recent survey study of physicians in Germany indicates widely differing opinions among practitioners about the importance of infection control measures for patients who have CF. The investigators submit that variation in recommendations from the health care team may contribute to increased patient fear and impaired quality of life in families who have an affected member [167]. A conflicting report from Melbourne, Australia indicates that segregation was broadly accepted by patients and families, particularly in the setting of local epidemics [168,169]. Despite all of the concerns about infection control at CF centers, the CF community should never lose sight of the importance of center-directed care, which has been shown to result in better clinical outcomes for patients who have the disease [170].

Future directions for infection control research

Clues in the Cystic Fibrosis National Registry

The health care community is armed with powerful tools that can be brought to bear in the fight against CF. One such instrument is the CF National Registry, which provides a wealth of information to direct future approaches to disease management and quality improvement. With respect to infection control, the registry tracks local prevalence of airway pathogens at the CF center level. Figs. 3–6 provide a picture of apparently wide regional variation in the prevalence of the most important CF pathogens. Are these figures hinting at regional epidemics? Do they point to local failures of infection control? Is there simply a wide distribution of various pathogens in different geographic locations? Could it be that some centers do not have appropriate protocols for handling CF sputum cultures (thus leading to underreporting of species that require special processing for proper growth)? A recent study indicates that CF centers are generally processing sputum specimens appropriately [171], although the investigation did not specifically address potential problems with data entry into the registry. Regardless, current information suggests that differences in regional prevalence are real and worthy of further investigation.

Strategies for local surveillance

Standards for local microbiologic surveillance have not been universally adopted by CF centers.

However, some guidelines have been advanced, including regular assessment of sputum cultures (at least once per year and preferably quarterly in stable patients [172]), targeting rates of particular epidemiologically important pathogens (eg, MDR-PA, MRSA, BCC), and regular communication with the local infection control team [32]. If a suspicious change in the pattern of sputum isolates seems to be emerging, then further evaluation can be performed, a practice increasingly embraced in Europe and Australia [173–175]. Particularly helpful for United States CF Centers is the CFF *Burkholderia cepacia* Research Laboratory and Repository at the University of Michigan. Molecular typing may identify an epidemic strain that warrants adjustment in local infection control practices to reduce the risk of spread, as was accomplished recently in Boston (David Waltz, personal communication, 2006). With advances in molecular technology, it may eventually be practical to "fingerprint" highly transmissible isolates rapidly at regional clinical microbiology facilities. Initial studies using the PAO1 genome chip [176] and polymerase chain reaction [177–179] have shown promising results.

A broader view of infection control

Discussion of infection control often focuses on reducing PTP spread of pathogenic organisms through direct contact. A comprehensive approach should include examination of the contribution of environmental acquisition from natural reservoirs (environmental factors), the pathogenesis of chronic infection rather than transient colonization (host and pathogen factors), and the contamination of local spaces (behavioral factors), which might affect other patients through indirect contact. This broader view is illustrated in schematic form in Fig. 7. A multipronged approach to infection control is promoted by this model and includes the following components: (1) Identify and reduce patient exposure to environmental reservoirs of respiratory pathogens; (2) reduce the frequency of direct contact with other patients who have CF; (3) eliminate opportunities for contaminated local environments to infect others; and (4) disengage these three mechanisms to further diminish the rate of infection. In most circumstances, the risk of acquisition of an airway pathogen seems to be far greater from environmental sources than via direct or indirect human contact. This suggests that efforts to better understand the factors influencing environmental

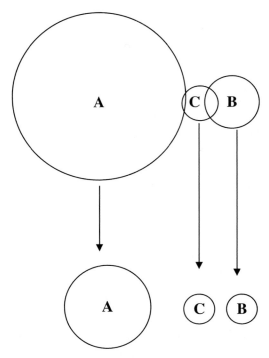

Fig. 7. Strategic approaches to infection control in CF. Venn diagram illustrating various mechanisms of infection in CF. The area of each circle represents its approximate contribution to the overall rate of infection in a population of patients who have CF. (*A*) Acquisition from environmental reservoirs (eg, soil, water sources). (*B*) Direct pathogen acquisition from human contact. (*C*) Infection through contact with local environments contaminated by infected individuals (eg, hospital room, clinic space). This schematic is for illustrative purposes only. The frequency of acquisition by these respective mechanisms (area of the circles) may vary due to local host, pathogen, and environmental factors.

acquisition might have a greater impact on infection control for most patients who have CF than, for example, whether or not HCWs wear gowns and gloves in the outpatient setting. The model predicts that high leverage areas for clinical research might include further development of vaccines against PA [180–182], evaluation of common environmental reservoirs for CF respiratory pathogens [183–185], and exploration of ways to improve hygienic care of respiratory equipment [186]. Research into the underpinnings of CF pathophysiology may yield the most effective control strategy by repairing local host defense machinery in the airway, thereby preventing the establishment of chronic infection.

Acknowledgments

The authors thank John LiPuma for instructive comments and suggestions during his review of the manuscript and David Waltz for his helpful input and provision of radiograph and pathology images.

References

[1] Cystic Fibrosis Foundation patient registry 2005. Cystic Fibrosis Foundation. Bethesda (MD); 2006.
[2] Moore JE, et al. Infection control and the significance of sputum and other respiratory secretions from adult patients with cystic fibrosis. Ann Clin Microbiol Antimicrob 2004;3:8–12.
[3] Isles A, et al. Pseudomonas cepacia infection in cystic fibrosis: an emerging problem. J Pediatr 1984; 104(2):206–10.
[4] Hardy KA, et al. Pseudomonas cepacia in the hospital setting: lack of transmission between cystic fibrosis patients. J Pediatr 1986;109(1):51–4.
[5] Thomassen MJ, et al. Pseudomonas cepacia: decrease in colonization in patients with cystic fibrosis. Am Rev Respir Dis 1986;134(4):669–71.
[6] LiPuma JJ, et al. Person-to-person transmission of Pseudomonas cepacia between patients with cystic fibrosis. Lancet 1990;336(8723):1094–6.
[7] Pegues DA, et al. Acquisition of Pseudomonas cepacia at summer camps for patients with cystic fibrosis. Summer Camp Study Group. J Pediatr 1994; 124(5 Pt 1):694–702.
[8] Johnson WM, Tyler SD, Rozee KR. Linkage analysis of geographic and clinical clusters in Pseudomonas cepacia infections by multilocus enzyme electrophoresis and ribotyping. J Clin Microbiol 1994;32(4):924–30.
[9] Govan JR, et al. Evidence for transmission of Pseudomonas cepacia by social contact in cystic fibrosis. Lancet 1993;342(8862):15–9.
[10] Jones AM, Dodd ME, Webb AK. Burkholderia cepacia: current clinical issues, environmental controversies and ethical dilemmas. Eur Respir J 2001; 17(2):295–301.
[11] Holmes A, et al. An epidemic of Burkholderia cepacia transmitted between patients with and without cystic fibrosis. J Infect Dis 1999;179(5):1197–205.
[12] Ledson MJ, et al. Cross infection between cystic fibrosis patients colonised with Burkholderia cepacia. Thorax 1998;53(5):432–6.
[13] Aris RM, et al. Lung transplantation for cystic fibrosis patients with Burkholderia cepacia complex: survival linked to genomovar type. Am J Respir Crit Care Med 2001;164(11):2102–6.
[14] Chaparro C, et al. Infection with Burkholderia cepacia in cystic fibrosis: outcome following lung transplantation. Am J Respir Crit Care Med 2001; 163(1):43–8.

[15] Webb AK, Egan J. Should patients with cystic fi-brosis infected with Burkholderia cepacia undergo lung transplantation? Thorax 1997;52(8):671–3.

[16] Chen JS, et al. Endemicity and inter-city spread of Burkholderia cepacia genomovar III in cystic fibro-sis. J Pediatr 2001;139(5):643–9.

[17] Speert DP, et al. Epidemiology of Pseudomonas aeruginosa in cystic fibrosis in British Columbia, Canada. Am J Respir Crit Care Med 2002;166(7): 988–93.

[18] Whiteford ML, et al. Outcome of Burkholderia (Pseudomonas) cepacia colonisation in children with cystic fibrosis following a hospital outbreak. Thorax 1995;50(11):1194–8.

[19] Segonds C, et al. Differentiation of Burkholderia species by PCR-restriction fragment length poly-morphism analysis of the 16S rRNA gene and application to cystic fibrosis isolates. J Clin Micro-biol 1999;37(7):2201–8.

[20] LiPuma JJ, et al. Disproportionate distribution of Burkholderia cepacia complex species and trans-missibility markers in cystic fibrosis. Am J Respir Crit Care Med 2001;164(1):92–6.

[21] Biddick R, et al. Evidence of transmission of Burkholderia cepacia, Burkholderia multivorans and Burkholderia dolosa among persons with cystic fibrosis. FEMS Microbiol Lett 2003;228(1): 57–62.

[22] Vermis K, et al. Proposal to accommodate Bur-kholderia cepacia genomovar VI as Burkholderia dolosa sp. nov. Int J Syst Evol Microbiol 2004; 54(Pt 3):689–91.

[23] Kalish LA, et al. Impact of Burkholderia dolosa on lung function and survival in cystic fibrosis. Am J Respir Crit Care Med 2006;173(4):421–5 [Epub 2005 Nov 4].

[24] Duff AJ. Psychological consequences of segrega-tion resulting from chronic Burkholderia cepacia infection in adults with CF. Thorax 2002;57(9): 756–8.

[25] Geddes DM. Of isolates and isolation: Pseudomo-nas aeruginosa in adults with cystic fibrosis. Lancet 2001;358(9281):522–3.

[26] Williams T. Evaluation of antimicrobial sensitivity patterns as markers of Pseudomonas aeruginosa cross-infection at a cystic fibrosis clinic. Br J Biomed Sci 1997;54(3):181–5.

[27] Tenover FC, et al. Interpreting chromosomal DNA restriction patterns produced by pulsed-field gel electrophoresis: criteria for bacterial strain typing. J Clin Microbiol 1995;33(9):2233–9.

[28] Sener B, et al. Epidemiology of chronic Pseudomo-nas aeruginosa infections in cystic fibrosis. Int J Med Microbiol 2001;291(5):387–93.

[29] Harris A, et al. Epidemiology and clinical outcomes of patients with multiresistant Pseudomonas aeru-ginosa. Clin Infect Dis 1999;28(5):1128–33.

[30] Struelens MJ, et al. Genome macrorestriction anal-ysis of diversity and variability of Pseudomonas aeruginosa strains infecting cystic fibrosis patients. J Clin Microbiol 1993;31(9):2320–6.

[31] Grothues D, et al. Genome fingerprinting of Pseu-domonas aeruginosa indicates colonization of cys-tic fibrosis siblings with closely related strains. J Clin Microbiol 1988;26(10):1973–7.

[32] Saiman L, Siegel J. Infection control recommenda-tions for patients with cystic fibrosis: microbiology, important pathogens, and infection control prac-tices to prevent patient-to-patient transmission. In-fect Control Hosp Epidemiol 2003;24(5 Suppl): S6–52.

[33] Renders N, Verbrugh H, Van Belkum A. Dynamics of bacterial colonisation in the respiratory tract of patients with cystic fibrosis. Infect Genet Evol 2001;1(1):29–39.

[34] Hoiby N. Prospects for the prevention and control of pseudomonal infection in children with cystic fibrosis. Paediatr Drugs 2000;2(6):451–63.

[35] West SE, et al. Respiratory infections with Pseudo-monas aeruginosa in children with cystic fibrosis: early detection by serology and assessment of risk factors. JAMA 2002;287(22):2958–67.

[36] Martin DW, et al. Mechanism of conversion to mucoidy in Pseudomonas aeruginosa infecting cys-tic fibrosis patients. Proc Natl Acad Sci U S A 1993; 90(18):8377–81.

[37] Worlitzsch D, et al. Effects of reduced mucus oxy-gen concentration in airway Pseudomonas infec-tions of cystic fibrosis patients. J Clin Invest 2002; 109(3):317–25.

[38] Govan JR, Deretic V. Microbial pathogenesis in cystic fibrosis: mucoid Pseudomonas aeruginosa and Burkholderia cepacia. Microbiol Rev 1996; 60(3):539–74.

[39] Pedersen SS. Lung infection with alginate-produc-ing, mucoid Pseudomonas aeruginosa in cystic fibrosis. APMIS Suppl 1992;28:1–79.

[40] Romling U, et al. Epidemiology of chronic Pseudo-monas aeruginosa infections in cystic fibrosis. J In-fect Dis 1994;170(6):1616–21.

[41] Kerem E, et al. Pulmonary function and clinical course in patients with cystic fibrosis after pulmo-nary colonization with Pseudomonas aeruginosa. J Pediatr 1990;116(5):714–9.

[42] Kosorok MR, et al. Acceleration of lung disease in children with cystic fibrosis after Pseudomonas aer-uginosa acquisition. Pediatr Pulmonol 2001;32(4): 277–87.

[43] Henry RL, Mellis CM, Petrovic L. Mucoid Pseudo-monas aeruginosa is a marker of poor survival in cystic fibrosis. Pediatr Pulmonol 1992;12(3): 158–61.

[44] Lechtzin N, et al. Outcomes of adults with cystic fi-brosis infected with antibiotic-resistant Pseudomo-nas aeruginosa. Respiration 2006;73(1):27–33 [Epub 2005 Aug 17].

[45] Jones AM, et al. Increased treatment requirements of patients with cystic fibrosis who harbour a highly

transmissible strain of Pseudomonas aeruginosa. Thorax 2002;57(11):924–5.

[46] Al-Aloul M, et al. Increased morbidity associated with chronic infection by an epidemic Pseudomonas aeruginosa strain in CF patients. Thorax 2004; 59(4):334–6.

[47] Zembrzuska-Sadkowska E, et al. Epidemiology of Pseudomonas aeruginosa infection and the role of contamination of the environment in the Danish Cystic Fibrosis Centre. J Hosp Infect 1995;29(1): 1–7.

[48] Tubbs D, et al. Pseudomonas aeruginosa in cystic fibrosis: cross-infection and the need for segregation. Respir Med 2001;95(2):147–52.

[49] da Silva Filho LV, et al. Molecular epidemiology of Pseudomonas aeruginosa infections in a cystic fibrosis outpatient clinic. J Med Microbiol 2001; 50(3):261–7.

[50] Kerr JR, et al. Evidence against transmission of Pseudomonas aeruginosa by hands and stethoscopes in a cystic fibrosis unit. J Hosp Infect 2002;50(4):324–6.

[51] Laraya-Cuasay LR, Cundy KR, Huang NN. Pseudomonas carrier rates of patients with cystic fibrosis and of members of their families. J Pediatr 1976; 89(1):23–6.

[52] Tummler B, et al. Nosocomial acquisition of Pseudomonas aeruginosa by cystic fibrosis patients. J Clin Microbiol 1991;29(6):1265–7.

[53] Bosshammer J, et al. Comparative hygienic surveillance of contamination with pseudomonads in a cystic fibrosis ward over a 4-year period. J Hosp Infect 1995;31(4):261–74.

[54] Ojeniyi B, Frederiksen B, Hoiby N. Pseudomonas aeruginosa cross-infection among patients with cystic fibrosis during a winter camp. Pediatr Pulmonol 2000;29(3):177–81.

[55] McCallum SJ, et al. Superinfection with a transmissible strain of Pseudomonas aeruginosa in adults with cystic fibrosis chronically colonised by P aeruginosa. Lancet 2001;358(9281):558–60.

[56] Jones AM, et al. Identification of airborne dissemination of epidemic multiresistant strains of Pseudomonas aeruginosa at a CF centre during a cross infection outbreak. Thorax 2003;58(6):525–7.

[57] Panagea S, et al. Environmental contamination with an epidemic strain of Pseudomonas aeruginosa in a Liverpool cystic fibrosis centre, and study of its survival on dry surfaces. J Hosp Infect 2005;59(2): 102–7.

[58] Scott FW, Pitt TL. Identification and characterization of transmissible Pseudomonas aeruginosa strains in cystic fibrosis patients in England and Wales. J Med Microbiol 2004;53(Pt 7):609–15.

[59] Farrell PM, et al. Acquisition of Pseudomonas aeruginosa in children with cystic fibrosis. Pediatrics 1997;100(5):E2.

[60] Kosorok MR, et al. Comprehensive analysis of risk factors for acquisition of Pseudomonas aeruginosa

in young children with cystic fibrosis. Pediatr Pulmonol 1998;26(2):81–8.

[61] Frederiksen B, Koch C, Hoiby N. Changing epidemiology of Pseudomonas aeruginosa infection in Danish cystic fibrosis patients (1974-1995). Pediatr Pulmonol 1999;28(3):159–66.

[62] Pedersen SS, et al. An epidemic spread of multiresistant Pseudomonas aeruginosa in a cystic fibrosis centre. J Antimicrob Chemother 1986;17(4): 505–16.

[63] Griffiths AL, et al. Effects of segregation on an epidemic Pseudomonas aeruginosa strain in a cystic fibrosis clinic. Am J Respir Crit Care Med 2005; 171(9):1020–5 [Epub 2005 Feb 11].

[64] Jones AM, et al. Prospective surveillance for Pseudomonas aeruginosa cross-infection at a cystic fibrosis center. Am J Respir Crit Care Med 2005; 171(3):257–60 [Epub 2004 Nov 12].

[65] Boukadida J, et al. Molecular epidemiology of chronic pulmonary colonisation by Pseudomonas aeruginosa in cystic fibrosis. J Med Microbiol 1993; 38(1):29–33.

[66] Hoogkamp-Korstanje JA, et al. Risk of cross-colonization and infection by Pseudomonas aeruginosa in a holiday camp for cystic fibrosis patients. J Clin Microbiol 1995;33(3):572–5.

[67] Cheng K, et al. Spread of beta-lactam-resistant Pseudomonas aeruginosa in a cystic fibrosis clinic. Lancet 1996;348(9028):639–42.

[68] Adams C, et al. Epidemiology and clinical impact of Pseudomonas aeruginosa infection in cystic fibrosis using AP-PCR fingerprinting. J Infect 1998; 37(2):151–8.

[69] Jones AM, et al. Spread of a multiresistant strain of Pseudomonas aeruginosa in an adult cystic fibrosis clinic. Lancet 2001;358(9281):557–8.

[70] Goering RV, et al. Staphylococcus aureus in patients with cystic fibrosis: an epidemiological analysis using a combination of traditional and molecular methods. Infection 1990;18(1):57–60.

[71] Foca M, et al. Endemic Pseudomonas aeruginosa infection in a neonatal intensive care unit. N Engl J Med 2000;343(10):695–700.

[72] Doring G, et al. Distribution and transmission of Pseudomonas aeruginosa and Burkholderia cepacia in a hospital ward. Pediatr Pulmonol 1996; 21(2):90–100.

[73] Barth AL, Pitt TL. The high amino-acid content of sputum from cystic fibrosis patients promotes growth of auxotrophic Pseudomonas aeruginosa. J Med Microbiol 1996;45(2):110–9.

[74] Zimakoff J, et al. Epidemiology of Pseudomonas aeruginosa infection and the role of contamination of the environment in a cystic fibrosis clinic. J Hosp Infect 1983;4(1):31–40.

[75] Doring G, et al. Generation of Pseudomonas aeruginosa aerosols during handwashing from contaminated sink drains, transmission to hands of hospital personnel, and its prevention by use of

a new heating device. Zentralbl Hyg Umweltmed 1991;191(5–6):494–505.

[76] Anaissie EJ, Penzak SR, Dignani MC. The hospital water supply as a source of nosocomial infections: a plea for action. Arch Intern Med 2002;162(13): 1483–92.

[77] Jensen ET, et al. Epidemiology of Pseudomonas aeruginosa in cystic fibrosis and the possible role of contamination by dental equipment. J Hosp Infect 1997;36(2):117–22.

[78] Rosenfeld M, et al. Cleaning home nebulizers used by patients with cystic fibrosis: is rinsing with tap water enough? J Hosp Infect 2001;49(3):229–30.

[79] Pitchford KC, et al. Pseudomonas species contamination of cystic fibrosis patients' home inhalation equipment. J Pediatr 1987;111(2):212–6.

[80] Jakobsson BM, et al. Low bacterial contamination of nebulizers in home treatment of cystic fibrosis patients. J Hosp Infect 1997;36(3):201–7.

[81] Jakobsson B, Hjelte L, Nystrom B. Low level of bacterial contamination of mist tents used in home treatment of cystic fibrosis patients. J Hosp Infect 2000;44(1):37–41.

[82] Berrouane YF, et al. Outbreak of severe Pseudomonas aeruginosa infections caused by a contaminated drain in a whirlpool bathtub. Clin Infect Dis 2000;31(6):1331–7 [Epub 2000 Nov 29].

[83] Kuehnert MJ, et al. Prevalence of Staphylococcus aureus nasal colonization in the United States, 2001–2002. J Infect Dis 2006;193(2):172–9 [Epub 2005 Dec 15].

[84] Kirby W. Extraction of a highly potent penicillin inactivator from penicillin resistant Staphylococci. Science 1944;99(2579):452–3.

[85] Barber M. Methicillin-resistant staphylococci. J Clin Pathol 1961;14:385–93.

[86] Hackbarth CJ, Chambers HF. Methicillin-resistant staphylococci: genetics and mechanisms of resistance. Antimicrob Agents Chemother 1989;33(7): 991–4.

[87] Katayama Y, Zhang HZ, Chambers HF. PBP 2a mutations producing very-high-level resistance to beta-lactams. Antimicrob Agents Chemother 2004;48(2):453–9.

[88] Boxerbaum B, Jacobs MR, Cechner RL. Prevalence and significance of methicillin-resistant Staphylococcus aureus in patients with cystic fibrosis. Pediatr Pulmonol 1988;4(3):159–63.

[89] Saravolatz LD, Pohlod DJ, Arking LM. Community-acquired methicillin-resistant Staphylococcus aureus infections: a new source for nosocomial outbreaks. Ann Intern Med 1982;97(3):325–9.

[90] Creech CB 2nd, et al. Increasing rates of nasal carriage of methicillin-resistant Staphylococcus aureus in healthy children. Pediatr Infect Dis J 2005; 24(7):617–21.

[91] Phaff SJ, et al. Macrolide resistance of Staphylococcus aureus and Haemophilus species associated with long-term azithromycin use in cystic fibrosis.

J Antimicrob Chemother 2006;57(4):741–6 [Epub 2006 Feb 9].

[92] Prunier AL, et al. Clinical isolates of Staphylococcus aureus with ribosomal mutations conferring resistance to macrolides. Antimicrob Agents Chemother 2002;46(9):3054–6.

[93] Prunier AL, et al. High rate of macrolide resistance in Staphylococcus aureus strains from patients with cystic fibrosis reveals high proportions of hypermutable strains. J Infect Dis 2003;187(11):1709–16 [Epub 2003 May 15].

[94] Goerke C, et al. Molecular epidemiology of community-acquired Staphylococcus aureus in families with and without cystic fibrosis patients. J Infect Dis 2000;181(3):984–9.

[95] Branger C, Gardye C, Lambert-Zechovsky N. Persistence of Staphylococcus aureus strains among cystic fibrosis patients over extended periods of time. J Med Microbiol 1996;45(4):294–301.

[96] Miall LS, et al. Methicillin resistant Staphylococcus aureus (MRSA) infection in cystic fibrosis. Arch Dis Child 2001;84(2):160–2.

[97] Liou TG, et al. Predictive 5-year survivorship model of cystic fibrosis. Am J Epidemiol 2001; 153(4):345–52.

[98] Looney WJ. Small-colony variants of Staphylococcus aureus. Br J Biomed Sci 2000;57(4):317–22.

[99] Schlichting C, et al. Typing of Staphylococcus aureus by pulsed-field gel electrophoresis, zymotyping, capsular typing, and phage typing: resolution of clonal relationships. J Clin Microbiol 1993; 31(2):227–32.

[100] Givney R, et al. Methicillin-resistant Staphylococcus aureus in a cystic fibrosis unit. J Hosp Infect 1997;35(1):27–36.

[101] Renders NH, et al. Molecular epidemiology of Staphylococcus aureus strains colonizing the lungs of related and unrelated cystic fibrosis patients. Clin Microbiol Infect 1997;3(2):216–21.

[102] Nadesalingam K, Conway SP, Denton M. Risk factors for acquisition of methicillin-resistant Staphylococcus aureus (MRSA) by patients with cystic fibrosis. J Cyst Fibros 2005;4(1):49–52.

[103] Burkholder WH. Sour skin, a bacterial rot of onion bulbs. Phytopathology 1950;40:115–7.

[104] Holmes A, Govan J, Goldstein R. Agricultural use of Burkholderia (Pseudomonas) cepacia: a threat to human health? Emerg Infect Dis 1998;4(2):221–7.

[105] Ramette A, LiPuma JJ, Tiedje JM. Species abundance and diversity of Burkholderia cepacia complex in the environment. Appl Environ Microbiol 2005;71(3):1193–201.

[106] Moore JE, et al. Occurrence of Burkholderia cepacia in foods and waters: clinical implications for patients with cystic fibrosis. J Food Prot 2001;64(7): 1076–8.

[107] LiPuma JJ, Mahenthiralingam E. Commercial use of Burkholderia cepacia. Emerg Infect Dis 1999; 5(2):305–6.

[108] Estivariz CF, et al. An outbreak of Burkholderia cepacia associated with contamination of albuterol and nasal spray. Chest 2006;130(5): 1346–53.

[109] Miller SC, LiPuma JJ, Parke JL. Culture-based and non-growth-dependent detection of the Burkholderia cepacia complex in soil environments. Appl Environ Microbiol 2002;68(8):3750–8.

[110] Lessie TG, et al. Genomic complexity and plasticity of Burkholderia cepacia. FEMS Microbiol Lett 1996;144(2–3):117–28.

[111] Vandamme P, Vanlaere E. Taxonomy and epidemiology of B. cepacia complex: where are we now? Pediatr Pulmonol 2006;S29:114–5.

[112] Winkelstein JA, et al. Chronic granulomatous disease: report on a national registry of 368 patients. Medicine (Baltimore) 2000;79(3):155–69.

[113] Reik R, Spilker T, Lipuma JJ. Distribution of Burkholderia cepacia complex species among isolates recovered from persons with or without cystic fibrosis. J Clin Microbiol 2005;43(6):2926–8.

[114] Martin DW, Mohr CD. Invasion and intracellular survival of Burkholderia cepacia. Infect Immun 2000;68(1):24–9.

[115] Schwab U, et al. Patterns of epithelial cell invasion by different species of the Burkholderia cepacia complex in well-differentiated human airway epithelia. Infect Immun 2002;70(8):4547–55.

[116] Baird RM, et al. Burkholderia cepacia is resistant to the antimicrobial activity of airway epithelial cells. Immunopharmacology 1999;44(3): 267–72.

[117] Maschmeyer G, Gobel UB. Stenotrophomonas maltophilia and Burkholderia cepacia. In: Mandel GL, Bennett JE, Dolin R, editors. Principles and Practices of Infectious Diseases. Philadelphia: Elsevier; 2005. p. 2515–22.

[118] McMenamin JD, et al. Misidentification of Burkholderia cepacia in US cystic fibrosis treatment centers: an analysis of 1,051 recent sputum isolates. Chest 2000;117(6):1661–5.

[119] Coenye T, LiPuma JJ. Molecular epidemiology of Burkholderia species. Front Biosci 2003;8:e55–67.

[120] LiPuma JJ. Burkholderia cepacia: management issues and new insights. Clin Chest Med 1998;19(3): 473–86, vi.

[121] Ledson MJ, et al. Outcome of Burkholderia cepacia colonisation in an adult cystic fibrosis centre. Thorax 2002;57(2):142–5.

[122] Corey M, Farewell V. Determinants of mortality from cystic fibrosis in Canada, 1970-1989. Am J Epidemiol 1996;143(10):1007–17.

[123] Courtney JM, et al. Clinical outcome of Burkholderia cepacia complex infection in cystic fibrosis adults. J Cyst Fibros 2004;3(2):93–8.

[124] Liou TG, Adler FR, Huang D. Use of lung transplantation survival models to refine patient selection in cystic fibrosis. Am J Respir Crit Care Med 2005;171(9):1053–9 [Epub 2005 Feb 1].

[125] Blackburn L, et al. 'Cepacia syndrome' with Burkholderia multivorans, 9 years after initial colonization. J Cyst Fibros 2004;3(2):133–4.

[126] Cunha MV, et al. Molecular analysis of Burkholderia cepacia complex isolates from a Portuguese cystic fibrosis center: a 7-year study. J Clin Microbiol 2003;41(9):4113–20.

[127] Lipuma JJ. Which is the "Bad Cepacia"? Pediatr Pulmonol 2006;S29:118–9.

[128] Pegues DA, et al. Possible nosocomial transmission of Pseudomonas cepacia in patients with cystic fibrosis. Arch Pediatr Adolesc Med 1994;148(8): 805–12.

[129] Tablan OC, et al. Colonization of the respiratory tract with Pseudomonas cepacia in cystic fibrosis: risk factors and outcomes. Chest 1987;91(4): 527–32.

[130] Burdge DR, Nakielna EM, Noble MA. Case-control and vector studies of nosocomial acquisition of Pseudomonas cepacia in adult patients with cystic fibrosis. Infect Control Hosp Epidemiol 1993; 14(3):127–30.

[131] LiPuma JJ, et al. Ribotype analysis of Pseudomonas cepacia from cystic fibrosis treatment centers. J Pediatr 1988;113(5):859–62.

[132] Smith DL, et al. Epidemic of Pseudomonas cepacia in an adult cystic fibrosis unit: evidence of person-to-person transmission. J Clin Microbiol 1993; 31(11):3017–22.

[133] Sun L, et al. The emergence of a highly transmissible lineage of cbl+ Pseudomonas (Burkholderia) cepacia causing CF centre epidemics in North America and Britain. Nat Med 1995;1(7):661–6.

[134] Mahenthiralingam E, et al. Epidemiology of Burkholderia cepacia infection in patients with cystic fibrosis: analysis by randomly amplified polymorphic DNA fingerprinting. J Clin Microbiol 1996; 34(12):2914–20.

[135] Segonds C, et al. Genotypic analysis of Burkholderia cepacia isolates from 13 French cystic fibrosis centers. J Clin Microbiol 1997;35(8):2055–60.

[136] Clode FE, Metherell LA, Pitt TL. Nosocomial acquisition of Burkholderia gladioli in patients with cystic fibrosis. Am J Respir Crit Care Med 1999; 160(1):374–5.

[137] Speert DP, et al. Epidemiology of Burkholderia cepacia complex in patients with cystic fibrosis, Canada. Emerg Infect Dis 2002;8(2):181–7.

[138] Campana S, et al. Transmission of Burkholderia cepacia complex: evidence for new epidemic clones infecting cystic fibrosis patients in Italy. J Clin Microbiol 2005;43(10):5136–42.

[139] Mahenthiralingam E, Simpson DA, Speert DP. Identification and characterization of a novel DNA marker associated with epidemic Burkholderia cepacia strains recovered from patients with cystic fibrosis. J Clin Microbiol 1997;35(4):808–16.

[140] Sajjan US, Forstner JF. Role of a 22-kilodalton pilin protein in binding of Pseudomonas cepacia

to buccal epithelial cells. Infect Immun 1993;61(8): 3157–63.

[141] McDowell A, et al. Epidemiology of Burkholderia cepacia complex species recovered from cystic fibrosis patients: issues related to patient segregation. J Med Microbiol 2004;53(Pt 7):663–8.

[142] Ramsey AH, et al. Burkholderia cepacia lower respiratory tract infection associated with exposure to a respiratory therapist. Infect Control Hosp Epidemiol 2001;22(7):423–6.

[143] Hutchinson GR, et al. Home-use nebulizers: a potential primary source of Burkholderia cepacia and other colistin-resistant, gram-negative bacteria in patients with cystic fibrosis. J Clin Microbiol 1996;34(3):584–7.

[144] Hamill RJ, et al. An outbreak of Burkholderia (formerly Pseudomonas) cepacia respiratory tract colonization and infection associated with nebulized albuterol therapy. Ann Intern Med 1995;122(10): 762–6.

[145] Reboli AC, et al. An outbreak of Burkholderia cepacia lower respiratory tract infection associated with contaminated albuterol nebulization solution. Infect Control Hosp Epidemiol 1996;17(11):741–3.

[146] Gravel D, et al. Outbreak of Burkholderia cepacia in the adult intensive care unit traced to contaminated indigo-carmine dye. Infect Control Hosp Epidemiol 2002;23(2):103–6.

[147] Saiman L, Siegel J. Infection control in cystic fibrosis. Clin Microbiol Rev 2004;17(1):57–71.

[148] Saiman L, et al. Infection control in cystic fibrosis: practical recommendations for the hospital, clinic, and social settings. Am J Infect Control 2000; 28(5):381–5.

[149] Olivier KN, et al. Nontuberculous mycobacteria. II: nested-cohort study of impact on cystic fibrosis lung disease. Am J Respir Crit Care Med 2003; 167(6):835–40 [Epub 2002 Nov 14].

[150] Ramsey BW, et al. The effect of respiratory viral infections on patients with cystic fibrosis. Am J Dis Child 1989;143(6):662–8.

[151] Wang EE, et al. Association of respiratory viral infections with pulmonary deterioration in patients with cystic fibrosis. N Engl J Med 1984;311(26): 1653–8.

[152] Tarran R, et al. Normal and cystic fibrosis airway surface liquid homeostasis: the effects of phasic shear stress and viral infections. J Biol Chem 2005;280(42):35751–9 [Epub 2005 Aug 8].

[153] Larson EL, et al. Effect of antiseptic handwashing vs alcohol sanitizer on health care-associated infections in neonatal intensive care units. Arch Pediatr Adolesc Med 2005;159(4):377–83.

[154] Garner JS. Guideline for isolation precautions in hospitals. Part I: evolution of isolation practices, Hospital Infection Control Practices Advisory Committee. Am J Infect Control 1996;24(1):24–31.

[155] Ensor E, et al. Is Burkholderia (Pseudomonas) cepacia disseminated from cystic fibrosis patients during physiotherapy? J Hosp Infect 1996;32(1): 9–15.

[156] Standaert TA, et al. Effects of repetitive use and cleaning techniques of disposable jet nebulizers on aerosol generation. Chest 1998;114(2):577–86.

[157] Reychler G, et al. In vitro evaluation of efficacy of 5 methods of disinfection on mouthpieces and facemasks contaminated by strains of cystic fibrosis patients. J Cyst Fibros 2005;4(3):183–7.

[158] Rutala WA, et al. Antimicrobial activity of home disinfectants and natural products against potential human pathogens. Infect Control Hosp Epidemiol 2000;21(1):33–8.

[159] Sanborn MR, Wan SK, Bulard R. Microwave sterilization of plastic tissue culture vessels for reuse. Appl Environ Microbiol 1982;44(4):960–4.

[160] Silva MM, et al. Effectiveness of microwave irradiation on the disinfection of complete dentures. Int J Prosthodont 2006;19(3):288–93.

[161] Rutala WA, et al. Efficacy of a washer-pasteurizer for disinfection of respiratory-care equipment. Infect Control Hosp Epidemiol 2000;21(5):333–6.

[162] Bartlett JG. Narrative review: the new epidemic of Clostridium difficile-associated enteric disease. Ann Intern Med 2006;145(10):758–64.

[163] Peach SL, et al. Asymptomatic carriage of Clostridium difficile in patients with cystic fibrosis. J Clin Pathol 1986;39(9):1013–8.

[164] Yahav J, Samra Z, Blau H, et al. Helicobacter pylori and Clostridium difficile in cystic fibrosis patients. Dig Dis Sci 2006;51(12):2274–9.

[165] Binkovitz LA, et al. Atypical presentation of Clostridium difficile colitis in patients with cystic fibrosis. AJR Am J Roentgenol 1999;172(2):517–21.

[166] Zuckerman JB, et al. Measurement of bacterial shedding in CF clinics. Pediatr Pulmonol 2005; (Suppl 28):301.

[167] Steinkamp G, Ullrich G. Different opinions of physicians on the importance of measures to prevent acquisition of Pseudomonas aeruginosa from the environment. J Cyst Fibros 2003;2(4):199–205.

[168] Griffiths AL, et al. Cystic fibrosis patients and families support cross-infection measures. Eur Respir J 2004;24(3):449–52.

[169] Russo K, Donnelly M, Reid AJ. Segregation: the perspectives of young patients and their parents. J Cyst Fibros 2006;5(2):93–9 [Epub 2006 Jan 31].

[170] Mahadeva R, et al. Clinical outcome in relation to care in centres specialising in cystic fibrosis: cross sectional study. Br Med J 1998;316(7147): 1771–5.

[171] Zhou J, et al. Compliance of clinical microbiology laboratories in the United States with current recommendations for processing respiratory tract specimens from patients with cystic fibrosis. J Clin Microbiol 2006;44(4):1547–9.

[172] Yankaskas JR, et al. Cystic fibrosis adult care: consensus conference report. Chest 2004;125(1 Suppl): 1S–39S.

[173] Armstrong DS, et al. Detection of a widespread clone of Pseudomonas aeruginosa in a pediatric cystic fibrosis clinic. Am J Respir Crit Care Med 2002;166(7):983–7.

[174] O'Carroll MR, et al. Clonal strains of Pseudomonas aeruginosa in paediatric and adult cystic fibrosis units. Eur Respir J 2004;24(1):101–6.

[175] Edenborough FP, et al. Genotyping of Pseudomonas aeruginosa in cystic fibrosis suggests need for segregation. J Cyst Fibros 2004;3(1):37–44.

[176] Lewis DA, et al. Identification of DNA markers for a transmissible Pseudomonas aeruginosa cystic fibrosis strain. Am J Respir Cell Mol Biol 2005; 33(1):56–64 [Epub 2005 Apr 15].

[177] Panagea S, et al. PCR-based detection of a cystic fibrosis epidemic strain of Pseudomonas aeruginosa. Mol Diagn 2003;7(3–4):195–200.

[178] Smart CH, et al. Development of a diagnostic test for the Midlands 1 cystic fibrosis epidemic strain of Pseudomonas aeruginosa. J Med Microbiol 2006;55(Pt 8):1085–91.

[179] Parsons YN, et al. Use of subtractive hybridization to identify a diagnostic probe for a cystic fibrosis epidemic strain of Pseudomonas aeruginosa. J Clin Microbiol 2002;40(12):4607–11.

[180] Zuercher AW, et al. Antibody responses induced by long-term vaccination with an octovalent conjugate Pseudomonas aeruginosa vaccine in children with cystic fibrosis. FEMS Immunol Med Microbiol 2006;47(2):302–8.

[181] Pier G. Application of vaccine technology to prevention of Pseudomonas aeruginosa infections. Expert Rev Vaccines 2005;4(5):645–56.

[182] Lang AB, et al. Vaccination of cystic fibrosis patients against Pseudomonas aeruginosa reduces the proportion of patients infected and delays time to infection. Pediatr Infect Dis J 2004;23(6): 504–10.

[183] Vianelli N, et al. Resolution of a Pseudomonas aeruginosa outbreak in a hematology unit with the use of disposable sterile water filters. Haematologica 2006;91(7):983–5 [Epub 2006 Jun 1].

[184] Exner M, et al. Prevention and control of health care-associated waterborne infections in health care facilities. Am J Infect Control 2005;33(5 Suppl 1):S26–40.

[185] Head NE, Yu H. Cross-sectional analysis of clinical and environmental isolates of Pseudomonas aeruginosa: biofilm formation, virulence, and genome diversity. Infect Immun 2004;72(1): 133–44.

[186] Lester MK, et al. Nebulizer use and maintenance by cystic fibrosis patients: a survey study. Respir Care 2004;49(12):1504–8.

**ELSEVIER
SAUNDERS**

Clin Chest Med 28 (2007) 405–421

**CLINICS
IN CHEST
MEDICINE**

Imaging of the Chest in Cystic Fibrosis

Terry E. Robinson, MD

*Department of Pediatrics, Center of Excellence in Pulmonary Biology (Pulmonary Division),
Stanford University Medical Center, 770 Welch Road, Suite 350, Palo Alto, CA 94304-5715, USA*

Cystic fibrosis (CF) is the most common lethal autosomal recessive disease in white populations, affecting nearly 60,000 people worldwide [1,2]. The predominant cause of morbidity and mortality is progressive obstructive lung disease and airway damage resulting from reduced mucociliary clearance, bronchiolar and bronchial obstruction, recurrent endobronchial infections, and persistent inflammation and destruction of the airways [3,4]. Although the lungs of children who have CF are essentially normal at birth, morphologic changes occur quite rapidly within the first year of life [5–7]. Early manifestations of CF lung disease include depletion of airway surface liquid, submucosal gland hypertrophy, and ineffective mucociliary clearance resulting in small and large airway obstruction, development of chronic bacterial infections, and the potential for ensuing chronic airway inflammation leading to airway damage even within the first year of life [5,6,8]. These processes continue throughout the life of the patient who has CF, ultimately leading to pervasive lung destruction and subsequent death.

In the last 2 decades significant strides have been made in the application of chest imaging modalities to assess CF lung disease. In addition, several chest radiograph, chest CT, and other imaging modality (eg, hyperpolarized Helium MRI) scoring systems have been developed, as well as new quantitative imaging outcome measures providing a greater understanding of initial and progressive structural damage that occurs in CF. A unique aspect of CF lung disease is the heterogeneous development of structural changes that occur adjacent to normal-appearing airways and lung parenchyma. Early CF lung disease may affect any lobe and is not distributed evenly

through the lungs [9], as elucidated by high-resolution CT (HRCT) chest imaging in the last 10 years [9–12]. These changes defined by CF CT scoring systems include regional air trapping, regional bronchial wall thickness and bronchiectasis, large and small airway mucus plugging (distal small airway bronchiolar mucus plugging often is manifested as centrilobular nodules), ground-glass opacities, and parenchymal opacities [7,12], which can include the potential for segmental and subsegmental atelectasis that can lead to possible chronic collapse and regional scarring. More severe disease includes these findings with additional cystic bronchiectasis, regional bullae, severe mucus plugging, and pervasive severe air trapping [7,12,13].

Chest imaging of CF lung disease has evolved over the last 2 decades, augmenting pulmonary function tests and traditional chest radiographs to provide a more comprehensive assessment of disease. Recent clinical research using HRCT chest imaging in children who have CF has shown that there is a prominent dissociation between progressive structural damage noted on chest CT scans and either stable or improved pulmonary function in many children who have CF [12–15]. This article covers current chest imaging modalities. It discusses CT, the research modality most commonly used to assess lung disease in CF, new insights regarding CF lung disease, and future directions in research and clinical care.

Chest imaging modalities in cystic fibrosis

Chest radiography

The Cystic Fibrosis Foundation currently recommends that chest radiographs be obtained every 2 to 4 years for routine monitoring of clinically stable patients who have CF and at least

E-mail address: ter@stanford.edu

annually for patients who have frequent infections or declining lung function [16]. To enhance the interpretation of radiographic findings in CF, several scoring systems have been developed over nearly 5 decades to monitor changes in lung disease. These scoring systems have been used either alone or as part of larger clinical scoring systems to evaluate progression of disease. The scoring systems most prominently used include the Schwachman-Kulczycki score [17], the Chrispin-Norman score [18], the Brasfield (BCXR) score [19], the adjusted Chrispin-Norman score [20], the Wisconsin (WCXR) score [21], and the Northern score [22]. All these systems use a variety of scoring methods to assess the distribution and severity of hyperinflation, linear markings, atelectasis, cysts, nodules, and large lesions or opacities found in CF [23]. Terheggen-Lagro and colleagues [24] compared these six scoring systems in 2003 and found low interobserver variability with good limits of agreement between two readers (radiologists) and also good correlation with all pulmonary function measurements. In addition, Cleveland and associates [25], evaluating more than 3000 serial chest radiographs in 230 patients who had CF, found that the BCXR scoring system had good intra- and interobserver reliability and could track the severity of disease reliably, demonstrating progressive disease with advancing age. More recently Farrell and colleagues [26–29] from the Wisconsin CF Neonatal Screening Project demonstrated that quantitative chest radiography was more useful than traditional pulmonary function measurements for following bronchopulmonary disease in children who had CF. In this project the WCXR and BCXR scoring systems were compared with forced expiratory volume in 1 second (FEV_1)/forced vital capacity (FVC), percent predicted FEV_1 and mean midexpiratory flow rate ($FEF_{25-75\%}$), and reserve volume (RV)/total lung capacity (TLC) in children who were followed over a 15-year period from initial diagnosis of CF to adolescence. In 64 patients diagnosed with CF at a median age of 6.71 weeks, time-to-event analysis revealed irreversible abnormalities (primarily peribronchial thickening and bronchiectasis) in quantitative chest radiograph scores in 50% of the patients by 2 years of age compared with initial abnormal airway obstruction on pulmonary function tests that occurred in 50% of the patients at ages 9.91, 15.0, and 10.5 years, respectively, for FEV_1/FVC, percent predicted FEV_1, and percent predicted $FEF_{25-75\%}$ [26]. By 5 years of age, 85% of the children had irreversible

lung disease defined by chest radiograph abnormalities. In this study using a generalized estimating equation, the WCXR score worsened significantly with age, with pancreatic insufficiency, and with the occurrence of two *Staphylococcus aureus*–positive respiratory cultures during the first 2 years of life. These results and other findings from this study suggest that bronchiectasis and other radiographic abnormalities occur before airway obstruction in this CF cohort, that increasing severity of lung disease is more attributable to chronic lower respiratory tract infection rather than to airway obstruction, and that quantitative chest radiograph scores are more sensitive than routine pulmonary function tests in picking up early and progressive lung disease. In a follow-up study that compared 49 neonatal patients screen-positive for CF (mean age at diagnosis, 13.1 weeks) with 40 nonscreened control patients who had CF (mean age at diagnosis, 107 weeks), the initial chest radiograph scores (WCXR and BCXR) were significantly better in the neonatally screened group than in the control group (Table 1) [27]. When defined discriminators of potentially irreversible lung disease (WCXR score ≥5 and BCXR score ≤21) were used, approximately 50% of the control group had reached this stage on the initial chest radiograph near the time of diagnosis, compared with about 25% of the neonatally screened group. In contrast, with longitudinal assessment of these two groups after age 5 years using a generalized estimating equation that accounted for patient group, CF Center, gender, and age, there were significantly worse WCXR and BCXR scores in the neonatally screened group than in the control group ($P = .017$ for WCXR, and $P = .041$ for BCXR) over time. When genotype, pancreatic status, and indicators of *Pseudomonas aeruginosa* infection were also included in a further model for the WCXR and BCXR scores, however, there were no significant differences between groups ($P = .10$ for WCXR, and $P = .20$ for BCXR). Further inspection of WCXR scores related to age demonstrated no obvious difference between groups before age 10 years but subsequent divergence thereafter with significantly higher scores in the neonatally screened group from age 12 years onward. Further analysis of these data evaluating subcomponent WCXR scores revealed significantly higher scores in the neonatally screen group than in the control group for structural airway changes (peribronchial thickness and bronchiectasis) but not in subcomponent scores reflecting hyperinflation (gas trapping). This finding, the authors concluded, suggests that

Table 1
Initial chest radiographic scores in the Wisconsin Cystic Fibrosis Neonatal Screening Project

	Screened group	Control group	P value
Number of patients[a]	49	40	—
Age at diagnosis (in weeks)	13.1 ± 6	107 ± 19	<.001
Age at first chest radiograph (in weeks)	14.3 ± 6	108 ± 19	<.001
WCXR scores (mean ± SEM)	4.2 ± 0.5	7.2 ± 1.0	.012
WCXR scores, age adjusted[b]	4.2 ± 0.7	7.0 ± 0.9	.014
WCXR scores adjusted for age, genotype, and pancreatic status[b]	4.3 ± 0.7	7.2 ± 0.9	.013
BCXR scores[b]	21.7 ± 0.3	20.6 ± 0.4	.022
WCXR scores >5 (%)	33	50	.097
BCXR scores <21 (%)	24	45	.042

WCXR scores (21) range from 0 (normal) to 100 (most severe), whereas the corresponding BCXR scores (19) range from 25 (normal) to 3 (most severe). Both methods quantitate a combination of hyperinflation measures associated with airways obstruction and indicators of infection such as peribronchial thickening and bronchiectasis. Table includes mean ± SEM.

Abbreviations: BCXR, Brasfield chest radiograph; WCXR, Wisconsin chest radiograph.

[a] Seven patients in the screened group and seven in the control group did not have a score for a chest radiograph within the first 6 months of diagnosis.

[b] Because some measures may be age dependent, and the mean ages of the two groups at the time of diagnosis were significantly different, the mean values were recalculated for each group after adjustment for age at the time of diagnosis. The age-adjusted means for the two groups were compared with an analysis of covariance.

Data from Farrell PM, Li Z, Kosorok MR, et al. Bronchopulmonary disease in children with cystic fibrosis after early and delayed diagnosis. Am J Respir Crit Care Med 2003;168:1103.

differences noted in the total WCXR scores were caused largely by indicators of apparent infection rather than by airway obstruction. In contrast, there were no significant differences noted between these two groups in pulmonary function measurements at 7 years of age and over time thereafter.

In a further follow-on study for this project, Li and associates [28] prospectively evaluated 56 patients who had CF from birth to age 16 years using initially obtained oropharyngeal culture swabs and subsequent expectorated sputum samples to assess the longitudinal development of *P aeruginosa* infection, specific antibody responses to *Pseudomonas*, and lung disease progression assessed by chest radiograph scores and pulmonary function measurements. In this study respiratory cultures were obtained from patients every 6 months and at all nonprotocol visits requiring cultures. Antibody titers to *P aeruginosa* were collected every 6 months coinciding with the sputum cultures. Chest radiographs were obtained every 6 months for the first 4 years and annually thereafter and were scored using the WCXR and BCXR scores. Spirometry was initiated around age 4 years and was obtained every 6 months thereafter. In the first 6 months of life, 29% of these patients acquired nonmucoid *P aeruginosa* by first positive result. Between 1 and 13 years of age, 50% of these

patients had their first positive nonmucoid and mucoid *P aeruginosa* cultures. Abrupt elevations in *P aeruginosa* antibody titers occurred with transition from no *P aeruginosa* to nonmucoid *P aeruginosa*, and a second elevation occurred with transition from nonmucoid *P aeruginosa* to mucoid *P aeruginosa*. Chest radiograph scores varied with *P aeruginosa* stage, remaining essentially normal over the non–*P aeruginosa* stage, worsening slightly with nonmucoid acquisition, and worsening significantly with transition from nonmucoid to mucoid *P aeruginosa* (Fig. 1) [28]. Pulmonary function also changed with *P aeruginosa* acquisition but was little affected by the transition from non–*P aeruginosa* to nonmucoid *P aeruginosa* stage and showed significant declines for percent predicted FEV_1, FVC, and $FEF_{25-75\%}$ at a later age. Because of the early acquisition and prevalence of *P aeruginosa* noted in this cohort, the authors concluded that there seems to be a critical window of opportunity within the first few years of life for suppression and possible eradication by antibiotic therapy of initial *P aeruginosa* infection. *Pseudomonas* antibody titers, cough scores, and chest radiograph scoring were more effective than pulmonary function measurements in picking up early signs of nonmucoid *P aeruginosa*.

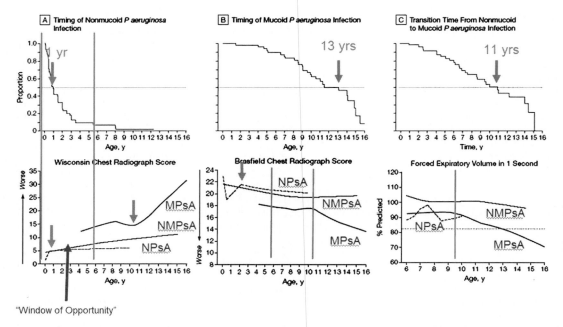

Fig. 1. Time to infection with nonmucoid *Pseudomonas aeruginosa* (NMPsA) and mucoid *Pseudomonas aeruginosa* (MpsA). (*Adapted from* Li Z, Kosorok MR, Farrell PM, et al. Longitudinal development of mucoid *Pseudomonas aeruginosa* infection and lung disease in children with cystic fibrosis. JAMA 2005;293(5):585–6; with permission.)

Recently Lording and colleagues [30] also have evaluated chest radiograph scoring in conjunction with pulmonary function measurements and lower respiratory tract infection in children who had mild variant CF gene mutations. This retrospective cohort study compared 11 patients who had mild CF genotypes (compound heterozygous ΔF508/mild mutation, mainly R117H) with a matched group of patients who had homozygous ΔF508 CF. The mild-variant group had a small but significant difference in the Chrispin-Norman chest radiograph score (median value, 5.1; range, 4–9) compared with the patients who had more severe CF genotypes (median value, 5.8; range, 3–10) (P = .04), a significantly higher Shwachman score (median value for mild variant CF, 94; range, 74–92, versus median value for severe CF, 88; range, 77–91; P < .005), but a non-significant difference in lung function measured by percent predicted FEV_1 (median value for mild-variant CF, 86.5; range, 68–87, versus median value for severe CF, 76.0; range, 65–88; P = .5). S aureus was isolated in 8 of 11 patients who had mild-variant disease, and P aeruginosa was found in seven of these patients as well. Positive cultures, however, were significantly less frequent in the mild-variant group (2.8/year) than in the

severe group (6.1/year) (P < .05). The authors concluded that most patients who have mild-variant CF have positive S aureus and P aeruginosa bacterial airway cultures requiring antibiotic therapy three to four times per year and that anti-Staphylococcal prophylaxis should be considered in the first 2 years of life.

These studies highlight the importance of routine monitoring of early and progressive bronchopulmonary disease in patients who have severe and mild CF genotypes using chest imaging, which is more sensitive than pulmonary function measurements. Optimally, chest imaging should be used in conjunction with pulmonary function tests in infants, preschool and older children, and adults to monitor the onset and progression of CF lung disease.

MRI and hyperpolarized 3-Helium MRI

There has been a growing interest in using chest MRI in patients who have CF because it is a radiation-free imaging modality that allows patients who have chronic conditions to be followed serially without concern for cumulative radiation exposure. MRI has the advantage of good contrast resolution allowing tissue characterization and is able to provide functional assessment of the heart and lungs (cardiac perfusion and lung ventilation studies).

Initial studies of MRI in patients who had CF suggested that it could be useful in assessing lung disease because it detected early mucus plugs and differentiated mucoid impaction from atelectasis [31], differentiated hilar adenopathy from enlarged hilar vessels [32,33], and had the ability to evaluate bronchiectasis [32]. In 1987 Fiel and colleagues [32] compared chest and abdominal MRIs with chest radiographs and abdominal ultrasounds in 16 young adults who had CF to evaluate the utility of MRI in a clinical context. They concluded that chest MRI is superior to chest radiography in detecting hilar and mediastinal adenopathy and differentiating nodes from prominent vascular structures and is useful in the evaluation of bronchiectasis but is less useful than chest radiographs in assessing infiltrates, hyperinflation, sternal bowing, volume loss, and hilar retractions.

In the last 2 decades chest MRI has been used less often than chest CT imaging for both clinical and research applications in patients who have CF because of its lower spatial resolution, longer required imaging acquisition times, and greater need for sedation. Several recent MRI innovations, including increased magnetic field strength (currently 3 Tesla clinically and 7 Tesla for research) to enhance the signal-to-noise ratio, faster acquisition protocols, and use of contrast agents such as gadolinium-dietheylenetriamine

penta-acetic acid (Gd-DTPA) or polarized ^{3}He gas, have addressed these issues to some extent. These innovations have allowed chest MRI to become a more viable option in the assessment of CF lung disease, especially in the realm of functional imaging (ventilation or perfusion studies). Despite these improvements, however, the spatial resolution for MRI continues to be lower than that of chest CT imaging (Fig. 2) and therefore has been used largely only in a research setting.

Several recent studies have used MRI to evaluate hemodynamic changes, pulmonary perfusion, and lung morphology in patients who have CF [34–36]. To evaluate hemodynamic changes that might contribute to pulmonary hypertension, 10 patients who had CF (six females, four males; mean age, 29 ± 6 years) were compared with 15 control volunteers (4 females, 11 males; mean age, 26 ± 6 years) using conventional phase-contrast MRI [34]. Hemodynamic MRI measurements revealed significantly lower flow measures for pulmonary arteries and a greater shunt volume in patients who had CF than in controls. These findings suggest that MRI can detect early signs of pulmonary hypertension in patients who have CF. The impact of structural abnormalities such as bronchiectasis, bronchial wall thickness, mucus plugging, and consolidation on lung perfusion have been studied further in 11 children and adolescents who had CF (9 females, 2 males; median age, 16 years; range, 11–19 years) with contrast-enhanced three-dimensional (3D) MRI using

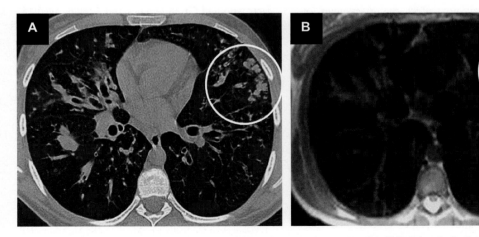

Fig. 2. Comparison between (*A*) inspiratory multislice CT and (*B*) transversal half-Fourier single-shot turbo spin-echo sequence MRI for matched images in the middle and lower lobes of a 16-year-old patient who has CF. Note the severe mucus plugging in segment four of the left lung (white circles). (*From* Puderbach M, Eichinger M, Gahr J, et al. Proton MRI appearance of cystic fibrosis: comparison to CT. Eur Radiol 2007;17(3):718; with permission.)

gadodiamide and specialized postprocessing algorithms to evaluate morphology and perfusion [35].
Two radiologists scored a total of 198 lung
segments for morphologic changes and perfusion
defects. There was good correlation between
normal lung parenchymal segments and normal
homogenous lung perfusion and between severe
morphologic segment changes and significant perfusion defects. Segments with moderate morphologic changes, however, demonstrated normal or
impaired perfusion and could not be differentiated
unless MRI perfusion studies were obtained.
These findings suggest that MRI measurements
of lung perfusion may be useful for earlier detection of vascular abnormalities in patients who
have CF. A recent study assessing the feasibility
of proton MRI in patients who have CF
compared contrast Gd-DTPA MRI and HRCT
imaging for diagnostic purposes in 30 patients
(18 females, 12 males; mean age, 16.9 years) who
had stable CF lung disease [36]. Comparable images by contrast MRI and HRCT imaging were
assessed and showed that morphologic changes
in the lung including bronchiectasis, bronchial
wall thickness, mucus plugging, air fluid levels,
consolidation, and segmental/lobar destruction
could be visualized by MRI, although with lower
spatial resolution than with HRCT. Mild morphologic changes such as peripheral bronchiectasis without bronchial wall thickening, discrete
mucus plugging of small airways, and regional
air trapping were not well visualized by MRI,
however. This limitation seriously affects the assessment of initial and early progressive CF lung
disease but may not affect the assessment of
more advanced disease; therefore MRI imaging
might be useful as a radiation-free imaging modality to monitor structure and function in more
advanced CF lung disease.

Given the low signal-to-noise ratio and low
proton density in the lung, spatial resolution
MRI is substantially lower than in CT imaging,
making evaluation of fine interstitial patterns
and morphologic changes difficult to ascertain.
To address this issue, inhalation of hyperpolarized
Helium (^{3}He) during MRI was used recently in
several studies of patients who had CF to increase
the signal-to-noise ratio, enhancing the detection
of ventilated areas within the lung [37–40]. In
1999 Donnelly and associates [37] studied four
young adults (two males, two females, mean age,
20 years; range, 18–24 years) who had stable
moderate-to-severe CF lung disease to evaluate
preliminary functional and anatomic findings

with combined ^{3}He and conventional proton
MRI. A functional MRI scoring system (Donnelly score) was used to determine the severity
of ventilatory defects based on ^{3}He MRI in these
four patients (Table 2) [37]. Each lung was divided into six zones (upper, middle, and lower
zones with anterior and posterior zones for
each major region) and was scored independently by two radiologists. A total score was
computed as the sum of all 12 zones for the
two lungs. The potential total score ranged
from 0 to 48, with higher scores representing
more severe disease leading to ventilation defects. A morphologic scoring system with a grading scale of 0 to 4 based on percentage of
involvement of bronchial abnormalities (peribronchial thickening, mucus plugging, and bronchiectasis) and acinar replacement (from lung
consolidation, collapse, or bullous change) was
used also, and additional separate grading (0–
4) was used for the presence of hilar, subcarinal,
or mediastinal lymphadenopathy. With this scoring system, the total score for all 12 zones was
144. Both scoring systems were compared with
percent predicted FEV_1 and BCXR scores in
the four patients (Table 3). Both morphologic
and ventilatory defects could be detected in all
four subjects (Fig. 3). There was general correlation between the total MRI scores, BCXR scores,
and percent predicted FEV_1 in the four subjects.
This report is the first to suggest that ventilation defects are related to structural abnormalities of the
lung in patients who have moderate-to-severe CF
lung disease. In a follow-up to this study, 15 subjects who had CF (8 females and 7 males aged 15–
33 years; mean age, 21 years) were compared with
16 healthy adult subjects (8 females and 8 males

Table 2
Scoring system for lung function based on percentage of
lung ventilated as seen on ^{3}He MRI

Grade	Percentage ventilation
0[a]	100
1	76–99
2	51–75
3	26–50
4[b]	1–25

[a] Normal.
[b] Severe disease.
Data from Donnelly LF, MacFall JR, McAdams HP,
et al. Cystic fibrosis: combined hyperpolarized 3He-
enhanced and conventional proton MR imaging in the
lung–preliminary observations. Radiology 1999;212(3):
886.

Table 3
Comparison between MRI scores, chest radiograph scores, and pulmonary function test results in four patients who have CF

Modality (maximum score)	Score (% maximum score)			
	Patient number			
	1	2	3	4
Total MRI imaging (maximum = 144)	39 (27)	50 (35)	52 (36)	66 (46)
Functional ³He MRI (maximum = 48)	29 (60)	25 (52)	31 (65)	25 (52)
Morphologic MRI (maximum = 96)	10 (10)	25 (26)	21 (22)	41 (43)
FEV₁ (percentage of predicted value)	62	29	39	30
Brasfield chest radiograph (maximum = 25)	8	16	12	17

Data from Donnelly LF, MacFall JR, McAdams HP, et al. Cystic fibrosis: combined hyperpolarized 3He-enhanced and conventional proton MR imaging in the lung–preliminary observations. Radiology 1999;212(3): 887.

aged 21–33 years; mean age, 21 years) using hyperpolarized ³He lung ventilation MRI and spirometry at baseline [38]. All subjects who had CF delayed airway clearance on the day of testing until after MRI. In eight patients from the CF group, additional follow-up ³He MRI scans were obtained after administration of nebulized Albuterol and again after recombinant human deoxyribonuclease (DNase) followed by chest physiotherapy. For each ³He MRI study, ventilation defects were identified as areas of the lung either completely lacking a gas signal (appearing black) or having decreased signal intensity compared with surrounding lung tissue. A reader counted these defects for each image, and the total number of all defects for all images was divided by the number of images to obtain the average number of ventilation defects per image (VDI). The VDI was compared with lung function measurements. Healthy subjects had homogenous distribution of ³He gas signal throughout both lungs with fewer defects than subjects who had CF (mean VDI, 1.6 ± 0.8 for normal subjects versus 8.2 ± 3.0 for subjects who had CF; $P < .05$) (Fig. 4). Similarly, the normal subjects had significantly higher percent predicted FEV₁ values (mean FEV₁, 103% ± 13% predicted for normal subjects versus 67% ± 27% predicted for subjects who had

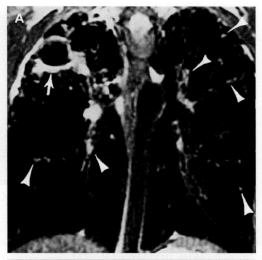
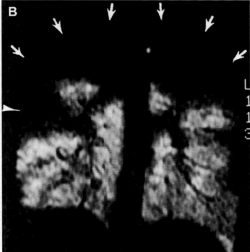

Fig. 3. (*A*) Conventional and (*B*) hyperpolarized 3-He MRI . (*A*) Bullous change (*arrow*) and increased linear nodular signal intensity (*arrowheads*) involving the upper and lower lobes bilaterally. (*B*) Complete absence of signal intensity (*arrows*) noted in upper lobes bilaterally. (*From* Donnelly LF, MacFall JR, McAdams HP, et al. Cystic fibrosis: combined hyperpolarized 3He-enhanced and conventional proton MR imaging in the lung—preliminary observations. Radiology 1999;212(3):888; with permission.)

CF; $P < .05$). In four subjects who had CF but who had normal FEV₁ values (>80% predicted), the number of ventilation defects still was significantly greater than in the normal subjects. For all subjects, there were moderate correlations between VDI and percent predicted FVC, FEV₁, and FEV₁/FVC (−0.59, −0.71,

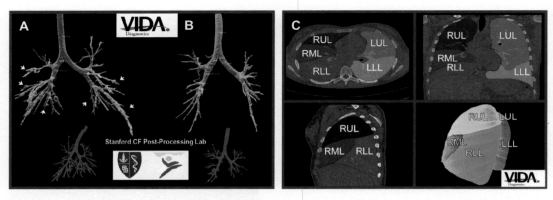

Fig. 4. 3D tracheobronchial airway segmentation (Vida Diagnostics, Inc. and Stanford CF Post-Processing Laboratory) with defined bronchial segments in two adolescents who have CF and 2D and 3D lobar segmentation in a 19-year-old adolescent who has CF. Note the diffuse lobar bronchiectasis (↓) with predominant lower lobe findings in (A) a 15-year-old adolescent who has more severe CF lung disease compared with (B) a 19-year-old adolescent who has mild CF lung disease. (C) Lobar segmentation in the 19-year-old adolescent who has mild CF lung disease. LLL, left lower lobe; LUL, left upper lobe; RLL, right lower lobe; RML. right middle lobe; RUL, right upper lobe.

and −0.65, respectively). There was a small but significant decrease from baseline in the mean VDI of seven of the eight subjects who had CF and who underwent additional ^{3}He MRI scans after administration of Albuterol aerosol. A mild increase in the mean VDI was driven by increases in six of the eight subjects after DNase and chest physiotherapy. This study demonstrated that hyperpolarized ^{3}He MRI correlates with spirometry, can detect changes with treatment, and can identify ventilation defects in patients who have CF and who have normal FEV$_1$ results. In addition, patients who had CF had more ventilation defects than age-matched healthy control subjects.

Two recent observational studies have compared ventilation defects seen using ^{3}He functional MRI and ventilation scores with chest HRCT scoring and spirometry results in eight adults who had CF [39] and with Shwachman and Chrispin-Norman scores and spirometry in 18 children who had CF [40]. In the eight adults who had moderate obstructive lung disease (mean FEV$_1$, 52% ± 29% predicted) there was a significantly strong correlation between the severity of the ventilation defects measured by a modified Donnelly ventilation score and the total modified Bhalla chest HRCT score (r value, −0.89). When individual components for this HRCT score were compared with the modified Donnelly ventilation score, there continued to be significantly strong correlations for the bronchiectasis score (r value, −0.95), the peribronchial thickening score (r value, −0.90), and the mucus

plugging score (r value, −0.85). There was poor correlation between the ventilation score and mosaic perfusion HRCT score (r value, −0.37). When spirometry was compared with the modified Donnelly ventilation score and total modified Bhalla score, there were higher correlations for ^{3}He MRI (^{3}He MRI versus FEV$_1$ and FVC, r = 0.86, r = 0.93, respectively) than for HRCT imaging (HRCT versus FEV$_1$ and FVC, r = −0.72, r = −0.81, respectively). In children who had mild obstructive CF lung disease (mean FEV$_1$, 70% ± 18.5% predicted), diminished but moderate correlations were noted between the Donnelly ventilation score and percent predicted FVC (r = −0.42, P <. 05) and FEV$_1$ (r = −0.41, P < .05). Lower correlations between the ventilation score and Schwachmann and Chrispin-Norman scores also were reported respectively (r = −0.38, P = .06; r = 0.25, P = .159, respectively). These studies demonstrate that functional ^{3}He MRI clearly detects ventilation defects and demonstrate strong correlations with pulmonary function measurements and chest CT imaging in older patients who have with more advanced CF disease. In children who have less obstructive CF lung disease, however, there are only moderate correlations with spirometry and even lower, nonsignificant correlations for Chrispin-Norman chest radiograph scores and Schwachman scores.

Positron emission tomography [^{18}F]-fluorodeoxyglucose

A study in 2006 demonstrated the feasibility of detecting and quantifying regional lung inflammation in adult patients who have CF [41]. This new imaging methodology probably will be used in the future to follow regional infection and early and progressive inflammation that ultimately lead to structural airway damage in patients who have CF. Twenty adult patients who had CF (11 females, 9 males; mean age, 28 ± 10 years) were compared with seven healthy volunteers (age >18 years) using the radionuclide, ^{18}F-fluorodeoxyglucose ([^{18}F]FDG) and positron emission tomography (PET), which is able to detect regional airway inflammation by the neutrophilic uptake of [^{18}F]FDG. In addition, a subset of seven patients who had CF also underwent bronchoscopy with bronchoalveolar lavage (BAL) on the day after initial PET scanning. The uptake of [^{18}F]FDG was measured by the net influx rate constant, K_i. Differences between the CF and normal groups were evaluated initially. Additionally the patients who had CF were stratified by rate of decline in pulmonary function measurements into stable, intermediate, and rapidly declining groups, and the net influx rate constant was compared among these groups. Finally, K_i was correlated against neutrophil concentrations in BAL fluid in the seven patients who had CF and who underwent bronchoscopy. K_i was significantly higher in patients who had CF than in healthy control subjects and in subjects who had CF with more rapidly declining pulmonary function. K_i also was correlated positively with the number of neutrophils in BAL fluid for the seven subjects in the CF group who underwent bronchoscopy. These findings suggest that FDG-PET imaging may be a useful new imaging modality to quantify lung inflammation in patients who have CF and to follow the response to specific anti-inflammatory treatments. With new PET/CT coregistration imaging, this technique could compare regional lung inflammation directly with structural lung damage assessed by HRCT/CT imaging.

CT

During the last decade HRCT has been recognized increasingly as the most effective imaging modality for following progressive CF lung disease. Because of its exquisite ability to detect disease in patients who have asymptomatic CF, normal chest radiographs, and normal pulmonary function measurements [42] and its ability to monitor the progression of disease more effectively than pulmonary function measurements in patients who have more advanced CF disease [43], it now is recognized as the imaging modality that can provide the most information for initial and progressive changes. With the recent understanding that structural lung disease in CF continues to progress despite improved or stable pulmonary function measurements [10,12], it is recognized further that CT indices from CF CT scoring systems and quantitative CT measurements may offer the most sensitive outcome measures for detecting early disease.

The Cystic Fibrosis Foundation has not issued current guidelines specifying the use of high-resolution or spiral CT imaging to monitor the progression of CF lung disease. This lack of guidelines in large part comes from this modality being used initially in a research setting to describe progression of CF lung disease and more recently in clinical trials to evaluate specific therapeutic interventions. Another major reason for the lack of current guidelines may be the concern that CT scanning, with higher radiation exposures than chest radiographs, may lead to significant cumulative exposure in children and adults as they are followed with serial scanning to monitor early and progressive disease. This issue is being addressed now with new low-dose CT scanning protocols on new-generation CT machines cable of adjusting the peak kilovolt, amperage, slice thickness, scan rotation, and pitch settings independently. Because of the technical advances that have occurred, especially with the advent of multidetector CT technology, it now is possible to obtain a low-dose chest inspiratory and expiratory HRCT scan that corresponds to approximately 0.3 mSv [44], or 10-fold less exposure than the annual background radiation at sea level. This exposure is close to that of a posteroanterior and lateral chest radiograph (approximately 0.1 mSv), which would allow patients who have CF to be followed serially by CT imaging every 2 years to monitor progression of disease.

CT technique

Current scanner designs allow the CT technologist to use either thin-slice HRCT imaging or continuous volumetric scans obtained by spiral CT imaging of the entire chest. HRCT techniques sample the lung by acquiring thin 0.5- to 1.5-mm slices every 0.5, 1, or 2 cm with gaps between slices. Scans are obtained from the apex to the base of the lung for inspiratory scans. For expiratory imaging, a smaller number of scans are acquired either evenly spaced or at anatomic determined locations. Typically 20 to 30 HRCT images are acquired during inspiration, and a variable number between 3 and 25 are obtained for expiratory scans. Inspiratory HRCT scans acquired at intervals greater than 10 mm result in significantly lower CF CT severity scores and limit the detection of worsening CT scores at 2 years compared with scans obtained every 10 mm [45]. For expiratory imaging, regional air trapping is assessed best with at least six HRCT images that sample the upper, middle, and lower lung regions [7,11,46–48]. Because the CT scanner must move and stop the patient for each slice, HRCT requires more time than spiral CT, approximately 2 seconds for each slice. For clinical evaluation of lung disease in infants, children, and adults who have CF, it is reasonable to obtain HRCT imaging every 0.5 to 1 cm for inspiratory and expiratory scans using a low-dose protocol (eg, 100 kVp; 30 to 50 mAs; slice thickness, 1.0; scan rotation time, 0.5 seconds). This protocol provides regional information but at low radiation exposures (approximately 0.2–0.3 mSv) corresponding to approximately two to three chest radiographs [44]. For more comprehensive assessments that allow precise serial matching of CT scans, it may be necessary to perform initial spiral volumetric inspiratory and expiratory CT imaging followed by subsequent limited HRCT scans in 2 years that can be matched to the original complete CT dataset. The total radiation exposure with this type of protocol is equivalent to approximately 6 months' background radiation exposure at sea level (1.5 mSv) with a Siemens Sensation 64 CT scanner (100 kVp; 30–50 mAs; slice thickness, 0.5 mm; pitch, 1.0–1.2) (ImPACT CT Patient Dosimetry Calculator {Version $0.99\times$ 20/01/06}, ImPACT scan Organization, London, UK) [49].

Advances in CT technology, particularly the advent of much finer-resolution multidetector scanners with subsecond rotation technology, have resulted in faster scan acquisition and higher resolution CT datasets allowing 3D reconstruction of the lungs and airways. Current multidetector scanners (typically 16–64 detectors) can provide complete volumetric datasets using continuous spiral CT scanning of the entire lung from apex to base in approximately 10 seconds, resulting in typically 800 to 1000 thin-slice images. The latest CT scanners now available offer even finer resolution with 128 detectors. The advantage of these higher detector scanners is chiefly in the greater resolution in the Z direction (head to toe) for 3D reconstructions of the lung and airways and shorter total scan times. Spiral volumetric

imaging facilitates better serial matching of airways and air trapping for evaluating therapeutic interventions, as well as providing comprehensive 3D assessments of lung parenchyma and airway abnormalities in CF [44]. With low-dose CT settings this technique can segment the lung into lobes, and can obtain airway measurements out to the fifth- and sixth-generation airways for each lobe (see Fig. 4).

Lung volume control

CT scans are acquired by volitional breath holds, typically directed by the CT technologist during inspiratory and expiratory imaging [9,10,12,13–15,23,42,43,45,50–65] or by standardized volume control techniques (controlled-ventilation CT scanning in infants [66–72] or spirometer-controlled CT in older children and adults [7,11,44,46–48]). CT scan acquisition, especially expiratory scans, is affected by the lung volume at which the scans are obtained. Previous research has shown that quantitative air trapping and global lung density are influenced by the lung volume at which the CT scans are acquired [11]. Expiratory scans obtained at near functional residual capacity lead to significantly higher quantitative air-trapping values and lower lung-density values than scans obtained in the same patient at lower lung volumes corresponding to near residual volume [7,11]. Expiratory CT scans at different lung volumes on serial studies therefore can lead to erroneously higher air-trapping and lower lung-attenuation values, limiting the ability of CT scanning to detect changes following an intervention. Quantitative airway measurements also are affected by the degree of lung inflation [73].

Controlled-ventilation CT scanning in infants requires deep conscious sedation. Respirations are controlled by a respiratory therapist using a positive-pressure facemask and a bias flow device at the scanner to obtain images at full inspiration ($+25$ cm H_2O) [74]. For expiratory images, no mask pressure is applied, and the lungs deflate to near functional residual capacity ($+0$ cm H_2O) [74]. For spirometer-controlled CT imaging, a portable spirometer unit is used adjacent to the scanner to inhibit airflow at preselected lung volumes corresponding to full inflation and near residual volume [75]. Inspiratory and expiratory thresholds are determined initially by supine lung volume measurements, which are used later for planned scanned acquisitions. For inspiratory scans, the threshold is set at 95% slow vital capacity (SVC) or higher. For expiratory scans, the threshold typically is set to lung volumes corresponding to 5% to 12% SVC. This technique allows standardization of CT measurements at comparable lung volumes for serial evaluations and objective quantitative CT measurements.

High-resolution CT scoring systems

In 1991, Bhalla and associates [50] published the first HRCT scoring system for CF. In the same year Nathanson and colleagues also published a CF HRCT scoring system [51]. Since then several modifications or alternative HRCT scoring systems have been developed that identify and assess the severity of CT features associated with CF lung disease (Table 4) [23]. All scoring systems include bronchiectasis, peribronchial thickening, mucus plugging, and parenchymal opacities [12]. Some of the scoring systems include small nodules, mosaic attenuation, sacculations, and air trapping on expiratory images. Scoring systems differ in how features are defined anatomically (eg, lobar regions versus zones) [12]. For all

these scoring systems, each component score is added to provide a final total CT score. Although there are inherent differences in scoring systems, comparisons of five of these HRCT scoring systems [50,54–56,76] showed good interobserver and intraobserver reproducibility and reliability, and all scoring systems had moderate-to-strong correlations with pulmonary function measurements [14,23]. Despite these promising results, the major limitations of HRCT scoring systems have been lower reproducibility with longer intervals of time (1–2 months) between repeat measurements, increased interobserver variability for low HRCT scores in healthier subjects, and the lack of clear definitions for some of the HRCT scoring components [14,77].

Two other scoring systems have been recently developed. One provides an approach for evaluating the extent and severity of CT features in CF lung disease by lobar distribution [78]. The other provides a method of combining different measures of HRCT component scores and lung

Table 4
CF HRCT scoring systems

Original system: first author (year) modification of system: first author (year)	Reference	No. of patients	Age range (in years)	Clinical status	No. of HRCT parameters assessed	Regional weighting
Bhalla (1991)	[50]	14	5–42	Not stated	9	BP
Santamaria (1998)	[54]	30	6.75–24 (mean = 13.9; median = 13.2)	Not stated	11 (AT)	BP
Helbich (1999)	[55]	107	2.8–32.3 (mean = 14.5 ± 7.3)	Stable/not infected	10	BP
Robinson (2001)	[46]	17	9–33 (mean = 17.3 ± 7.2)	During acute exacerbation	6 (AT)	SL/sl
Oikonomou (2002)	[59]	47	6.42–23.3 (mean = 13.6 ± 4.8)	During remission	11	SL/sl and BP
Nathanson (1991)	[51]	28	0.5–35 (mean = 14.1 ± 1.7)	Not stated	2	Z
Maffessanti (1996)	[52]	36	5–28 (mean = 13)	Stable	7	R
Brody (1999)	[56]	8	5–16 (mean = 12.7, median = 13.3)	During acute exacerbation	7	SL/sl
Castile (2000)	[76]	31	0.2–5.5 (mean = 2.3 ± 1.3)	Not stated	8 (AT)	R

Abbreviations: AT, air trapping (includes air trapping in assessment); BP, anatomic bronchopulmonary segments (18 total: 10 right, 8 left); R, each lung divided into superior and inferior halves; SL/sl, CT at six levels (SL) in six lobes (sl) with lingula of left upper lobe considered a separate lobe; Z, each lung divided into upper, middle, and lower regions and each region further divided into anterior and posterior areas.

Data from Moskowitz SM, Gibson RL, Effmann EL. Cystic fibrosis lung disease: genetic influences, microbial interactions, and radiological assessment. Pediatr Radiol 2005;35:750.

function to obtain a more sensitive outcome measure to discriminate treatment effects in young patients who have mild CF disease [79]. The first scoring system was evaluated in 16 HRCT scans obtained in children who had CF and who were participating in the Wisconsin CF Neonatal Screening Project [78]. This scoring system demonstrated good agreement and sensitivity and demonstrated excellent reproducibility. The second scoring system, the composite CT/pulmonary function test score, demonstrated that by combining different measures of structure and function in CF assessment, a more sensitive outcome measure could be developed that better discriminated treatment effects in young patients who had mild CF disease [79]. In this 1-year, double-blind, placebo-controlled study of rhDNase in children, the largest treatment effect measured by change from baseline was in the composite CT/pulmonary function test score (30% change), compared with 13% for $FEF_{25-75\%}$ and 6% for the total HRCT score.

Despite the promising results for HRCT scoring systems in the past 10 years, only one study using an HRCT scoring system demonstrated a significant difference in the total HRCT score after a specific therapeutic intervention other than antibiotic therapy for a pulmonary exacerbation in patients who had CF [58]. In five clinical interventions, including two rhDNase studies in children who had mild CF lung disease [15,79], gene therapy using an adeno-associated virus vector in children and adults who had CF [61], a P_2Y_2 chloride-channel receptor agonist (Inspire) in children and adults who had CF [62], and the use of tobramycin solution for inhalation in children and adults who had CF [65], total HRCT scores have shown no significant difference in treatment effects between groups.

Quantitative CT measurements

Computer analysis of CT datasets offers an objective, reproducible method for quantifying structural changes in CF lung disease. Computer programs have been developed to evaluate both lung parenchyma and airway morphology. Quantitative CT programs that evaluate lung parenchyma assess either (1) global lung hyperinflation, typically obtained from lung density measurements noted on segmented expiratory lung images [11,47,70], or (2) regional air trapping, determined by obtaining the percentage of segmented expiratory lung that is considered air trapped (quantitative air trapping) [11,47,48]. In CF, the best-studied parameter using computerized analysis of CT scans is quantitative air trapping [11,47,48]. Regional air trapping, a finding present in early CF lung disease, reflects small airway obstruction that can be measured indirectly from quantitative CT techniques. In a study comparing 25 subjects who had mild CF lung disease with 10 normal subjects, only the RV/TLC was statistically different ($P = .011$) between groups for all pulmonary function test measurements [47]. When these two groups were compared further with quantitative CT measurements, however, the quantitative air-trapping measurement showed a far greater statistical difference between groups, demonstrating much greater sensitivity ($P = .0003$). These 25 subjects who had CF were studied further in a 1-year, randomized, double-blind, placebo-controlled trial evaluating rhDNase in children who had mild CF lung disease [48]. No significant differences were noted between rhDNase and placebo aerosol groups for any pulmonary function test measurements after 3 and 12 months of treatment. There was a significant difference in quantitative air-trapping measurements between groups at 3 months and a nearly significant difference between groups at 12 months despite a smaller number of participating subjects [48].

Computer programs also have been developed to quantify airway morphology for single-slice axial CT images [14,80–84] and 3D volumetric datasets that involve initial airway segmentation and subsequent airway measurements [84–88]. Previous validation studies of airway measurements [80,89–91] show reasonable correlations between quantitative CT determined airway measures and corresponding pathologic airway measurements down to airway sizes of 2 to 3.5 mm in diameter [83,89]. In cross-sectional data of infants who have CF, quantitative airway measurements obtained from single-slice axial CT images have shown an increase in airway wall thickness and lumen area (bronchiectasis) in infants who have CF compared with normal control infants [69,92]. In infants who have CF, the severity of the bronchiectasis as measured by the dilatation of the airway lumen also increased significantly with age, whereas in the control subjects there was no significant increase with age. In a further cross-sectional study of older children who have CF, de Jong and associates [14] did not find a correlation between quantitative airway measurements and pulmonary function tests.

In an additional longitudinal study in children who have CF (baseline mean age, 11.1 years) in which quantitative CT airway measurements and pulmonary function tests were obtained at baseline and after a 2-year interval, quantitative airway wall thickness increased without increases in lumen area, and increases in airway wall thickness correlated with decreases in percent predicted $FEF_{25-75\%}$ [82]. This study suggests that although bronchial dilatation in these school-aged children did not progress (bronchiectasis stable), there was still progression of airway wall thickness that impacted airway function. In a similar fashion, Martinez and associates [70] recently have demonstrated that in infants who have CF, airway walls are thickened and airway lumens are narrowed compared with age-matched normal control infants. Among infants who have CF, there was a greater ratio of airway wall:lumen area, which also correlated with lower airway function as measured by $FEV_{0.5}$ values.

New insights on progression of cystic fibrosis structural lung disease

Cumulative chest imaging research during the last decade in infants, children, and adults who have CF has provided a better understanding of early and progressive lung disease.

In CF, a continuum of progressive lung changes occurs over time, with different structural components emphasized, depending on the developmental phase of the disease (Fig. 5). In early disease, regional air trapping (pulmonary lobular air trapping), bronchial wall thickness, and possibly limited mucus plugging in peripheral small airways (centrolobular nodules) can be demonstrated. In more progressed disease, more extensive bronchial wall thickness, cylindrical bronchiectasis, and increased air trapping (subsegmental and segmental to lobar air trapping) can be demonstrated. Additional large airway mucus plugging can also be present. As the disease progresses, bronchiectasis continues to evolve from initial cylindrical to ultimate cystic bronchiectasis, and severe mucus plugging occurs. More severe disease also is manifested by global air trapping and chronic atelectasis and consolidation. Unique to CF is the characteristic heterogeneous distribution of these structural changes that occur regionally and can be demonstrated at different stages of progressive lung damage. In the last 5 years CT scans in infants and children who have CF have unmasked early, previously undetectable, changes in lung structure that precede detectable changes in pulmonary function. Early disease is manifested primarily by regional air trapping and bronchial wall thickness that impacts hyperinflation (RV/TLC) and probably contributes to the initial finding of elevated lung clearance index noted in young children who have mild CF disease. Recent research further suggests that acute and chronic lower respiratory tract infections with *Haemophilus influenzae, S aureus, P aeruginosa*, and other bacteria probably leads to persistent airway

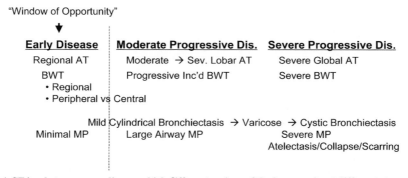

Progression of CF Structural Lung Disease

"Window of Opportunity"

Early Disease	Moderate Progressive Dis.	Severe Progressive Dis.
Regional AT	Moderate → Sev. Lobar AT	Severe Global AT
BWT	Progressive Inc'd BWT	Severe BWT
• Regional		
• Peripheral vs Central		

Mild Cylindrical Bronchiectasis → Varicose → Cystic Bronchiectasis

| Minimal MP | Large Airway MP | Severe MP |
| | | Atelectasis/Collapse/Scarring |

* CF is a heterogenous disease which different regions of the lung can be at different stages of early/moderate to more advanced/severe disease.

Fig. 5. CF is a heterogeneous disease in which different regions of the lung can be at different stages of early/moderate to more advanced/severe disease. CF lung disease is a continuum of progressive structural lung changes that occur over time and have different emphasized structural components depending on the developmental phase of the lung disease. AT, airway trapping; BWT, bronchial wall thickness; MP, mucus plugging.

damage from chronic airway inflammation [72,93,94]. Work by Farrell and associates [26–28] from the Wisconsin Neonatal screening project indicates there is a critical window of opportunity to address early changes in CF disease to prevent or possibly reverse early structural damage that ultimately leads to irreversible bronchiectasis. This possibility requires a paradigm shift from routine treatment of CF lung disease to treatment strategies directed at prevention or reversal of early lung disease: early implementation of therapies directed at mucociliary clearance (hypertonic saline, Pulmozyme aerosol) and potential prophylactic or eradication strategies for identified lower respiratory tract bacteria. To address these early changes, sensitive outcome measures that can assess early structure and functional changes must be studied, and closer surveillance protocols must be developed to follow progression of early and advancing disease more closely.

Summary

In the last 2 decades significant strides have been made in the application of chest imaging modalities to assess CF lung disease. Current imaging modalities are able to localize lung inflammation (PET imaging with 18-FDG), provide functional assessment of the heart and lungs (MRI), delineate initial and progressive structural lung disease (chest CT, chest radiography), and detect regional lung damage (chest CT, other modalities) before changes are seen in global spirometry measurements. During the next decade strategies must be implemented to monitor early and progressive disease by optimizing imaging and functional assessments, and strategies must be developed for optimal treatment of CF lung disease.

References

[1] Davis PB, Drumm M, Konstan MW. Cystic fibrosis. Am J Respir Crit Care Med 1996;154:1229–56.

[2] Moss RB. Long-term benefits of inhaled tobramycin in adolescent patients with cystic fibrosis. Chest 2002; 121:55–63.

[3] Esterly JR, Oppenheimer EH. Observations in cystic fibrosis of the pancreas, 3: pulmonary lesions. Johns Hopkins Med J 1968;122:94–101.

[4] Lynch D, Brasch R, Hardy K, et al. Pediatric pulmonary disease: assessment with high-resolution ultrafast CT. Radiology 1990;176:243–8.

[5] Boucher RC. New concepts of the pathogenesis of cystic fibrosis lung disease. Eur Respir J 2004;23: 146–58.

[6] Brody AS. Early morphologic changes in the lungs of asymptomatic infants and young children with cystic fibrosis. J Pediatr 2004;144:145–6.

[7] Robinson TE. High-resolution CT scanning: potential outcome measure. Curr Opin Pulm Med 2004; 10(6):537–41.

[8] Mall M, Grubb BR, Harkema JR, et al. Increased airway epithelial Na$^+$ absorption produces cystic fibrosis-like lung disease in mice. Nat Med 2004; 10(5):487–93.

[9] Helbich TH, Heinz-Peer G, Eichler I, et al. Cystic fibrosis: CT assessment of lung involvement in children and adults. Radiology 1999;213:537–44.

[10] Tiddens HA. Detecting early structural lung damage in cystic fibrosis. Pediatr Pulmonol 2002;34(3):228–31.

[11] Bonnel AS, Song SM, Kesavaraju K, et al. Quantitative air trapping analysis in children with mild cystic fibrosis pulmonary disease. Pediatr Pulmonol 2004; 38:396–405.

[12] Brody AS, Tiddens HA, Castile RG, et al. Computed tomography in the evaluation of cystic fibrosis lung disease. Am J Respir Crit Care Med 2005; 172(10):1246–52.

[13] Tiddens HA, de Jong PA. Update on the application of chest computed tomography scanning to cystic fibrosis. Curr Opin Pulm Med 2006;12(6):433–9.

[14] de Jong PA, Ottink MD, Robben SG, et al. Pulmonary disease assessment in cystic fibrosis: comparison of CT scoring systems and value of bronchial and arterial dimension measurements. Radiology 2004;231(2):434–9.

[15] Brody AS, Klein JS, Molina PL, et al. High-resolution computed tomography in young patients with cystic fibrosis: distribution of abnormalities and correlation with pulmonary function tests. J Pediatr 2004;145(1):32–8.

[16] Clinical practice guidelines for cystic fibrosis. Bethesda (MD): Cystic Fibrosis Foundation; 1997.

[17] Shwachman H, Kulczycki LL. Long term study of 105 patients with CF. Am J Dis Child 1958;96:6–15.

[18] Chrispin AR, Norman AP. The systematic evaluation of a chest radiograph in CF. Pediatr Radiol 1974;2:101–6.

[19] Brasfield D, Hicks G, Soong S, et al. The chest roentgenogram in CF: a new scoring system. Pediatrics 1979;63:24–9.

[20] van der Put JM, Meradji M, Danosastro D, et al. Chest radiographs in cystic fibrosis. A follow-up study with application of a quantitative scoring system. Pediatr Radiol 1982;12:57–61.

[21] Weatherly MR, Palmer CGS, Peters ME, et al. Wisconsin cystic fibrosis chest radiograph scoring system. Pediatrics 1993;91:488–95.

[22] Conway SP, Pond MN, Bowler I, et al. The chest radiograph in CF, a new scoring system compared with the Chrispin-Norman and Brasfield scores. Thorax 1994;49:860–2.

[23] Moskowitz SM, Gibson RL, Effmann EL. Cystic fibrosis lung disease: genetic influences, microbial

interactions, and radiological assessment. Pediatr Radiol 2005;35:739–57.

[24] Terheggen-Lagro S, Truijens N, van Poppel N, et al. Correlation of six different cystic fibrosis chest radiograph scoring systems with clinical parameters. Pediatr Pulmonol 2002;35:441–5.

[25] Cleveland RH, Neish AS, Zurakowski D, et al. Cystic fibrosis: a system for assessing and predicting progression. AJR 1998;170:1067–72.

[26] Farrell PM, Li Z, Kosorok MR, et al. Longitudinal evaluation of bronchopulmonary disease in children with cystic fibrosis. Pediatr Pulmonol 2003;36:230–40.

[27] Farrell PM, Li Z, Kosorok MR, et al. Bronchopulmonay disease in children with cystic fibrosis after early and delayed diagnosis. Am J Respir Crit Care Med 2003;168:1100–8.

[28] Li Z, Kosorok MR, Farrell PM, et al. Longitudinal development of mucoid Pseudomonas aeruginosa infection and lung disease in children with cystic fibrosis. JAMA 2005;293(5):581–8.

[29] Farrell PM, Lai HJ, Li Z, et al. Evidence on improved outcomes with early diagnosis of cystic fibrosis through neonatal screening: enough is enough. J Pediatr 2005;147:S30–6.

[30] Lording A, McGaw J, Dalton A, et al. Pulmonary infection in mild variant cystic fibrosis: implications for care. J Cyst Fibros 2006;5(2):101–4.

[31] Gooding CA, Lallemand DP, Brasch RC, et al. Magnetic resonance imaging in cystic fibrosis. J Pediatr 1984;105:384–8.

[32] Fiel SB, Friedman AC, Caroline DF, et al. Magnetic resonance imaging in young adults with cystic fibrosis. Chest 1987;91:181–4.

[33] Kinsella D, Hamilton A, Goddard P, et al. The role of magnetic resonance imaging in cystic fibrosis. Clin Radiol 1991;44:23–6.

[34] Ley S, Puderbach M, Eichinger M, et al. Assessment of hemodynamic changes in the systemic and pulmonary arterial circulation in patients with cystic fibrosis using phase-contrast MRI. Eur Radiol 2005;15:1575–80.

[35] Eichinger M, Puderbach M, Fink C, et al. Contrast-enhance 3D MRI of lung perfusion in children with cystic fibrosis—initial results. Eur Radiol 2006;16:2147–52.

[36] Puderbach M, Eichinger M, Gahr J, et al. Proton MRI appearance of cystic fibrosis: comparison to CT. Eur Radiol 2007;17(3):716–24.

[37] Donnelly LF, MacFall JR, McAdams HP, et al. Cystic fibrosis: combined hyperpolarized 3He-enhanced and conventional proton MR imaging in the lung–preliminary observations. Radiology 1999;212(3):885–9.

[38] Mentore K, Froh DK, de Lange EE, et al. Hyperpolarized He 3 MRI of the lung in cystic fibrosis: assessment at baseline and after bronchodilator and airway clearance treatment. Acad Radiol 2005;12(11):1423–9.

[39] McMahon CJ, Dodd JD, Hill C, et al. Hyperpolarized (3)helium magnetic resonance ventilation imaging of the lung in cystic fibrosis: comparison with high resolution CT and spirometry. Eur Radiol 2006;16(11):2483–90.

[40] van Beek EJ, Hill C, Woodhouse N, et al. Assessment of lung disease in children with cystic fibrosis using hyperpolarized 3-Helium MRI: comparison with Shwachman score, Chrispin-Norman score and spirometry. Eur Radiol 2007;17(4):1018–24.

[41] Chen DL, Ferkol TW, Mintun MA, et al. Quantifying pulmonary inflammation in cystic fibrosis with positron emission tomography. Am J Respir Crit Care Med 2006;173(12):1363–9.

[42] de Jong PA, Nakano Y, Lequin MH, et al. Progressive damage on high resolution computed tomography despite stable lung function in cystic fibrosis. Eur Respir J 2004;23:93–7.

[43] Judge EP, Dodd JD, Masterson JB, et al. Pulmonary abnormalities on high-resolution CT demonstrates more rapid decline than FEV$_1$ in adults with cystic fibrosis. Chest 2006;130:1424–32.

[44] Robinson TE. CT scanning techniques for the evaluation of cystic fibrosis lung disease. Proceedings of the American Thoracic Society 2007, accepted for publication.

[45] de Jong PA, Nakano Y, Lequin MH, et al. Dose reduction for CT in children with cystic fibrosis: is it feasible to reduce the number of images per scan. Pediatr Radiol 2006;36:50–3.

[46] Robinson TE, Leung AN, Northway WH, et al. Spirometer-triggered high-resolution computed tomography and pulmonary function measurements during an acute exacerbation in patients with cystic fibrosis. J Pediatr 2001;138:553–9.

[47] Goris ML, Zhu HJ, Blankenberg F, et al. An automated approach to quantitative air trapping measurements in mild cystic fibrosis. Chest 2003;123:1655–63.

[48] Robinson TE, Goris ML, Zhu HJ, et al. Changes in quantitative air trapping, pulmonary function, and chest HRCT scores in CF children during a Pulmozyme intervention study. Chest 2005;128:2327–35.

[49] Jones D, PC Shrimpton. Survey of CT practice in the UK: normalised organ doses for x-ray computed tomography calculated using Monte Carlo techniques. National Radiological Protection Board. Harwell UK 1991. Available at: www.impactscan.org/ctdosimetry.htm.

[50] Bhalla M, Turcios N, Aponte V, et al. Cystic fibrosis: scoring system with thin-section CT. Radiology 1991;179:783–8.

[51] Nathanson I, Conboy K, Murphy S, et al. Ultrafast computerized tomography of the chest in cystic fibrosis: a new scoring system. Pediatr Pulmonol 1991;11:81–6.

[52] Maffessanti M, Candusso M, Brizzi F, et al. Cystic fibrosis in children: HRCT findings and distribution of disease. J Thorac Imaging 1996;11:27–38.

[53] Shah RM, Sexauer W, Ostrum BJ, et al. High-resolution CT in the acute exacerbation of cystic fibrosis:
evaluation of acute findings, reversibility of those
findings, and clinical correlation. AJR Am J Roentgenol 1997;169:375–80.

[54] Santamaria F, Grillo G, Guidi G, et al. Cystic fibrosis: when should high-resolution computed tomography of the chest be obtained? Pediatrics 1998;
101:908–13.

[55] Helbich TH, Heinz-Peer G, Fleischmann D, et al.
Evolution of CT findings in patients with cystic
fibrosis. AJR Am J Roentgenol 1999;173:81–8.

[56] Brody AS, Molina PL, Klein JS, et al. High-resolution computed tomography of the chest in children
with cystic fibrosis: support for use as an outcome
surrogate. Pediatr Radiol 1999;29:731–5.

[57] Demirkazik FB, Ariyurek OM, Ozcelik U, et al.
High resolution CT in children with cystic fibrosis:
correlation with pulmonary functions and radiographic scores. Eur J Radiol 2001;37:54–9.

[58] Nasr SZ, Kuhns LR, Brown RW, et al. Use of computerized tomography and chest x-rays in evaluating
efficacy of aerosolized recombinant human DNase
in cystic fibrosis patients younger than age 5 years:
a preliminary study. Pediatr Pulmonol 2001;31:
377–82.

[59] Oikonomou A, Manavis J, Karagianni P, et al. Loss
of FEV1 in cystic fibrosis: correlation with HRCT
features. Eur Radiol 2002;12:2229–35.

[60] Dakin CJ, Pereira JK, Henry RL, et al. Relationship
between sputum inflammatory markers, lung function, and lung pathology on high-resolution computed tomography in children with cystic fibrosis.
Pediatr Pulmonol 2002;33:475–82.

[61] Moss RB, Rodman D, Spencer LT, et al. Repeated
adeno-associated virus serotype 2 aerosol-mediated
cystic fibrosis transmembrane regulator gene transfer to the lungs of patients with cystic fibrosis: a multicenter, doubleblind, placebo-controlled trial. Chest
2004;125:509–21.

[62] Brody AS, Robinson TE, Knowles MR, et al. The
use of high-resolution CT in intervention studies of
cystic fibrosis. Pediatr Pulmonol 2004;27(Suppl):
298.

[63] Brody AS, Sucharew H, Campbell JD, et al.
Computed tomography correlates with pulmonary
exacerbations in children with cystic fibrosis. Am J
Respir Crit Care Med 2005;172:1128–32.

[64] de Jong PA, Lindblad A, Rubin L, et al. Progression
of lung disease on computed tomography and pulmonary function tests in children and adults with
cystic fibrosis. Thorax 2006;61:80–5.

[65] Nasr SZ, Gordon D, Sakmar E, et al. High resolution computerized tomography of the chest and
pulmonary function testing in evaluating the effect
of tobramycin solution for inhalation in cystic fibrosis patients. Pediatr Pulmonol 2006;41:1129–37.

[66] Long FR, Castile RG, Brody AS, et al. Lungs in infants and young children: improved thin-section CT

with a noninvasive controlled-ventilation technique—
initial experience. Radiology 1999;212:588–93.

[67] Long FR, Castile RG. Technique and clinical
application of full-inflation and end-exhalation
controlled-ventilation chest CT in infants and young
children. Pediatr Radiol 2001;31:413–22.

[68] Long FR. High-resolution CT of the lungs in infants
and young children. J Thorac Imaging 2001;16:
184–96.

[69] Long FR, Williams RS, Castile RG. Structural airway abnormalities in infants and young children
with cystic fibrosis. J Pediatr 2004;144:154–61.

[70] Martinez TM, Llapur CJ, Williams TH, et al. High-
resolution tomography imaging of airway disease in
infants with cystic fibrosis. Am J Respir Crit Care
Med 2005;172:1133–8.

[71] Long FR, Williams RS, Adler BH, et al. Comparison of quiet breathing and controlled ventilation in
the high-resolution CT assessment of airway disease
in infants with cystic fibrosis. Pediatr Radiol 2005;
35:1075–80.

[72] Davis S, Fordham L, Brody AS, et al. Computed tomography reflects lower airway inflammation and
tracks changes in early cystic fibrosis. Am J Respir
Crit Care Med February 15, 2007 [epub ahead of
print].

[73] Brown RH, Mitzner W, Wagner E, et al. Airway distention with lung inflation measured by HRCT.
Acad Radiol 2003;10:1097–103.

[74] Long FR. Imaging evolution of airway disorders in
children. Radiol Clin North Am 2005;43:371–89.

[75] Robinson TE, Leung AN, Moss RB, et al. Standardized high-resolution CT of the lung using a spirometer-triggered electron beam CT scanner. AJR Am J
Roentgenol 1999;172:1636–8.

[76] Castile RG, Long FR, Flucke RL, et al. Correlation
of structural and functional abnormalities in the
lungs of infants with cystic fibrosis. Pediatr Pulmonol Suppl 2000;20:295.

[77] Oikonomou A, Hansell DM. Recent advances in imaging. In: Bush A, Alton EW, Davies JD, et al, editors. Cystic fibrosis in the 21st century. (Progress in
respiratory research, vol. 34). 1st edition. Basel
(Switzerland): S Karger AG; 2006. p. 203–11.

[78] Brody AS, Kosorok MR, Li Z, et al. Reproducibility
of a scoring system for computed tomography scanning in cystic fibrosis. J Thorac Imaging 2006;21:
14–21.

[79] Robinson TE, Leung AN, Northway WH, et al.
Composite spirometric-computed tomography out-
come measure in early cystic fibrosis lung disease.
Am J Respir Crit Care Med 2003;168:588–93.

[80] King GG, Muller NL, Whittall KP, et al. An analysis algorithm for measuring airway lumen and
wall areas from high-resolution computed tomography data. Am J Respir Crit Care Med 2000;161:
574–80.

[81] Nakano Y, Whittall KP, Kalloger SE, et al. Development and validation of human airway analysis

algorithm using multidetector row CT. Proc SPIE 2002;4683:460–9.

[82] de Jong PA, Nakano Y, Hop WC, et al. Changes in airway dimension on computed tomography scans of children with cystic fibrosis. Am J Respir Crit Care Med 2005;172:218–24.

[83] Dame Carroll JR, Chandra A, Jones AS, et al. Airway dimensions measured from micro-computed tomography and high-resolution computed tomography. Eur Respir J 2006;28(4):712–20.

[84] Raman R, Raman P, Venkatraman R, et al. A quantitative algorithm to compare 2D and 3D bronchial airway morphology from chest CT datasets. J Digit Imaging, submitted for publication.

[85] Tschirren J, Palagyi K, Hoffman EA, et al. Segmentation, skeletonization, and branchpoint matching; a fully automated quantitative evaluation of human intrathoracic airway trees. In: Dohi T, Kikinis R, editors. Proceedings of the Fifth International Conference on Medical Image Computing and Computer Assisted Intervention, 2002, Tokyo, Japan. Berlin: Springer-Verlag; 2002. p. 12–9.

[86] Tschirren J, Hoffman EA, McLennan L, et al. Branchpoint labeling and matching in human airway trees. In: Clough AVA, Amir A, editors. Proceedings of the SPIE Medical Imaging 2003. San Diego (CA): Proc International Society of Optical Engineers; 2003. p. 187–94.

[87] Tschirren J, Hoffman EA, McLennan L, et al. Intrathoracic airway trees: segmentation and airway morphology analysis from low dose CT scans. IEEE Trans Med Imaging 2005;24:1529–39.

[88] Venkatraman R, Raman R, Raman B, et al. Fully automated system for three-dimensional bronchial morphology analysis using volumetric multidetector computed tomography of the chest. J Digit Imaging 2006;19(2):132–9.

[89] Nakano Y, Muller NL, King GG, et al. Quantitative assessment of airway remodeling using high-resolution CT. Chest 2002;122:271S–5S.

[90] McNitt-Gray MF, Goldin JG, Johnson TD, et al. Development and testing of image processing methods for the quantitative assessment of airway hyperresponsiveness from high-resolution CT images. J Comput Assist Tomogr 1997;21:939–47.

[91] Reinhardt JM, D'Souza ND, Hoffman EA. Accurate measurement of intrathoracic airways. IEEE Trans Med Imaging 1997;16:820–7.

[92] de Jong PA, Muller NL, Pare PD, et al. Computed tomographic imaging of the airways: relationship to structure and function. Eur Respir J 2005;26:140–52.

[93] Armstrong DS, Hook SM, Jamsen KM, et al. Lower airway inflammation in infants with cystic fibrosis detected by newborn screening. Pediatr Pulmonol 2005;40(6):500–10.

[94] Robinson TE, Emond M, Chen X, et al. Chest HRCT discriminates bacterial infection effects on disease severity in children with mild cystic fibrosis. Am J Respir Crit Care Med 2007, submitted for publication.

CLINICS
IN CHEST
MEDICINE

Clin Chest Med 28 (2007) 423–432

Transition and Transfer of Patients Who Have Cystic Fibrosis to Adult Care

H. Worth Parker, MD

Dartmouth-Hitchcock Medical Center, 1 Medical Center Drive, Lebanon, NH 03756, USA

"We must remember, however, that adolescence is, one hopes, a self limiting disorder."

George Vaillant, M.D. [1].

Twenty-five years ago I was asked to consult on a 34-year-old man who had cystic fibrosis (CF) who had been admitted to the adult patient floor by one of our allergists. He was a practicing lawyer in our community and was in the midst of a CF pulmonary exacerbation. He was wary of what I knew about CF and made the statement, "Am I going to have to teach you about CF too?" We became partners in his CF care and developed a strong relationship over the next decade. He taught me about how he had taken responsibility for his own care and about what the ingredients to a successful life with CF might be. Regardless of what system of transition of care our CF centers adopt, the persisting challenge is to share responsibility for developing skills to help adult patients who have CF attain their best quality of life (Box 1).

There is a growing body of literature about transition from pediatric to adult care, but the data remain mostly anecdotal [2–4]. We know something about the characteristics of the successful transitioned patient with chronic illness [5]. But what are the characteristics of families and health care systems that promote success in this area? Is there any evidence that transitioning to adult care improves outcomes? Only some of these questions have been answered.

The exciting transition of patients who have CF to adult care, which is a result of healthier young

adults who have CF, has become a significant issue facing CF clinicians. This story of improved outcomes in CF care is elegantly displayed in the histograms developed by the Cystic Fibrosis Foundation (CFF) using data from a registry that has been kept by the CFF for the past 23 years (Cystic Fibrosis Foundation Registry [CFFR]) [6]. From 1985 to 2005, there was a 10-year improvement in median survival with CF, and further improvements are expected (Fig. 1). The age distribution of the CF patient population continues to expand (Fig. 2), and, if this trend continues, there will soon be more patients older than 18 years than younger. The ages from birth to 6 years seem to be key years for maximizing the pulmonary function in adolescence. The first forced expiratory volume in 1 second measurement at age 6 years has improved during the last 15 years of the CFFR (Fig. 3). However, the slope of decline from that improved starting point has not changed since 1990, and the natural history of CF throughout childhood and adolescence continues to be a gradual decline in lung function despite adherence to an evidence-based best practice regimen. Once a patient enters the age where lung function can be measured, a gap already exists between the best and other outcomes.

As a result of this knowledge, the goal of pediatric clinicians and families is to make the diagnosis early (newborn screening) and redouble efforts toward early aggressive care for lung and nutritional issues before age 6. Fig. 4 shows that the slope of decline of lung function in a cohort of patients who was born between 1995 and 1999 may see a slower rate of decline when compared with their counterparts in the group born in between 1980 and 1984. The hope of all involved is that this CF lung function decline will

This article was supported by the Cystic Fibrosis Foundation Center grant.

E-mail address: h.worth.parker@hitchcock.org

plateau and that more and more adolescents will enter the adult-oriented care system with better overall health.

These dramatic advances in CF care are a call to action for the CF community. It is our responsibility to ensure that our systems of care are ready to bring these ever healthier young people into their adult lives with the proper tools to cope with ever more complex treatment regimens.

From the pediatric into the adult cystic fibrosis clinic

Transition is defined by the American Academy of Pediatrics as "the purposeful, planned movement of adolescents and young adults with chronic physical and medical conditions from child-centered to adult-oriented health care system" [7]. Previous surveys of young adults reveal that patients who have chronic illness who are not severely ill transition to adult care with ease. The most severely ill patients experience limits in functioning [8].

Transition to the care of practitioners who deal with problems that are age specific is a sound strategy [9]. Pediatric systems of care are not geared toward some adult issues. As one pediatric resident put it, "As a (pediatric) resident I once took care of a 30-some-year old man with Down's syndrome who had heart disease, it was clear that our expertise was not in his best interest any longer" [8].

The improving life expectancy in CF focused the CF community on the issue of transition, and in 1998 the CFF announced that they would require each accredited CF center to have

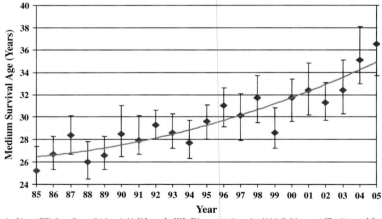

As of August 2006, the median predicted survival is 36.5 years for 2005. This represents the age by which half of the current CF registry population would be expected to be dead, given the ages of the patients in the registry and the mortality distribution of the deaths in 2005. The whiskers represent the 95 percent confidence bounds for the survival estimates, so the 2005 median predicted survival is between 33.7 and 40.0 years.

Fig. 1. Median predicted survival age, 1985–2005 (with 95% confidence intervals). The median predicted survival was 36.5 years for 2005. This represents the age by which half of the current CF registry population would be expected to be dead, given the ages of the patients in the registry and the mortality distribution of the deaths in 2005. The whiskers represent the 95% confidence intervals for the survival estimates, so the 2005 median predicted survival is between 33.7 and 40.0 years. (*From* 2005 Annual Data Report to the Center Directors. Cystic Fibrosis Patient Registry, Bethesda, MD; used with permission.)

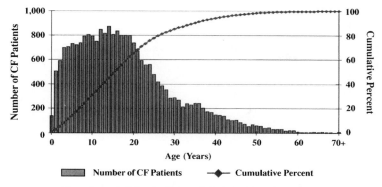

Fig. 2. Age distribution of the CF patient population, 2005. The median age is 15.9 years. The range is from birth to more than 70 years. (*From* 2005 Annual Data Report to the Center Directors. Cystic Fibrosis Patient Registry, Bethesda, MD; used with permission.)

identified an adult CF team by the year 2000 [10]. This was an important stance because it forced many programs to formally engage their adult care colleagues in a partnership. Before this announcement, there were only 44 CFF-approved adult care programs out of the 110 approved CF centers in the United States [11]. In a 1998 survey published in 2001, 22% of 66 remaining CF centers reported having an adult program, but they were not approved by the CFF, and another 39% had no adult program. A late push by the CF community led to most centers having adult teams in place by the 2000 deadline.

What were some of the issues that arose in the community of CF caregivers? Some centers (20%) could not identify an adult CF caregiver. Pediatric caregivers feared that some adult practitioners, although well trained in their parent specialty, had no specific training in CF and would not be ready to care for the specifics of CF and that the patient might suffer. Barriers to the transfer of care identified in one study included patient/family resistance (51.4%), disease severity (50.5%), and developmental delay (46.7%) [11]. Another study by Boyle and colleagues [2] suggested that patients and parents were overwhelmingly positive toward the development of adult CF programs.

The CFF responded to these concerns with a multilayered administrative and education strategy. They established a mentorship program where newly identified adult care providers could spend time with experienced CF adult care teams. Educational sessions were developed for new adult program providers at the annual North American Cystic Fibrosis Conference. The CFF earmarked financial support for adult centers so

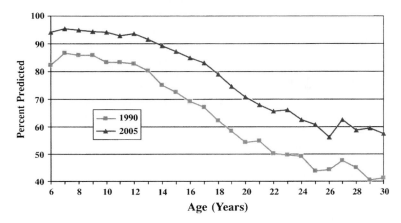

Fig. 3. Median percent predicted forced expiratory volume in 1 second (FEV$_1$) versus age, 1990 and 2005. (*From* 2005 Annual Data Report to the Center Directors. Cystic Fibrosis Patient Registry, Bethesda, MD; used with permission.)

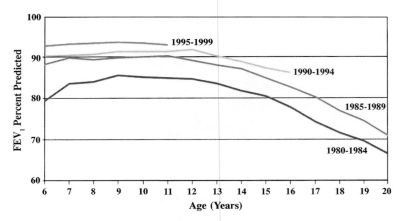

Fig. 4. Median forced expiratory volume in 1 second (FEV$_1$) percent predicted versus age by birth cohort. (*From* 2005 Annual Data Report to the Center Directors. Cystic Fibrosis Patient Registry, Bethesda, MD; used with permission.)

that these centers could be recognized by deans, chairs, division chiefs, and practice colleagues as separate and important viable entities. The CFF established a permanent position on its Center Committee for an adult caregiver representative to give the adult center directors a permanent voice in the clinical care governance structure of the Foundation. Site visitors from the CFF are now looking for evidence of a transition plan with each center visit every 3 to 5 years.

Internationally, transition was also a topic of interest. The Royal Brompton Hospital in London, with 350 pediatric and approximately 600 adult patients, had approximately 100 patients who were approaching transition in June 2000 [12]. They standardized collaboration between the pediatric and adult services and measured the impact of this standard process, noting that "there was an improvement in the process of transfer from pediatric to adult care." They recognized that further work was necessary.

What model of health care transition is best for your site?

Several models for transition have been described in the CF and other disease-specific states [4,13–15]. Models range from separate pediatric and adult clinics that are housed in unique facilities with unique staff to special home site teen clinics hosted by joint staff from pediatric and adult clinics. Although models of CF care are limited by the available physical plant and knowledgeable staff, all models need to address communication between pediatric and adult clinics, avoiding in-hospital transition, age of transition, and the differences between pediatric and adult systems of care.

Physical proximity of the pediatric and adult cystic fibrosis clinics: a study in micro-systems

Each CF clinic has to define a method of communication between pediatric and adult provider that works for their center or "micro-system." When our medical center recently underwent renovations, separating the pediatric and adult CF clinics, we realized how much we relied on physical proximity to help with the transition from pediatric to adult CF care. The previous arrangement allowed patients to be seen in age-appropriate areas within close proximity to each other. The nurse coordinator in the pediatric CF clinic could easily walk to the adult pulmonary clinic for a consult, creating a natural "transition moment." The pediatric and adult CF clinics have moved to new spaces within the same complex and are separated by a short walk. With the move to the new space, the spontaneity of the drop-in appearance (which facilitated familiarity of patients and families with a face on the adult team) has vanished. We have since developed a system where the pediatric patients show up on the adult CF providers' daily schedule, and a member of the adult team can go to the pediatric clinic.

Transition can be challenging when an adult team is separated from the pediatric team by a campus or town. At our site, after the patient reaches 16 years of age, members of the adult team begin to formally see the patient as the primary caregiver once a year in the adult or pediatric clinic.

We also have attempted to see all teen patients when they are admitted to the pediatric inpatient service and have attempted a transition clinic with variable success. Schidlow and Fiel [9] stated in their 1990 article on transition that if a transitioning teen has to move from one institution to another, it can be considered a "rite of passage" and that physical separation between sites can help to minimize attempts to pit care teams against each other. On the other hand, an unfamiliar venue with new faces is potentially frightening to the patient and parent and could lead to ambivalence or reluctance to follow through.

In-hospital transition

Those in the CF community try to avoid in-hospital transition to adult services whenever possible. In general, an ill patient in a foreign hospital room would be less likely to trust a new care team. In-hospital transitions do occur, but they should be viewed as red flags that one's system is not identifying patients early enough to facilitate a less abrupt transition.

One method that some groups find successful is to have the transition-age patient and family take a tour of the adult inpatient facility when the patient is well. This tour can be led by the appropriate CF adult care team member and the lead CF inpatient nurse. Sometimes the patient and family see familiar faces of respiratory care or nutrition members of the CF inpatient pediatric team while visiting the adult care inpatient center. Often, however, the venues are new, increasing the importance that members of the adult team have an outpatient connection with the patient and family that can decrease the anxiety of their first inpatient experience. Infection control guidelines also mandated the placement of signs outside the patient's room that alert all that enter that the patient has an illness that demands special treatment (eg, gowns on entry, gloves if touching). This can be frightening to some patients who do not want others to know that they are infected or need special treatment. Managing education about infection control prospectively can reduce anxiety. On the other hand, infection control has reduced fears of having to share a room with an elderly patient because private rooms have become the norm for CF inpatient care.

At our facility, families have had input into how to make this part of transition easier, and we have incorporated their suggestions into our practice. Some patient suggestions have been to have a refrigerator to store snacks and shakes like they have on the pediatric inpatient service and to make available electronic games that can be used through the patient's television (mimicking the scene in the children's hospital.)

Age of transition

There is no definite age when transition should occur. Ideally, transition should be competency based, and skills should be evident before transfer is complete. Viner [16] describes how adolescents do best if they understand relevant therapies and know how to respond. This competency-based approach is inadequate if other systems issues force a certain age of transfer. Other experts suggest that the timing of transfer to adult care should be linked to developmental milestones, such as the end of secondary education. Most survey-based references suggest that caregivers, patients, and families would not transition patients with special needs until there is evidence of adequate resources post-transfer and that patients near death should not be transferred [11]. Models of transition deal with young adults who are in college away from home in differing ways. Some patients in transition from the end of high school and to college are embraced by the adult team, and other centers continue to care for these late teens in their pediatrics center. Some centers such as ours pick the age of transfer of care by inpatient admission age cutoffs, mandating patients 19 or older to be admitted to the adult care floors.

Differences in pediatric versus adult systems of care

The child who has CF usually has adequate resources for care with support from state and federal agencies. In contrast, adults who have CF often have incomplete health care coverage from government payers. Forty-three percent of adults older than 18 years of age had Medicaid/State or Federal insurance coverage in 2005 [6]. The fact that Medicaid reimburses at such a low rate may limit the number and enthusiasm of adult clinicians willing to become engaged in CF care. The adult pulmonary community can choose to focus on areas of their specialty that are better remunerated for the amount of effort spent. The time spent in the office visit with a complex, ill patient who has CF (not to mention the hours of follow-up work) are not reimbursed at the same level and carry lower currency than a procedure or the same amount of effort spent with a critical care patient.

This potential disincentive is magnified by the fact that most adult CF practitioners may be members of cross-coverage groups where on the same day they are seeing the chronically and acutely ill patients. Thus, maintenance care and ongoing office educational needs of the chronically ill patient who has CF could be cut short by other acutely ill patient needs. The life of the adult pulmonary, gastroenterology, or infectious disease specialist working in CF care is often one where they are doing in-hospital ICU or consultative work, leading to a feeling of a faster pace of office visits. Patients feel the difference between these models. Reiss [17] found in focus groups of transitioning patients that patients felt distinctive differences between pediatric and adult clinics. He called them "different medical subcultures."

The complexity and pace of care brings into focus the need for a strong interdisciplinary team effort, where education regarding maintenance care, medication use, and exacerbation prevention are performed by all on the team. Care management nurses are supported (in some institutions) to prospectively manage this population of patients so that admission to the hospital is minimized. This concept may gain more support by hospital administrators as they look to fill beds with patients whose illness or elective surgical needs (eg, cardiac catheterization, joint replacement) brings higher levels of remuneration. Thus, the challenge to the CF community is to document the judicious use of inpatient resources that may lead to better patient health outcomes.

Interdisciplinary team care can become a challenge during transition because as the patient who has CF ages, the chance of developing CF-related diabetes is more likely. Expanding the team to include pediatric and adult endocrine physicians and nurses has brought expertise in treating types I and II diabetes and bone health to the CF-related diabetes clinic, improving the lives of patients who have CF and underscoring the need for good communication between teams. Once the endocrine team bonds with the patient, their familiar faces help during transitions to adult care.

Psychosocial and developmental issues during transition

Adolescence and chronic illness collide

The confluence of adolescence and a chronic disease like CF brings with it a complex emotional landscape. Delayed physical development due to CF disease (eg, delayed growth, delayed menarche) may lead to poor body image, low self-esteem, and isolation. Depression in patients who have CF who are older than 18 years of age was 15.9% in 2005 but may range to as high as 50% in some centers [6]. Most CF teams have counselors in the form of social workers or psychologists, but some patients do not have coverage for these services.

CF-related diabetes raises difficult emotional issues. The patient can be ambivalent about this discovery and its treatment. The misinformation and unknowns of having CF-related diabetes may push the young adult into a tailspin, so emotional issues need to be addressed proactively when diabetes is diagnosed. The complexity of checking blood sugars and correctly using insulin can be overwhelming to patient and family. Literature regarding the transition of the juvenile onset diabetic reads much like that of CF: "...young adults with diabetes are a forgotten group, whose special needs seem to fall outside the primary focus of both pediatric and adult medicine. Many challenges are confronted at this critical transition when young adults take over the responsibility of their own self-care" [18]. CF-related diabetes calls on the teen to wonder if it is all worth the effort. Some teens need to make choices regarding which treatment or which medication they can find time to do. For treatment to be fully successful, their CF is brought "out in the open" because they are checking blood sugars at school or at work instead of doing their treatments at home privately. It leads to questions from peers regarding their illness that they have previously not wanted or have not had to confront. Many of their peers understand more about what diabetes is than what CF is. This can cut both ways to bring friends into the caring subgroup or to force further isolation.

Isolation, acceptance, being different

The teen who has CF fights to be normal, yet when one has to take enzymes with each meal or use an inhaler before one exercises, it can draw the wrong kind of attention to one's body and foster stigma. Sometimes people do not understand that CF is not infectious, so the teen is excluded for fear of being infectious to others. The patient who has CF also has absences from school that force them to miss activities and opportunities for friendships. Later in young adulthood, meaningful long-term relationships are flavored by concerns about prognosis and fear of rejection if the patient becomes ill.

Developmental issues

Wolpert and Anderson [18], in their editorial in Diabetes Care in 2001, state, "the overwhelming changes in the first phase of the young-adult period (including graduating from high school, moving away from home, beginning new educational directions and beginning to work and to be self supporting) are often a distraction from the demands of managing diabetes. However, later, the developmental focus shifts toward making choices and plans about relationships, work directions and lifestyle behaviors. This second phase of the young-adult period, when the life-long routines of self-care are set, can present a window of opportunity for the provider to intervene and to influence habits that will help to determine the future health of young adults with diabetes." These two phases of young adult development confront the CF practitioner and team with similar challenges but a slightly different urgency. Fig. 5 shows that the average age of death for the patient who has CF is 26 years [6]. In contrast, 15% of patients who have type I diabetes die by age 40 [19]. Therefore, the pace of illness in CF means that waiting until the teenager or young adult is ready to follow a regimen for success for care could be lethal. Witnessing this biologic, predictable maturation delay is the greatest challenge about caring for adolescent and young adult patients who have CF.

Pediatric development experts note that older teenagers have a sense of "invulnerability" and tend to discount risks to their future health and need for medical care [20]. How can we not become concerned about patients who do not follow evidence-based regimens for care and who do ot take medications or do recommended nutritional or airway clearance therapies? How does one sit by and watch without being paternalistic, by reverting to our own doctoring behavior that was successful when the young person was under the influence of parental control? How does the team remain engaged with the patient who is not caring for their own CF?

Promoting self-care

The traditional model of top-down medical care delivery where the practitioner prescribes a regimen and the patient is expected to follow is a bad match for adolescence. We need to nurture further development of this concept in the pediatric and adult CF care clinics. In survey studies about transition in all chronic conditions, including CF, one parent stated that her child's practitioner "...always included some discussion of what my daughter will need to do for herself as she gets older. I see more and more of the conversations regarding her health being directed to her (my daughter)" [8].

The care delivery team must present a constant theme that includes thinking about the future. Another parent in this same survey applauded "...two exceptional physicians who really care(d)

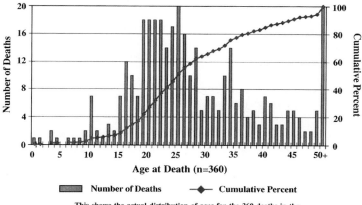

This shows the actual distribution of ages for the 360 deaths in the CF registry for 2005, with a median of 25.3 years (as of August 2006).

Fig. 5. Age at death, 2005. This shows the actual distribution of ages for the 360 deaths in the CF registry for 2005, with a median of 25.3 years (as of August 2006). (*From* 2005 Annual Data Report to the Center Directors. Cystic Fibrosis Patient Registry, Bethesda, MD; used with permission.)

about our daughter's wellness...and future within the community" [8]. At the transition to adult care, there is an opportunity for the pediatrician and the adult provider to help the patient envision their future life.

Patients who have CF may ask, "Why should I do these treatments if I am going to die anyway" or may say "You don't know how hard these treatments are to do!" They express a common complaint of even our most engaged young adults: There is not enough time to do all the treatments and to still have a life. This growing issue will hopefully be addressed in the future by trials that compare current treatments head to head to eliminate less effective but time-consuming therapies.

To inject reality, give helpful hints. and provide hope, CF Family Night at our center hosts a panel of young adults who present a vignette about themselves and then answer questions from the audience. The CF team does not script this session but facilitates the discussion. Some of these young adults have had the usual bumpy road through ages 17 to 22 where they did not pay attention or have a care plan that they actually followed. Some have always paid attention and speak to the challenges that they faced. Some are well, and some are sick, wearing oxygen and becoming breathless as they speak. Evaluations from the audience have stated the value of this approach. Predictably, some parents are frightened and feel that we are trying to put a damper on the celebration of successes in CF care. The feedback is overwhelmingly positive, with requests to that have regular return panels.

Challenges to transitioning from pediatric to adult cystic fibrosis care

From a patient's viewpoint

Boyle and colleagues [2] did an anonymous 22-question pretransition questionnaire and post-transition interviews with 60 patients who had CF and their parents as they went through the transition for pediatric to adult CF care. The two most important concerns (scale 1–5, with 5 most concerning) identified by the patients before transition to adult care were potential exposure to infection (3.4 ± 1.1) and having to leave their previous caregivers (3.4 ± 1.0). Introduction to the adult CF team before transition was associated with significantly lower levels of concern in all areas, particularly about having to leave previous

caregivers (3.9 ± 0.7 versus 2.5 ± 0.6; $P < .004$). Age, gender, severity of lung disease, and age at diagnosis were not predictive of the level of patient concern for any area. The most important expectations for patients were ready phone access to a nurse (4.9 ± 0.6) and education about adult CF issues (4.6 ± 0.7).

Several other investigators have written about the concerns of patients who have CF regarding transfer to adult care. In a study looking at the perceptions of young adults who have CF regarding the impact the disease had on their lives, Palmer and Boisen [21] noted that concerns were raised regarding health insurance, finances, achievement of independence, and lack of optimism for the future. In another survey study of teens who had CF, Madge and Bryon [3] discovered that respondents felt that transition to an adult service was necessary and accepted, provided that "good preparation is given from the pediatric setting." Anderson and colleagues [22] showed that 334 patients who were members of the International Association of CF Adults felt that their level of concern about transfer to an adult center was minimal. The investigators note that this is far less than their CF physicians had reported in a previous published survey [11].

From a parent's viewpoint

From the parents' perspective, one transition concern was the ability of their child to care for their CF independently, a concern their children did not share (4.0 ± 1.1 versus 1.5 ± 0.5; $P < .0001$) [2]. This response speaks to the parents' ongoing anxiety about their child's chronic illness and the unknowns ahead in life but also reflects the need for greater parental education about the issues that teens who have CF are facing in transitioning from pediatric to adult care.

Challenges to transition from a practitioner's viewpoint

Pediatricians may resist the transition process if they lack confidence in their adult colleagues. In the past, the adolescent has not been adequately represented as a consumer of health care, and few providers are experts in adolescent health. Pediatricians have filled this void and provide care to this group of young adults who have chronic illnesses well beyond the traditional age of pediatric care [9]. Anderson and colleagues [22] make the point in their two studies that the pediatric team overestimates the patients' concerns regarding transition. They also report that non-physician team members felt that age (37.4%), marriage (16.2%), and pregnancy (27.1%) should be criteria for transfer.

Legal issues facing transitioning adults

Sufian and Passamano [23] reported the experience of the CFF Legal information hotline, a repository of data for legal issues for patients who have CF. This hotline received 6378 calls from 1998 to May 2006. Issues regarding health insurance and social security issues predominate in these calls, with education and employment making up the bulk of the rest of the calls. She concluded that "knowledge is the key to making sure young adults with CF have health insurance coverage that is needed. Teens and parents need to know that non-adherence to a medical regimen may have a negative effect on the ability to receive Social Security benefits or health insurance coverage once a child reaches a limiting age on the parent's policy. The ability to access legal rights concerning future employment or education can prove invaluable."

The transition is a great time to discuss the cost of each treatment that the patient is receiving. This "sticker shock" awareness is important for the young adult to understand why they should carefully consider each life change in the context of insurance coverage. This includes new jobs where insurance may not be offered or where coverage is less comprehensive. Getting married may result in the loss of Medicaid coverage when a spouse's income is accounted for. Patients who have CF who are in transition need to be knowledgeable about legislation related to privacy and portability of medical information and insurance, including COBRA and the definitions of pre-existing condition clauses. The patient needs access to information regarding Social Security Income/Disability application processes when poor health restricts their work options. There is information from the CFF legal hotline at 1-800-622-0385 for patients who have questions when applying for SSI/SSDI.

Approximately 25% of patients who have CF in the recent CFF Registry reported seeking higher education [6]. The Rehabilitation Act of 1973-Section 504 provides for protection in colleges and universities that receive federal funds. This can help the young person who has CF to devise a personal plan of learning that takes into consideration things like multiple absences or missing exams, layout and proximity of dorm rooms, and access to the Office of Students with Disabilities.

Vocational rehabilitation is available for patients who have CF and can lead to testing, training, and support for higher education and young adults who have CF. Pre-employment counseling regarding potential harmful job conditions is also important for lung health. Access to knowledge about the American with Disabilities Act, The Family and Medical Leave Act, and Medicare Parts B and D are important at certain times in their lives.

Measuring transition outcomes

In his recent review of transitions, Rosen [24] states, "There remains a paucity of outcome data, no long-term outcome data at all and no agreement even as to which long-term outcomes ought to be studied." The CFF has the ability to ask each center for a copy of their specific transition plan as part of its oversight of the quality of clinic care. This enables centers that have no formal transition plan to create one and may lead to benchmarking or at least literature review to provide this plan. It also promotes formal discussion between the transition teams in that center. Most CF centers should have this document.

The CF community has a robust registry of annual data from a large portion of the patients who have CF in the United States. There are several data points that, if earmarked, could give a "transition scorecard." This would have to be carefully constructed because many variables are at play in the transfer of care. Patients and families should be brought into the development of such a tool. A quality of life questionnaire could be used to augment objective data in this area.

Summary

Transition to age-appropriate care and transfer of care is a process that best occurs over time. Models to accomplish this are best designed at the local level because local factors weigh heavily on the model a center chooses. Ingredients for the successful transition must include focus on self-care and communication between CF teams, between patients who have CF and the teams, and between parents of patients who have CF and the teams. A timeline for transition should begin years before transfer with the realization that one plan may not accommodate all patients' needs.

Agreement within the CF community regarding the appropriate outcome measures for successful transition will be necessary going forward.

References

[1] Vaillant G. Ripeness is all: social and emotional maturation. In: Aging well. New York: Little, Brown and Company; 2002. p. 39–82.

[2] Boyle M, Farukhi Z, Nosky M. Strategies for improving transition to adult cystic fibrosis care, based on patient and parent views. Pediatr Pulmonol 2001; 32:428–36.

[3] Madge S, Bryon M. A model for transition from pediatric to adult care in cystic fibrosis. J Pediatr Nurs 2002;17(4):283–8.

[4] Viner R. Barriers and good practice in transition from paediatric to adult care. J R Soc Med 2001;94:2–4.

[5] Callahan S, Winitzer R, Keenan P. Transition from pediatric to adult-oriented health care: a challenge for patients with chronic disease. Current Opinion in Pediatrics 2001;13:310-16.

[6] Cystic Fibrosis Foundation. Cystic fibrosis patient registry 2005. Annual data report to the center directors. Bethesda (MD); 2006.

[7] American Academy of Pediatrics, Committee on children with disabilities and committee on adolescence. Transition of care provided for adolescents with special health care needs. Pediatrics 2002;110:1304–6.

[8] Scal P. Transition for youth with chronic conditions: primary care physicians' approaches. Pediatrics 2002;110:1315–21.

[9] Schidlow D. Life beyond pediatrics: transition of chronically ill adolescents from pediatrics to adult health care systems. Med Clin North Am 1990;75: 1113–20.

[10] Cystic Fibrosis Foundation. Guidelines for implementation of adult CF programs. Bethesda (MD); 1998.

[11] Flume P, Anderson D, Hardy K, et al. Transition programs in cystic fibrosis centers: perceptions of pediatric and adult program directors. Pediatr Pulmonol 2001;31(6):443–50.

[12] Cowlard J. Cystic fibrosis: transition from paediatric to adult care. Nurs Stand 2003;18(4):39–41.

[13] Rosen D, Blum R, Britto M, et al. Transition to adult health care for adolescents and young adults with chronic conditions. J Adolsc Health 2003;33: 309–11.

[14] Conway S, Stafleforth D, Webb A. The failing health care system for adult patients with cystic fibrosis. Thorax 1998;53:3–4.

[15] Yankaskas J, Marshall B, Sufian J. Cystic fibrosis adult care consensus conference report. Chest 2004;125:1S–39S.

[16] Viner R. Effective transition from pediatric to adult services. Hospital Medicine 2000;61:341–3.

[17] Reiss J, Gibson R, Walker L. Health care transition: youth, family, and provider perspectives. Pediatrics 2005;115:112–20.

[18] Wolpert H, Anderson B. Young adults with diabetes: need for a new treatment paradigm. Diabetes Care 2001;24(9):1513–4.

[19] Portuese E, Orchard T. Mortality in insulin-dependent diabetes. In: Harris MI, editor. Diabetes in America. 2nd edition. Bethesda (MD): National Institutes of Health; 1995. p. 221.

[20] Wysocki T, Hough B, Ward K, et al. Diabetes mellitus in the transition to adulthood: adjustment, self-care, and health care status. J Dev Behav Pediatr 1992;13:194–201.

[21] Palmer M, Boisen L. Cystic fibrosis and the transition to adulthood. Soc Work Health Care 2002; 36(1):45–58.

[22] Anderson D, Flume P, Hardy K, et al. Transition programs in cystic fibrosis centers: perceptions of patients. Pediatr Pulmonol 2002;33(5):327–31.

[23] Sufian B, Passamano J. Transitioning young adults face complex legal issues [abstract 561]. In: Program and abstracts of the Twentieth Annual North American Cystic Fibrosis Conference. Pediatr Pulmonol 2006, Suppl 29: 411.

[24] Rosen D. Transition of young people with respiratory disease to adult health care. Paediatr Respir Rev 2004;5:124–31.

ELSEVIER
SAUNDERS

CLINICS
IN CHEST
MEDICINE

Clin Chest Med 28 (2007) 433–443

Fertility and Pregnancy: Common Concerns of the Aging Cystic Fibrosis Population

Viranuj Sueblinvong, MD[a,*],
Laurie A. Whittaker, MD[b,c]

[a]Division of Pulmonary and Critical Care Medicine, The University of Vermont and Fletcher
Allen Health Care, 149 Beaumont Avenue, HSRF 231, Burlington, VT 05405, USA
[b]Department of Medicine, University of Vermont, 149 Beaumont Avenue, Burlington, VT 05405, USA
[c]Adult Cystic Fibrosis Program, Division of Pulmonary and Critical Care Medicine, The University of Vermont
and Fletcher Allen Health Care, Burlington, VT 05405, USA

Cystic fibrosis (CF) is a genetic disease arising from mutations in the cystic fibrosis transmembrane conductance regulator (CFTR) gene. CF is a multisystem disorder, with the most clinically significant disease arising in the lungs, gastrointestinal tract, and pancreas; however, any organ with a significant exocrine component may be affected by mutations in CFTR, including the reproductive systems of men and women.

Infertility has become a concern for men and women who have CF as quality of life and survival improves [1]. Obstructive azoospermia renders most CF men infertile, whereas 50% of women who have CF are able to conceive a child. Improved procedures of sperm retrieval and oocyte fertilization have provided men who have CF an opportunity at biologic fatherhood, and women who have CF are having children with much greater frequency and with better maternal and fetal outcomes than once anticipated. Successful pregnancies have even been reported after lung transplantation.

In this article, the authors discuss how mutations in CFTR affect the reproductive tracts of men and women and how this impacts fertility. The authors also discuss infertility treatment options in men who have CF and key considerations surrounding pregnancy and childbirth in women who have CF.

* Corresponding author.
E-mail address: viranuj.sueblinvong@med.uvm.edu (V. Sueblinvong).

Pathogenesis of infertility

Male infertility in cystic fibrosis

Multiple sites within the male reproductive tract are affected by mutations in CFTR, causing most men who have CF to be infertile (>98%) [2]. Obstructive azoospermia is the most common cause of infertility in these men [3]; however, all men who have CF should be offered a semen analysis because a small percentage are fertile, especially those who have a class V mutation of CFTR [4]. The causes of obstructive azoospermia include cystic dilatation of seminal vesicles, absence of ejaculatory ducts, and hypoplasia, aplasia, or congenital bilateral absence of the vas deferens (CBAVD) (Fig. 1) [5,6]. The presence of CBAVD is strongly associated with ΔF508 and R117H mutations of CFTR [6]. CFTR protein may be required during embryogenic development of the vas deferens; however, it remains unclear whether CBAVD is a direct result of a CFTR mutation or a consequence of structural atresia resulting from obstruction of the vas deferens with viscous mucus [7,8].

Although obstruction of the genitourinary tract leads to the vast majority of male CF infertility, nonobstructive causes have also been recognized. These include reduced spermatogenesis, reduced semen volume, and low semen pH [6,8,9]. In addition, carrying a CFTR mutation alone has been associated with an increased risk of male infertility despite a nonobstructed reproductive tract, suggesting that CFTR mutations

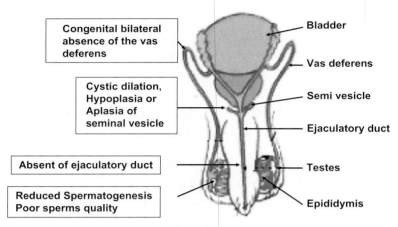

Fig. 1. Schematic drawing of the male reproductive system highlighting abnormalities that may lead to infertility in men who have CF. (*Adapted from* World Health Organization Reproductive Health and Research. Sexually transmitted and other reproductive tract infections—a guide to essential practice. Geneva: World Health Organization; 2005. p. 13. Available at http://www.who.int/reproductive-health/publications/rtis_gep/index.htm. Accessed March 3, 2007. Used with permission.)

may impact spermatogenesis by altering electrolyte and fluid transport in the epididymis [9,10].

Previously, infertility in men who had CF was untreatable. Over the past decade, however, sperm harvesting techniques have dramatically improved [11]. These techniques include microsurgical epididymal sperm aspiration (MESA), percutaneous epididymal sperm aspiration, testicular sperm aspiration, and testicular sperm extraction. MESA is the preferred method of sperm harvest because it has a lower complication rate and a higher sperm yield compared with other techniques [4]. MESA is an open surgical procedure performed under a local anesthetic whereby epididymal tubules are isolated followed by sperm aspiration. The sperm are cryopreserved or used immediately in assisted reproductive technology (ie, in vitro fertilization (IVF) or intracytoplasmic sperm injection (ICSI) followed by IVF) (Fig. 2).

Conventional IVF entails placing sperm directly into the vagina after it is collected; however, ICSI followed by IVF is a preferred option with improved fertilization and live birth rates because it overcomes issues surrounding reduced sperm motility [12]. ICSI is done by directly injecting sperm into the cytoplasm of an oocyte. Following the injection, the gamete is cultured until it reaches the blastomere stage. It is then injected into the uterus (see Fig. 2). This technique has the additional advantage of allowing sperm and oocytes to be collected and cryopreserved for multiple future attempts at ICSI. The pregnancy rate

with IVF/ICSI is about 30% to 50%, with a live birth rate of 30% to 40% [13]. A similar success rate can be expected with sperm from men who have CF [14,15].

Infant outcomes following ICSI remain a major concern for health care providers and potential parents [16]. Infant chromosomal abnormalities and neural tube defects initially attributed to oocyte injury during the ICSI procedure have been shown to be caused by the transfer of abnormal genetic material [17,18]. A recent meta-analysis found no significant increases in cardiovascular defects, musculoskeletal defects, hypospadias, neural tube defects, oral clefts, or impaired mental development following ICSI, suggesting that this technique is a safe and viable alternative for infertile men [18]. Little is known, however, about long-term fetal outcomes following ICSI on embryos derived from cryopreserved sperm and oocytes [16].

Female infertility in cystic fibrosis

Much of the female reproductive tract is lined by epithelial cells and is therefore potentially affected by mutations in CFTR [19]. Unlike men who have CF, up to 50% of women who have CF are able to conceive a child [20–22]; however, female infertility remains a significant problem for many women who have CF. Previously, ovulation disturbances and tenacious cervical mucous were believed to be major contributing factors, especially in patients who had severe lung disease

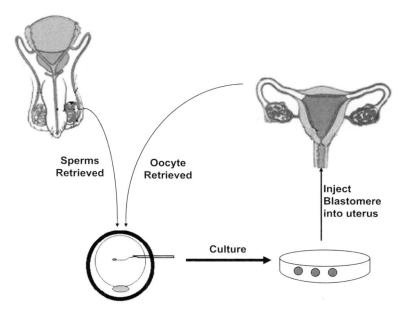

Fig. 2. Schematic drawing of the ICSI and IVF procedures. (*Adapted from* World Health Organization Reproductive Health and Research. Sexually transmitted and other reproductive tract infections—a guide to essential practice. Geneva: World Health Organization; 2005. p. 13. Available at http://www.who.int/reproductive-health/publications/rtis_gep/index.htm. Accessed March 3, 2007. Used with permission.)

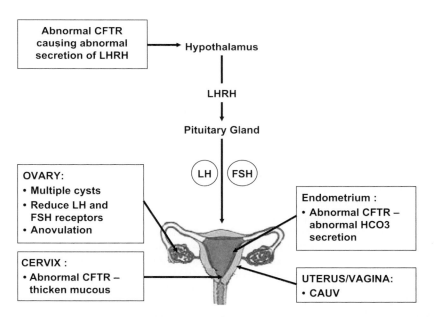

Fig. 3. Schematic drawing of the female reproductive tract highlighting abnormalities that may lead to infertility in women who have CF. CAUV, congenital absence of the uterus and vagina; FSH, follicle stimulating hormone; LH, luteinizing hormone; LHRH, luteinizing hormone-releasing hormone. (*Adapted from* World Health Organization Reproductive Health and Research. Sexually transmitted and other reproductive tract infections—a guide to essential practice. Geneva: World Health Organization; 2005. p. 13. Available at http://www.who.int/reproductive-health/publications/rtis_gep/index.htm. Accessed March 3, 2007. Used with permission.)

and/or nutritional failure. It is now recognized that there are other contributors including abnormal secretion of gonadotropin from the hypothalamus, alterations of uterine bicarbonate, and anatomic abnormalities (Fig. 3) [23–26].

Cervical mucus

Cervical mucus in women who have CF, similar to airway mucus, lacks appropriate water content, presumably due to enhanced sodium reabsorption in the absence of functional CFTR [19]. Dehydrated and thickened cervical mucus impairs cervical sperm penetration and ultimately results in failed egg fertilization. Women who have CF also have impaired midcycle "thinning" of cervical mucus, which typically occurs around the time of ovulation to favor sperm penetration of the cervical os [4,19,27].

Abnormal bicarbonate transportation

CFTR is a camp-regulated chloride channel with many functions including chloride and bicarbonate (HCO_3^-) secretion [28]. The clinical significance of altered HCO_3^- secretion has been unclear until recently [24]. Uterine fluids contain a high concentration of HCO_3^- [24], which is important in sperm capacitation [29], a poorly understood but essential process that renders a sperm able to fertilize an egg in the female reproductive tract [29]. In CF, defective CFTR within the endometrial epithelium results in altered HCO_3^- secretion, defective sperm capacitation, and failed egg fertilization [23,24]. The relative contribution of altered uterine HCO_3^- to CF female infertility is not known.

Anatomic abnormalities

Unlike men who have CF, women who have CF typically have anatomically normal reproductive tracts. Structural abnormalities, however, can sometimes arise and contribute to infertility. Ovarian cysts, redundant follicular cysts, and reduced follicle numbers have all been observed [19,25]. In addition, there is an association between CFTR mutations and congenital absence of the uterus and vagina (CAUV). In a study of 25 patients who had CAUV, CFTR mutations were twice as common compared with people who did not have CAUV (8% versus 4%) [30]. The association of CBAVD and CAUV with mutations in CFTR supports the notion that CFTR itself may be important in the embryogenic development of the male and the female reproductive tracts.

Ovulation disturbances

Delayed menarche is common in women who have CF, although the exact mechanism is not well understood. It likely results from a variety of factors directly and indirectly related to defects in CFTR. Poor nutritional and clinical health are potentially major contributors; however, a study by Johannesson and colleagues showed that delayed menarche is common even in healthy, well nourished women who have CF [31]. In their retrospective study, they found the mean age at puberty was delayed in women who had CF compared with normal control subjects (14.9 versus 13 years, respectively). The greatest delay occurred in those homozygous for the ΔF508 mutation and in those who had an abnormal oral glucose tolerance test (OGTT), even in the absence of overt diabetes [25,31]. The investigators speculated that these findings could potentially be explained by a variety of mechanisms. For instance, altered CFTR expression in the hypothalamus may lead to dysregulated neuroendocrine secretion of hormones and thereby delayed sexual maturation [31]. Increased energy consumption causing delayed menarche in women who have CF is also well recognized and can vary significantly between genotypes [31,32]. Furthermore, an abnormal OGTT in CF suggests a relative insulin deficiency that may contribute to altered ovulation by influencing ovarian follicle stimulating hormone and luteinizing hormone receptor expression [31]. Regardless of the mechanism, it appears clear that despite improving nutritional and clinical health, delayed menarche and impaired ovulation are problems likely to persist in some women who have CF.

Pregnancy in cystic fibrosis

As survival and quality of life improve in women who have CF, the numbers of CF pregnancies and live births have increased (Figs. 4 and 5) [33]. The first woman who had CF to carry a child to term was reported in 1960 [34]. Since that time, pregnancy has become a fairly common event, with better than expected maternal and fetal outcomes [35]. The Cystic Fibrosis Foundation started tracking CF pregnancies and births through its national patient registry in 1986; over the last 18 years, the number of annual CF pregnancies has increased from 45 in 1986 to 191 in 2004 (see Fig. 4). Despite these successes, the care of a pregnant woman who has CF presents many unique issues often best managed by a multidisciplinary team–based approach [33,36].

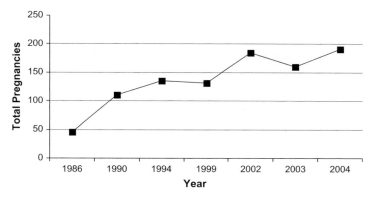

Fig. 4. Number of CF pregnancies from 1986 to 2004 reported in the United States. (*Data from* Cystic Fibrosis Foundation Patient Registry. Annual data report 1986–2004. Bethesda, MD.)

Prenatal considerations

Women who have CF who are considering pregnancy are encouraged to discuss their plans with their CF care provider. Discussions should be initiated to plan care during the pregnancy and to determine the key members of the multidisciplinary care team. It is especially important to find a high-risk obstetrician who has experience with CF and the unique issues that may arise during pregnancy [20]. Additional members of the team should include a CF physician, a respiratory therapist, a social worker, and a nutritionist. Using a multidisciplinary approach allows issues relating to nutrition, cardiopulmonary health, and psychologic well-being to be efficiently identified and addressed.

Some women who have CF are undernourished before pregnancy and may have difficulties with weight gain; therefore, nutritional status during pregnancy is often a major concern. Oral or nasogastric supplementation may be required before, during, and after the pregnancy to help women who have CF meet their caloric needs [37]. Adequate nutritional support should also include screening and management of CF-related diabetes mellitus (CFRD). CFRD is common in adults who have CF [38]. It is associated with increased mortality in women who have CF [39] and may be exacerbated by the physical and hormonal stress of pregnancy. Therefore, tight control before and throughout the pregnancy is desired to optimize maternal and fetal outcomes [40]. In addition, nutritional status assessment should include appropriate supplementation of fat-soluble vitamins and the establishment of goals for weight gain during the pregnancy [41].

Cardiopulmonary health is another important preconception consideration. Low lung function (forced expiratory volume in 1 second [FEV$_1$]

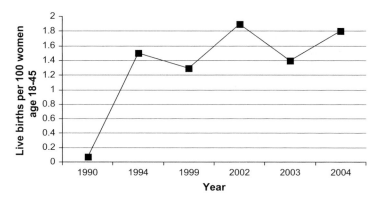

Fig. 5. Rate of CF pregnancies resulting in live births from 1990 to 2004 in the United States. (*Data from* Cystic Fibrosis Foundation Patient Registry. Annual data report 1990–2004. Bethesda, MD.)

< 50%) has been linked to lower infant birth weight [37], emphasizing the importance of maximizing lung health before pregnancy. Cardiac status should be assessed by an echocardiogram to determine whether significant pulmonary hypertension is present. A sputum culture should also be performed to look for evidence of *Burkholderia cepacia* and to determine the sensitivities of colonizing organisms. In addition, lung function should be monitored before pregnancy and monthly throughout pregnancy because an acute deterioration of pulmonary function is associated with poor maternal and fetal outcomes [20,42].

From the prepartum period forward, communication between the primary CF care team and the obstetric team is essential. Close maternal monitoring and aggressive treatment of medical issues during pregnancy is critical and may help minimize the impact of pregnancy on maternal health [43]. Although survival is improving in CF, it remains far from that of the general population. As a result, women who have CF and their partners must face the expectation of their unborn child prematurely losing a parent. In addition, these women should be counseled regarding the stress that accompanies parenthood, especially when added to the stresses of chronic illness [33]. Women who have CF should also be made aware that although it appears that pregnancy outcomes are better than once expected [33,37,43], it remains difficult to predict how an individual patient will tolerate pregnancy [37]. The possibility of significant clinical decline during pregnancy should be considered and a plan of action outlined, including early termination of the pregnancy [8].

Genetic screening of partners for CFTR mutations is another important preconception consideration. Women who have CF should be educated about the possibility of having a child who has CF if their partner is a carrier of a CFTR mutation [41]. Because CF is an autosomal recessive disorder, if the partner is a carrier, the chance of having a child who has CF is 50%. If the partner does not have mutations identified, it does not definitively exclude carrier status (not all mutations are routinely screened) but decreases the risk significantly. Expecting parents who have CF should be informed that all offspring will be carriers of a single CFTR mutation [21].

Safety of pregnancy

As previously mentioned, the first CF pregnancy resulting in a live birth was reported in 1960;

however, the mother died 6 weeks following delivery [34]. Since then, pregnancy is a much more common event, and outcomes for mother and child have improved. Multiple studies have demonstrated that pregnancy is safe and well tolerated by women who have CF in stable condition and under close medical monitoring, even in those who have severely impaired lung function and CFRD [2,14,20,22,35,36,44]. Pulmonary function may decline during pregnancy (as it does even in women who do not have CF) [45,46], but it appears that this is transient and that pregnancy itself does not result in significant irreversible loss of lung function [20,35]. Data from the Cystic Fibrosis Foundation Patient Registry and subsequent studies, comparing women who underwent pregnancy with those who did not, demonstrated similar rates of hospital admissions, use of home intravenous antibiotics, supplemental oxygen, and supplemental nutrition at 1 year following pregnancy [8,36, 44]. A recent study of 216 pregnant women who had CF found that compared with never-pregnant women who had CF, pregnancy was associated with similar respiratory and health trends but an increased number of therapies and more intensive monitoring of health [43]. These studies suggest that pregnancy can be safe and well tolerated when close medical monitoring and intensive treatments are part of the care plan.

Physiologic changes during pregnancy

Multiple physiologic changes occur during the course of pregnancy. These changes include hormonal, cardiovascular, pulmonary, and metabolic alterations. Although healthy women can often tolerate these changes without limitation, they may cause significant impairment in women who have CF. Although special attention is directed to pulmonary considerations, the other physiologic alterations coupled with multiorgan system dysfunction in CF are particularly important during pregnancy.

Estrogen levels change significantly during pregnancy and result in capillary congestion and mucus hypersecretion. Increases in progesterone stimulate respiratory drive and can result in significant hyperventilation [42]. The clinical symptoms associated with these changes may result in only minor annoyances in healthy pregnant women. In women who have CF, however, these symptoms may lead to increased airway clearance needs, sinus congestion, and worsening dyspnea, especially in those who have ventilatory limitation [42,47].

Cardiovascular alterations include increased circulating blood volume and increased cardiac output [20], which help to offset the increased oxygen consumption that accompanies pregnancy [47]. These changes may be poorly tolerated in patients who have severe lung disease, especially those who have coexisting pulmonary hypertension. Significant pulmonary hypertension can potentially impair the right heart's ability to adequately increase cardiac output and, in the most extreme instances, result in right heart failure and cardiovascular collapse [48]. These issues may become most apparent during delivery when cardiac output requirements are further increased. Compared to healthy women, women who have primary pulmonary hypertension have a poor prognosis with pregnancy [49], although they fare better than once thought if their disease is well controlled [50,51]. Women who have CF and severely impaired lung function (and presumably some degree of pulmonary hypertension) [52] are able to tolerate pregnancy [44], suggesting that pulmonary hypertension in the context of lung disease has a better pregnancy-related prognosis; however, the extent to which pulmonary hypertension is an independent risk factor for poor outcomes in CF pregnancy is not known [53].

Respiratory physiology is also affected by pregnancy. As the gravid uterus increases in size, it limits diaphragmatic excursion and decreases functional residual capacity. The decline in functional residual capacity starts during the second trimester, whereas forced vital capacity and FEV_1 are maintained. These changes may result in atelectasis and impairment of mucus clearance, which may worsen ventilation–perfusion mismatch and lead to impaired gas exchange [42,47]. Furthermore, the increased intraperitoneal pressure from the gravid uterus may result in worsening gastroesophageal reflux, which in turn may lead to more impaired pulmonary function [42]. It is essential to closely monitor pregnant women who have CF for evidence of changing lung function or further impairment of gas exchange and to intervene at the first sign of clinical decline.

Metabolic needs increase dramatically during pregnancy and may present a significant problem for women who have CF, especially if their nutritional status is suboptimal before conception [37]. Severe lung impairment, CFRD, and pancreatic insufficiency with fat malabsorption are several of the factors that make weight gain challenging for many CF patients. Maximizing the treatment of these conditions and considering patients for early intervention for supplemental oral or enteral nutrition is essential for adequate weight gain during pregnancy [37].

Medications during pregnancy

Although definitive pharmacologic studies are often lacking, the use of medications during pregnancy should be carefully considered for teratogenic effects and maternal benefit. Treatment with antibiotics is often necessary during a CF pregnancy. Quinolones are frequently used, particularly as outpatient therapy, and have been associated with arthropathy in animals, raising concern over possible teratogenic effects [54]. In humans however, the use of quinolones during pregnancy has not resulted in negative outcomes, suggesting that they are a safe choice [55]. Parenteral therapy with aminoglycosides, another important class of anti-*Pseudomonal* therapy with known nephrotoxic and ototoxic effects, has not been shown to increase teratogenic risk and, with close monitoring of drug levels, is believed to be safe to use during pregnancy [56,57]. Inhaled forms of aminoglycosides such as tobramycin (Tobi) and colistin (Polymyxin E, colestimethate, Coly-Mycin M) have little systemic absorption and are thought to be safe throughout pregnancy [58]. Very little is known about the effects of recombinant DNAase dornase alfa (Pulmozyme) in pregnancy. As a result, its use should be avoided, if possible [20]. Hypertonic saline is unlikely to have any teratogenic effects and may be a good alternative in appropriate patients because it aids in airway clearance and decreases the incidence pulmonary exacerbations [59]. As with any pregnancy, however, the most important concern is the care and well-being of the mother. As a result, if clinical symptoms worsen, all potentially beneficial therapies should be considered.

Cystic fibrosis–related diabetes mellitus and pregnancy

Gestational diabetes is a common complication of CF pregnancies [35]. The high prevalence of gestational diabetes can be explained in part by the high prevalence of diabetes in the population of adults who have CF [38]. Adults who have CF, however, often have impaired insulin secretion long before clinical diabetes develops and may initially show difficulties with glucose tolerance only at times of stress and decreased tissue insulin sensitivity [38]. Pregnancy alters tissue sensitivity to insulin; therefore, it is very important to screen all

pregnant women who have CF with an OGTT before pregnancy and at the end of each trimester to
identify those who have gestational diabetes [60].
Control of diabetes during pregnancy is important
to achieve successful maternal weight gain and to
decrease the risk of preterm delivery, low birth
weight, and fetal cardiovascular, renal, and neural
tube defects [61–63]. Early treatment with insulin
or oral hypoglycemic agents has been shown to improve maternal and fetal outcomes [60].

Infant outcome

The number of live births following a CF
pregnancy has dramatically increased over the
last 15 years (see Fig. 5). Women who have CF,
however, remain at risk for preterm labor and delivery [2,36]. The rate of preterm infant births is about
6% in the general population but can be as high as
18% to 24% in women who have CF [2] and is associated with a number of clinical predictors. These
predictors include severe lung disease (FEV_1
< 50%, forced vital capacity < 60%), *Burkholderia
cepacia* colonization, pancreatic insufficiency, malnutrition, and poorly controlled CFRD [19,21,53].
The signs and symptoms of preterm labor should be
discussed with high-risk women to reduce the risk
of preterm delivery [36].

Delivery and postnatal issues

Vaginal delivery with optimal pain control and
supplemental oxygen is recommended in pregnant
women who have CF. Given the risks of anesthe-
sia and surgery, cesarean section should be used
only for obstetric indications, with an attempt
made for early postoperative mobilization [20,21].
Decreased adherence to a medical regimen is
common in new mothers who have CF and may
contribute to postpartum lung function decline
[33]. Mothers who have CF should be monitored
closely following childbirth, with aggressive management of pulmonary exacerbations [37]. Nutritional status should also be monitored closely
during the postpartum period. Successful breastfeeding in mothers who have CF is possible and
may be a desired option for some women [64].
Breast milk from women who have CF has normal
sodium and protein levels, with lipid levels sufficient
for the nursing needs of the infant [65]. Pregnancy,
however, exerts a nutritional strain on mothers who
have CF, which is intensified by breastfeeding. To
minimize the risk of malnutrition, advice regarding
infant feeding should be tailored to fit each
mother's individual needs.

Pregnancy post lung transplantation

Lung transplantation has emerged as a treatment option for patients who have end-stage lung
diseases, including CF. Although survival after
bilateral lung transplantation has improved, it
remains much lower than other solid organ transplants, with 5-year and 10-year survival rates of
only 59% and 38%, respectively [66]. Successful
pregnancies have been reported in women following lung transplant [67,68]; however, it remains
a risky proposition [69]. Data from the National
Transplantation Pregnancy Registry shows that
23% of lung transplant recipients experience loss
of graft function within 2 years of delivery [70].
These findings are supported by a recent study
comparing renal and lung transplant recipient
outcomes after pregnancy. The study showed
that renal transplant recipients had a lower rate
of rejection (4% versus 40%) and graft loss
(13% versus 30%) than lung transplant recipients
[69]. Several case reports suggest that pregnancy
post lung transplant does not affect overall disease
severity or maternal survival in women who have
CF compared with no pregnancy post lung transplant in women who have CF [70–72]. These data
suggest that although pregnancy post lung transplant may have a higher complication rate compared with other solid organ transplants, it does
not change overall maternal outcome in CF. The
current recommendation is to postpone pregnancy
for at least 2 years after transplant to allow for adequate time to assess lung graft function, rejection, and immunosuppressive regimen [51,73].
Although increased risk of congenital malformations associated with the use of immunosuppression has not been reported, female lung
recipients have a high incidence of premature
and low birth weight newborns [73]. In addition,
potentially poor outcomes post lung transplant
and post pregnancy and lung transplant raise the
ethical question of whether patients who have
a limited survival should have children. Because
these patients may not survive to see their child
grow up, these issues should be discussed with
CF patients who are considering pregnancy.

Summary

In summary, fertility issues are of increasing
importance as the CF patient population ages and
as long-term quality of life improves. Most men
who have CF are infertile due to obstructive
azoospermia; however, a small percentage of these

men retain fertility. It is therefore important to discuss fertility with men who have CF as early as the teenage years and to offer them semen analyses. Those who are infertile and wish to start families should be informed of the various options including adoption and ICSI/IVF.

Unlike men who have CF, women who have CF are often fertile. They should be counseled during their adolescent years about fertility and pregnancy and the appropriate use of contraception when pregnancy is not desired. When pregnancy is desired, it is important to educate all women who have CF and their partners about genetic screening for CFTR mutations and the possibility of having a child who has CF. There is growing evidence suggesting that pregnancy is safe in women who have CF and that maternal and fetal outcomes are better than once anticipated. Pregnancy, however, should be planned so that lung and nutritional health may be maximized before conception. Care during the pregnancy is best delivered using a multidisciplinary approach that involves the entire CF care team and an obstetrician familiar with the unique issues that may arise during a CF pregnancy. Meticulous attention to maternal health during pregnancy is essential in maximizing maternal and fetal outcomes. The number of successful CF pregnancies has increased significantly over the last 19 years, and continued successes are anticipated as overall survival continues to improve. Despite successful pregnancies in many women who have CF, it remains difficult to predict who will be best able to tolerate pregnancy, and the possibility of clinical decline should be discussed with all women who have CF before conception.

CF is no longer a disease limited to childhood and is best described as a chronic disease of adulthood. Our understanding of fertility and pregnancy in CF has increased tremendously over the last decade as our experience in caring for adults who have CF has increased. Technology has also played an important role in offering fertility options where none previously existed. The next decade holds the opportunity for even greater advances as adults who have CF live longer and fuller lives.

References

[1] Cystic Fibrosis Foundation Patient Registry. Annual data report 2005. Available at: http://www.cff.org/ID=4573/TYPE=2676/2005%20Patient%20Registry%20Report.pdf.

[2] Boyd JM, Mehta A, Murphy DJ. Fertility and pregnancy outcomes in men and women with cystic fibrosis in the United Kingdom. Hum Reprod 2004; 19(10):2238–43.

[3] Lyon A, Bilton D. Fertility issues in cystic fibrosis. Paediatr Respir Rev 2002;3(3):236–40.

[4] Tullis E. Reproductive issues in cystic fibrosis. A primer for adult-trained physicians and caregivers to develop special expertise in CF. Presented at the 2005 North America CF Conference.

[5] Chillon M, Casals T, Mercier B, et al. Mutations in the cystic fibrosis gene in patients with congenital absence of the vas deferens. N Engl J Med 1995; 332(22):1475–80.

[6] Stuhrmann M, Dork T. CFTR gene mutations and male infertility. Andrologia 2000;32(2):71–83.

[7] Dork T, Dworniczak B, Aulehla-Scholz C, et al. Distinct spectrum of CFTR gene mutations in congenital absence of vas deferens. Hum Genet 1997; 100(3–4):365–77.

[8] Kotloff RM, FitzSimmons SC, Fiel SB. Fertility and pregnancy in patients with cystic fibrosis. Clin Chest Med 1992;13(4):623–35.

[9] Wong PY. CFTR gene and male fertility. Mol Hum Reprod 1998;4(2):107–10.

[10] van der Ven K, Messer L, van der Ven H, et al. Cystic fibrosis mutation screening in healthy men with reduced sperm quality. Hum Reprod 1996;11(3): 513–7.

[11] Van Peperstraten A, Proctor ML, Johnson NP, et al. Techniques for surgical retrieval of sperm prior to ICSI for azoospermia. Cochrane Database Syst Rev 2006;3:CD002807.

[12] Peeraer K, Nijs M, Raick D, et al. Pregnancy after ICSI with ejaculated immotile spermatozoa from a patient with immotile cilia syndrome: a case report and review of the literature. Reprod Biomed Online 2004;9(6):659–63.

[13] Schlegel PN, Girardi SK. Clinical review 87: in vitro fertilization for male factor infertility. J Clin Endocrinol Metab 1997;82(3):709–16.

[14] McCallum TJ, Milunsky JM, Cunningham DL, et al. Fertility in men with cystic fibrosis: an update on current surgical practices and outcomes. Chest 2000;118(4):1059–62.

[15] Phillipson GT, Petrucco OM, Matthews CD. Congenital bilateral absence of the vas deferens, cystic fibrosis mutation analysis and intracytoplasmic sperm injection. Hum Reprod 2000;15(2):431–5.

[16] Nikolettos N, Asimakopoulos B, Papastefanou IS. Intracytoplasmic sperm injection—an assisted reproduction technique that should make us cautious about imprinting deregulation. J Soc Gynecol Investig 2006;13(5):317–28.

[17] Ericson A, Kallen B. Congenital malformations in infants born after IVF: a population-based study. Hum Reprod 2001;16(3):504–9.

[18] Lie RT, Lyngstadaas A, Orstavik KH, et al. Birth defects in children conceived by ICSI compared with

children conceived by other IVF-methods: a meta-analysis. Int J Epidemiol 2005;34(3):696–701.

[19] Edenborough FP. Women with cystic fibrosis and their potential for reproduction. Thorax 2001;56(8):649–55.

[20] Johannesson M. Effects of pregnancy on health: certain aspects of importance for women with cystic fibrosis. J Cyst Fibros 2002;1(1):9–12.

[21] Odegaard I, Stray-Pedersen B, Hallberg K, et al. Maternal and fetal morbidity in pregnancies of Norwegian and Swedish women with cystic fibrosis. Acta Obstet Gynecol Scand 2002;81(8):698–705.

[22] Odegaard I, Stray-Pedersen B, Hallberg K, et al. Prevalence and outcome of pregnancies in Norwegian and Swedish women with cystic fibrosis. Acta Obstet Gynecol Scand 2002;81(8):693–7.

[23] Chan HC, Shi QX, Zhou CX, et al. Critical role of CFTR in uterine bicarbonate secretion and the fertilizing capacity of sperm. Mol Cell Endocrinol 2006;250(1–2):106–13.

[24] Wang XF, Zhou CX, Shi QX, et al. Involvement of CFTR in uterine bicarbonate secretion and the fertilizing capacity of sperm. Nat Cell Biol 2003;5(10):902–6.

[25] Johannesson M, Landgren BM, Csemiczky G, et al. Female patients with cystic fibrosis suffer from reproductive endocrinological disorders despite good clinical status. Hum Reprod 1998;13(8):2092–7.

[26] Kopito LE, Kosasky HJ, Shwachman H. Water and electrolytes in cervical mucus from patients with cystic fibrosis. Fertil Steril 1973;24(7):512–6.

[27] Jarzabek K, Zbucka M, Pepinski W, et al. Cystic fibrosis as a cause of infertility. Reprod Biol 2004;4(2):119–29.

[28] Rowe SM, Miller S, Sorscher EJ. Cystic fibrosis. N Engl J Med 2005;352(19):1992–2001.

[29] Visconti PE, Kopf GS. Regulation of protein phosphorylation during sperm capacitation. Biol Reprod 1998;59(1):1–6.

[30] Timmreck LS, Gray MR, Handelin B, et al. Analysis of cystic fibrosis transmembrane conductance regulator gene mutations in patients with congenital absence of the uterus and vagina. Am J Med Genet A 2003;120(1):72–6.

[31] Johannesson M, Bogdanovic N, Nordqvist AC, et al. Cystic fibrosis mRNA expression in rat brain: cerebral cortex and medial preoptic area. Neuroreport 1997;8(2):535–9.

[32] Stallings VA, Tomezsko JL, Schall JI, et al. Adolescent development and energy expenditure in females with cystic fibrosis. Clin Nutr 2005;24(5):737–45.

[33] Wexler I, Johannesson M, Edenborough FP, et al. Pregnancy and chronic progressive pulmonary disease. Am J Respir Crit Care Med 2006; [Epub ahead of print].

[34] Siegel B, Siegel S. Pregnancy and delivery in a patient with cystic fibrosis of the pancreas. Obstet Gynecol 1960;(16):438–40.

[35] Gilljam M, Antoniou M, Shin J, et al. Pregnancy in cystic fibrosis. Fetal and maternal outcome. Chest 2000;118(1):85–91.

[36] Barak A, Dulitzki M, Efrati O, et al. Pregnancies and outcome in women with cystic fibrosis. Isr Med Assoc J 2005;7(2):95–8.

[37] Cheng EY, Goss CH, McKone EF, et al. Aggressive prenatal care results in successful fetal outcomes in CF women. J Cyst Fibros 2006;5(2):85–91.

[38] Moran A, Doherty L, Wang X, et al. Abnormal glucose metabolism in cystic fibrosis. J Pediatr 1998;133(1):10–7.

[39] Milla CE, Billings J, Moran A. Diabetes is associated with dramatically decreased survival in female but not male subjects with cystic fibrosis. Diabetes Care 2005;28(9):2141–4.

[40] Hardin DS, Rice J, Cohen RC, et al. The metabolic effects of pregnancy in cystic fibrosis. Obstet Gynecol 2005;106(2):367–75.

[41] Bush A, Alton EWFW, Davies JC, et al. Cystic fibrosis in the 21st century. Progr Respir Res 2006;34.

[42] Fiel SB. Pulmonary function during pregnancy in cystic fibrosis: implications for counseling. Curr Opin Pulm Med 1996;2(6):462–5.

[43] McMullen AH, Pasta DJ, Frederick PD, et al. Impact of pregnancy on women with cystic fibrosis. Chest 2006;129(3):706–11.

[44] Goss CH, Rubenfeld GD, Otto K, et al. The effect of pregnancy on survival in women with cystic fibrosis. Chest 2003;124(4):1460–8.

[45] Edenborough FP, Stableforth DE, Webb AK, et al. Outcome of pregnancy in women with cystic fibrosis. Thorax 1995;50(2):170–4.

[46] Jankelson D, Robinson M, Parsons S, et al. Cystic fibrosis and pregnancy. Aust N Z J Obstet Gynaecol 1998;38(2):180–4.

[47] Connors PM, Ulles MM. The physical, psychological, and social implications of caring for the pregnant patient and newborn with cystic fibrosis. J Perinat Neonatal Nurs 2005;19(4):301–15.

[48] Weiss BM, Hess OM. Pulmonary vascular disease and pregnancy: current controversies, management strategies, and perspectives. Eur Heart J 2000;21(2):104–15.

[49] Weiss BM, Zemp L, Seifert B, et al. Outcome of pulmonary vascular disease in pregnancy: a systematic overview from 1978 through 1996. J Am Coll Cardiol 1998;31(7):1650–7.

[50] Bendayan D, Hod M, Oron G, et al. Pregnancy outcome in patients with pulmonary arterial hypertension receiving prostacyclin therapy. Obstet Gynecol 2005;106(5 Pt 2):1206–10.

[51] Budev MM, Arroliga AC, Emery S. Exacerbation of underlying pulmonary disease in pregnancy. Crit Care Med 2005;33(10 Suppl):S313–8.

[52] Fraser KL, Tullis DE, Sasson Z, et al. Pulmonary hypertension and cardiac function in adult cystic fibrosis: role of hypoxemia. Chest 1999;115(5):1321–8.

[53] Edenborough FP, Mackenzie WE, Stableforth DE. The outcome of 72 pregnancies in 55 women with cystic fibrosis in the United Kingdom 1977–1996. BJOG 2000;107(2):254–61.

[54] Burkhardt JE, Walterspiel JN, Schaad UB. Quinolone arthropathy in animals versus children. Clin Infect Dis 1997;25(5):1196–204.

[55] Loebstein R, Addis A, Ho E, et al. Pregnancy outcome following gestational exposure to fluoroquinolones: a multicenter prospective controlled study. Antimicrob Agents Chemother 1998;42(6): 1336–9.

[56] Czeizel AE, Rockenbauer M, Olsen J, et al. A teratological study of aminoglycoside antibiotic treatment during pregnancy. Scand J Infect Dis 2000;32(3): 309–13.

[57] Canny GJ. Pregnancy in patients with cystic fibrosis. CMAJ 1993;149(6):805–6.

[58] Geller DE, Pitlick WH, Nardella PA, et al. Pharmacokinetics and bioavailability of aerosolized tobramycin in cystic fibrosis. Chest 2002;122(1):219–26.

[59] Elkins MR, Robinson M, Rose BR, et al. A controlled trial of long-term inhaled hypertonic saline in patients with cystic fibrosis. N Engl J Med 2006; 354(3):229–40.

[60] Hardin DS, Rice J, Cohen RC, et al. The metabolic effects of pregnancy in cystic fibrosis. Obstet Gynecol 2005;106(2):367–75.

[61] Becerra JE, Khoury MJ, Cordero JF, et al. Diabetes mellitus during pregnancy and the risks for specific birth defects: a population-based case-control study. Pediatrics 1990;85(1):1–9.

[62] Mills JL. Malformations in infants of diabetic mothers. Teratology 1982;25(3):385–94.

[63] Mace S, Hirschfield SS, Riggs T, et al. Echocardiographic abnormalities in infants of diabetic mothers. J Pediatr 1979;95(6):1013–9.

[64] Michel SH, Mueller DH. Impact of lactation on women with cystic fibrosis and their infants: a review of five cases. J Am Diet Assoc 1994;94(2):159–65.

[65] Kent NE, Farquharson DF. Cystic fibrosis in pregnancy. CMAJ 1993;149(6):809–13.

[66] Egan TM, Detterbeck FC, Mill MR, et al. Long term results of lung transplantation for cystic fibrosis. Eur J Cardiothorac Surg 2002;22(4):602–9.

[67] Scott JP, Dennis C, Mullins P. Heart-lung transplantation for end-stage respiratory disease in cystic fibrosis patients. J R Soc Med 1993;86(Suppl 20): 19–22.

[68] Parry D, Hextall A, Robinson VP, et al. Pregnancy following a single lung transplant. Thorax 1996; 51(11):1162–4 [discussion: 1164–5].

[69] Gyi KM, Hodson ME, Yacoub MY. Pregnancy in cystic fibrosis lung transplant recipients: case series and review. J Cyst Fibros 2006;5(3):171–5.

[70] Armenti VT, Radomski JS, Moritz MJ, et al. Report from the National Transplantation Pregnancy Registry (NTPR): outcomes of pregnancy after transplantation. Clin Transpl 2002;16:121–30.

[71] Gertner G, Coscia L, McGrory C, et al. Pregnancy in lung transplant recipients. Prog Transplant 2000; 10(2):109–12.

[72] Parry D, Hextall A, Banner N, et al. Pregnancy following lung transplantation. Transplant Proc 1997; 29(1–2):629.

[73] McKay DB, Josephson MA. Pregnancy in recipients of solid organs—effects on mother and child. N Engl J Med 2006;354(12):1281–93.

ELSEVIER
SAUNDERS

Clin Chest Med 28 (2007) 445–457

CLINICS
IN CHEST
MEDICINE

Advances in Lung Transplantation for Patients Who Have Cystic Fibrosis

Hilary J. Goldberg, MD[a,b,*], Aaron Deykin, MD[a,b]

[a]*Department of Medicine, Harvard Medical School, PBB Clinics-3, 75 Francis Street, Boston, MA 02115, USA*
[b]*Division of Pulmonary and Critical Care Medicine, Brigham and Women's Hospital,
PBB Clinics-3, 75 Francis Street, Boston, MA 02115, USA*

Using innovative approaches to the management of cystic fibrosis (CF), practitioners and patients have worked together to improve survivorship, with predicted survival now reaching beyond 30 years of age [1]. Despite these accomplishments, CF remains a chronic, progressive illness, with CF-associated lung disease being the primary cause of death. Although progress in outcomes related to lung transplantation has not been as rapidly achieved, this modality remains an important therapeutic option for patients who have CF with deteriorating lung function. Transplantation in patients who have CF presents important challenges regarding appropriate candidate selection and preoperative management, technical obstacles in the perioperative period, the postoperative management of medical comorbidities related to CF, and the psychosocial impact of transplantation. This article outlines some of these challenges and describes recent advances in approaching this endeavor in patients who have CF.

Selection of appropriate candidates for lung transplantation is an important factor contributing to posttransplant outcomes. Regardless of their underlying lung diseases, recipients should be well conditioned so as to be able to participate in postprocedure rehabilitation, have adequate coping skills and social supports to meet the challenges of this undertaking, and have adequate

working relationships with practitioners to ensure compliance with the complicated protocols of posttransplant care. The unique aspects of their systemic illness also affect patients who have CF. The need for high doses of steroids posttransplant affects blood sugar control, and the presence of cirrhosis with portal hypertension is considered a contraindication to transplantation. Patients should be able to maintain 80% to 100% of ideal body weight. Colonization with resistant organisms should also be considered (Box 1). Such issues are addressed in more detail in this article.

Preoperative considerations

Patient selection and timing of referral

In light of improving survival in the CF population (Fig. 1) and limited gains in survival after lung transplantation (Fig. 2), initiating consideration for lung transplantation in the CF population has become more challenging. Patients and practitioners frequently attempt to delay the procedure as long as possible without allowing the patient to deteriorate to the point that they are no longer safe candidates. In this regard, there has been considerable interest in identifying accurate prognostic markers in CF that can be used to establish the appropriate timing for transplant referral. Historically, the forced expiratory volume in 1 second (FEV_1) is the most frequently used parameter for assessment of this goal. In 1992, Kerem and colleagues [3] reported that FEV_1 less than 30% predicted, along with hypoxemia and hypercapnia, were significant predictors of poor survival at 2 years in patients who have

---

* Corresponding author. Division of Pulmonary and Critical Care Medicine, Brigham and Women's Hospital, PBB Clinics-3, 75 Francis Street, Boston, MA 02115.
E-mail address: hjgoldberg@partners.org (H.J. Goldberg).

CF. The findings of Mayer-Hamblett and colleagues [4] support the use of FEV_1 as a predictor of mortality while awaiting transplantation. The authors compared FEV_1 percent predicted with a multicomponent model derived from CF Foundation National Patient Registry data. Despite the incorporation of age, the presence or absence of specific infectious organisms in culture, the need for hospitalization or intravenous antibiotics,

mean height, and mean FEV_1, the model was not superior to FEV_1% (at a threshold of 30%) with respect to predicting 2-year mortality. Because some data suggest that patients who have CF with FEV_1 less than 30% predicted who did not undergo transplantation survived longer than those who had similar FEV_1 measurements who did undergo transplant, the use of FEV_1% as a strict indication for lung transplantation is not universally accepted [5].

Although initial multicomponent prediction models for survival in CF were not robust enough to inform a clinical decision to proceed with transplant referral, subsequent prediction models developed for the CF population provided better assessments of mortality among patients who have CF. Incorporation of the rate of decline of FEV_1 and age led to a more successful predictive model of mortality for these patients [6,7]. Rosenbluth and colleagues [8], suggest that use of the rate of decline in lung function would not only prevent referral for patients with a higher likelihood of survival without transplant but might also allow for earlier referral of patients who have more rapid courses of deterioration. Some authors postulate that the duration of FEV_1 below 30% should be followed before committing patients to lung transplantation [9].

Hypercapnia has been found to be a significant predictor of mortality in patients who have CF, independent of spirometric data [3,10]. The 6-minute walk test may also help to identify appropriate timing of referral [11], with a distance of less than 400 m suggested as a threshold [12]. Pulmonary

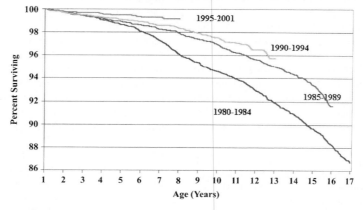

Fig. 1. Survival from age one by birth cohort. (*From* 2004 Annual Data Report to the Center Directors. Cystic Fibrosis Patient Registry, Bethesda, MD; used with permission.)

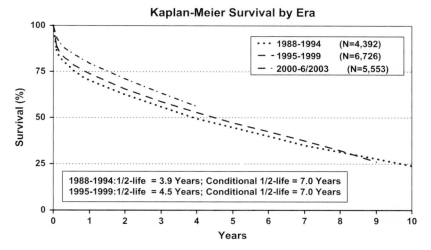

Fig. 2. Survival after lung transplantation by era from January 1988 to June 2003. (*From* 2004 Annual Data Report to the Center Directors. Cystic Fibrosis Patient Registry, Bethesda, MD; used with permission.)

hemodynamics are significant determinants of patient deterioration while awaiting transplantation. Mortality in patients who have CF is higher when pulmonary artery systolic pressure is elevated (>35 mm Hg) whether or not the pulmonary hypertension is clinically evident [13]. Venuta and colleagues [14] documented a significant deterioration in pulmonary hemodynamics in patients who had CF while awaiting transplantation. Disparity in perfusion between lungs as seen on ventilation-perfusion scans may identify a subset of patients who have CF with more severe pulmonary disease than is evident on pulmonary function testing alone [15].

The decision to proceed with transplantation for an individual patient involves consideration of mortality without transplant and the likelihood of an acceptable transplant outcome. In this regard, Liou and colleagues [16] found younger age at transplantation, the presence of *Berkholderia cepacia*, and the presence of CF-related arthropathy to be independent predictors of poor outcomes after transplant. Pretransplant clinical status, as determined by such parameters as minimum oxygen saturation during 12-minute walk testing, age-adjusted heart rate, and blood hemoglobin concentration and serum albumin, was not predictive of posttransplant survival in pediatric patients who had CF [17]. Bartz and colleagues [18] also found that the need for mechanical ventilation did not lead to suboptimal posttransplant outcomes, suggesting that the use of ventilatory support is not in

and of itself a contraindication to transplantation in patients who have CF. Caution should be used in advising transplantation for patients on mechanical ventilation who have limited mobility, significant deconditioning, and a low likelihood of participation in posttransplant rehabilitation.

In referral for transplant evaluation, the percent predicted FEV_1 should be considered in conjunction with other factors, such as rate of decline of pulmonary function, other medical comorbidities, and quality of life, in determining the optimal timing for evaluation. Although data suggest that percent predicted FEV_1 is a useful marker to follow, the urgency with which to consider transplantation cannot be determined by this marker alone. A recent consensus statement on lung transplantation in CF supports this comprehensive approach to timing discussions regarding lung transplantation (Box 1) [2].

The majority of the studies examining the timing of referral of patients who have CF for lung transplantation were conducted in the era of allocation based upon time served on the transplant list. Since May 2005, the United Network for Organ Sharing has instituted a new method of listing for lung transplantation. Potential recipients are now assigned Lung Allocation System (LAS) scores based upon objective data acquired at the time of listing (Box 2) [19]. The goal of the LAS scoring system is to minimize mortality for listed patients and to maximize posttransplant survival. Although underlying lung disease is factored

Box 2. Components of lung allocation score

Diagnosis
Age
Body mass index
Presence or absence of diabetes mellitus
Supplemental oxygen use
Six-minute walk distance
Pulmonary artery systolic pressure
Pulmonary capillary wedge pressure
Forced vital capacity
Serum creatinine (mg/dl)
Functional status
Presence or absence of assisted
  ventilation

Data from Information for transplant professionals about the lung allocation scoring system. Available at: http://www.unos.org/SharedContentDocuments/lung_allocation.professionalv4.pdf. Accessed November 13, 2006.

into the LAS calculation, the remaining criteria for listing are generic to all transplant recipients. Some of the components of the LAS score are predictive of survival for patients who have CF in particular, although forced vital capacity, and not FEV_1, is used to reflect lung function (Box 2). The aim of the LAS system is to shorten time to transplant for patients who have the most rapid deterioration in status, although outcome studies of the effectiveness of the system have not been conducted. Thus, recommendations for referral of patients who have CF to transplant centers will likely require modification in light of this new listing system.

Infectious considerations

Numerous organisms can colonize or infect the lungs of patients who have CF. Although any organism that is cultured preoperatively has the potential to complicate the patient's postoperative course, resistant gram-negative organisms pose the greatest threat to the transplanted lungs of patients who have CF and have been studied most extensively in the literature. Person-to-person transmission of organisms is also a concern, leading to the detailed investigation of infection control mechanisms in this population.

Specific infectious considerations

B cepacia and other Burkholderia infections. Because lung transplantation has become more common for patients who have CF and because their outcomes have been explored in more detail, CF centers have noted significant posttransplant complications related to *B cepacia* infection. As of 2004, the United States Cystic Fibrosis Foundation Patient Registry Report indicated that 2.9% of patients who have CF have positive cultures for *B cepacia* [1]. Although the majority of patients who have CF harbor the same strains of *B cepacia* pre- and posttransplantation [20], person-to-person transmission of this organism has been described at lung transplant referral centers [21]. Ramirez and colleagues [22] were the first to describe the impact of *B cepacia* on posttransplant outcomes in lung transplant recipients who have CF. In a retrospective study of 17 patients transplanted at the University of Toronto for CF lung disease, the most common cause of postprocedure morbidity and mortality was found to be *B cepacia*–related pneumonia. In a follow-up study, Snell and colleagues [23] found that of 24 patients transplanted for CF, 10 were colonized with *B cepacia* before transplant, and five subsequently acquired the organism. Of these 15 patients, seven died. More significantly, the median time to death was 28 days for those who were *B cepacia* positive, and five of the seven patients died as a direct result of the organism. The noted complications related to *B cepacia* included pneumonia, sepsis, empyema, abscess, pericarditis, and sinusitis. An example of *B cepacia*–related mediastinal infection is depicted in Fig. 3.

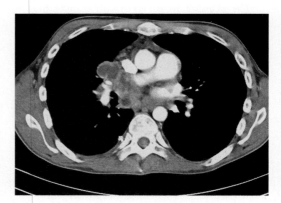

Fig. 3. Multilobular soft tissue densities in the mediastinum and right hilum representing *B cepacia* abscess formation in a patient who has CF 2 months after lung transplantation.

In contrast to the Toronto experience, early reports from the University of North Carolina [24] and the United Kingdom [25] failed to demonstrate an increased risk of complications related to *B cepacia* infection. Despite these discrepancies, numerous transplant programs in the United States identified the presence of *B cepacia* in pretransplant cultures to be an absolute contraindication to lung transplantation. Because the epidemiology of this organism has been elucidated, this decision has come under reconsideration.

As a result of recent studies, *B cepacia* has been identified as a complex divided into nine genomovars (I–IX), with distinct names for each strain (Table 1) [26]. In 2001, LiPuma and colleagues [27] demonstrated that epidemic strains were found only rarely in infected patients who have CF in the United States. *B cenocepacia* is most closely identified with complications in patients who have CF whether or not they undergo transplantation. In 2001, the North Carolina group reported increased mortality at 6 months and at 1, 3, and 5 years posttransplant in patients infected with *B cepacia* pretransplant [28]. All deaths occurred in patients infected with *B cenocepacia*. Similarly, in an update to the United Kingdom experience, De Soyza and colleagues [29] reported an almost 50% mortality risk in patients who had preoperative *B cepacia* infection. The authors attributed four of their five reported deaths to *B cenocepacia*; the fifth strain was unidentified. All deaths at their institution were associated with an epidemic strain that was highly prevalent at their center [30]. Investigators from Italy and Belgium also reported frequent infection with epidemic strains

Table 1
Taxonomy of the *Burkholderia cepacia* complex

Genomovar	Strain
I	*B cepacia*
II	*B multivorans*
III	*B cenocepacia*
IV	*B stabiliz*
V	*B vietnamiensis*
VI	*B dolosa*
VII	*B ambifaria*
VIII	*B anthina*
IX	*B pyrrocinia*

Data from Reik R, Spilker T, Lipuma JJ. Distribution of Burkholderia cepacia complex species among isolates recovered from persons with or without cystic fibrosis. J Clin Microbiol 2005;43(6):2926–8, and Refs. [26,27].

of *B cenocepacia* associated with a high mortality rate in patients who had CF who did not undergo transplantation [31,32].

The findings of these studies suggest that although deaths have been associated with other *B cepacia* strains [32], infection with *B cenocepacia* provides the greatest risk of morbidity and mortality among patients who have CF, particularly those who undergo lung transplantation. The high prevalence of an epidemic strain in Toronto may account for the findings reported by that transplant program [33]. In light of the low infection rate with this strain in other North American centers, other heterogenous strains and other virulence factors likely contribute to the poor outcomes associated with *B cenocepacia* infection.

As a result of the recent association of *B cenocepacia* with the majority of morbidity and mortality in patients who have CF who undergo lung transplantation, some investigators suggest that the use of genomovar typing may allow for the identification and safe transplantation of individuals infected with strains other than *B cenocepacia* [34]. Moreover, the Toronto and North Carolina groups have reported significant improvements in outcomes after alteration of their protocols for transplantation of individuals colonized with *B cenocepacia* [35,36]. Specifically, the Toronto protocol involves altered immunosuppression with the omission of antilymphocyte induction and a broadened prophylactic antibiotic regimen including intravenous chloramphenicol for all patients colonized with *B cepacia* [35]. In North Carolina, patients undergo pleural washouts with taurolidine [34]. Both institutions report improved outcomes, although few patients have been observed. Thus, although many transplant centers consider *B cepacia* infection as a relative contraindication to lung transplantation, patients who have CF with positive cultures should be referred for evaluation at programs with significant experience in transplantation in the setting of *B cepacia* infection if local centers defer transplantation for such patients. The morbidity associated with this infection posttransplantation independent of mortality must also be considered, and individualized decisions regarding transplantation should be used.

Burkholderia gladioli is another *Burkholderia* species associated with morbidity in lung transplant recipients who have CF. Two of 21 patients transplanted for CF at Duke University Medical Center were culture positive for *B gladioli* preprocedure [36]. Both patients suffered *B glad-ioli* wound infections and bacteremia posttransplant. Khan and colleagues [37] reported a case of death secondary to *B gladioli* infection after transplantation and suggested that this infection be considered in selection criteria for lung transplantation. This infection is much less common than *B cepacia* and is therefore less well studied in patients who have CF, regardless of their transplant status.

P aeruginosa. According to the Cystic Fibrosis Foundation Registry, over 57% of patients who have CF are colonized with *P aeruginosa* [1]. As a result of frequent exposure to antimicrobial agents, these patients often grow pan-resistant pseudomonas in culture, with one study identifying a greater than 75% incidence of pan-resistant strains [36], a pattern of concern in assessing posttransplant risk. In the immunosuppressed patient in particular, such organisms can become pathogenic, leading to infectious complications and contributing to the development of rejection in association with inflammatory pneumonic processes.

The majority of patients who have CF retain their original strains of *P aeruginosa* after transplantation [38]. In comparison with recipients of lung transplants for other indications, studies show that although patients who have CF demonstrate positive cultures for *P aeruginosa* earlier and more frequently after transplantation, patients who have CF are not at increased risk of mortality related to this organism [24,39]. This fact may result from the inadequacy of in vitro susceptibility testing to determine the realities of microbial sensitivities in vivo [40]. Despite this, infection with *P aeruginosa* seems to produce increased inflammation in the lung in CF and non-CF lung transplant recipients [39]. The impact of this increased level of inflammation on the development of acute rejection has not been well elucidated.

With the advent of synergy testing to determine the susceptibility of particular *P aeruginosa* strains to combination antibiotic regimens, the comfort level related to the acceptance of patients who have CF who are colonized with pan-resistant organisms has increased. The implementation of synergy testing into the selection of patients who have CF for transplantation has been advocated in guidelines for patient selection [41]. As a result, colonization with pan-resistant *P aeruginosa* is not considered a contraindication to lung transplantation.

Fungal infections. Colonization with fungi, such as *Aspergillus* species, is common in patients who have CF. One study assessed a 33% prevalence of aspergillus in sinus aspirates from patients who have CF [42]. In comparison with recipients who have other underlying lung diseases, patients who have CF do not seem to be at increased risk for invasive fungal pneumonia [43,44]. Patients who have CF are at risk for early anastomotic involvement with fungus, particularly if colonized pretransplant [4]. Such infections may require systemic treatment [44]. The role of fungal prophylaxis in the prevention of anastomotic and invasive fungal disease continues to be investigated, with many transplant programs incorporating prophylaxis into transplant protocols.

Other infections. Other microbial infections common to patients who have CF include *Staphylococcus aureus*, *Stenotrophomonas*, and atypical mycobacteria. Any pretransplant colonizing organism has the potential to become pathogenic posttransplantation, and prophylactic measures to prevent such complications, especially in the setting of mycobacterial infection, should be considered before proceeding with the procedure.

Infection control

In light of the ubiquitous nature of infectious organisms in patients who have CF and the significant risk and impact of person-to-person transmission, specific guidelines have been published for infection control in this group [45]. These include the use of contact precautions for patients infected or colonized with Methicillin resistant *Staphylococcus aureus*, *B cepacia*, multidrug-resistant *P aeruginosa*, or Vancomycin resistant *Enterococcus*; placement of lung transplant recipients in single rooms; and scheduling of testing and procedures for patients who have CF to minimize contact with each other. Patients who have cepacia in particular should be segregated from other patients who have CF, evaluated on separate clinic days or at the end of the day, and isolated from common waiting areas [46]. Such practices should be implemented in all transplant centers servicing patients who have CF.

Other preoperative considerations

Sinus colonization with infectious organisms can contribute to the development of posttransplant infections. As a result, pretransplant sinus evaluations with CT scans and ENT referrals should be considered in patients who have CF. Although to our knowledge no studies examining the impact of pretransplant sinus interventions have been published, postprocedure intervention produced a significant correlation between negative sinus aspirates and negative bronchoalveolar lavage cultures in one publication [46].

As a result of the effect of immune suppressive medications on the liver, pretransplant liver function should be assessed before transplantation. Although lung transplantation is contraindicated in patients who have cirrhosis and portal hypertension, for select patients, consideration can be made for combined lung–liver transplantation, with referral to a transplant center experienced in such procedures [47].

Studies suggest a more rapid deterioration in lung function in diabetic patients who have CF as compared with patients free of CF-related diabetes [48,49]. As a result, the presence of CF-related diabetes mellitus is one marker used for consideration of transplant referral. Transplantation is likely to exacerbate hyperglycemia, most significantly due to the high doses of corticosteroids administered postprocedure, and blood sugar control should be optimized before listing. Enhancement of glucose control pretransplant will also likely improve nutritional status in patients who have CF awaiting transplantation. Published guidelines on the management of diabetes mellitus in patients who have CF should be implemented in this population [50].

Nutritional status is another important consideration in patients who have CF who are under evaluation for lung transplantation. Although data on the impact of nutritional status on survival in patients who have CF are conflicting, at least one study of risk factors for death in patients who have CF who are awaiting lung transplantation demonstrated a correlation between the need for nutritional intervention and an increased risk of death [10]. This conclusion verifies the finding of an association between lean body mass and mortality in a cohort of patients with end-stage lung diseases of various types (including CF) awaiting lung transplantation [51]. Moreover, in patients requiring ICU stays of more than 5 days postsurgery, body mass index below the 25th percentile predicted an increased risk of death in another study [52]. Many transplant programs require patients to achieve at least 80% of ideal body weight before listing. Thus, nutritional interventions should be undertaken for patients who have CF who are below this threshold. One study of candidates for lung transplantation showed that a single session of individual dietary counseling was enough to achieve a significant increase in energy intake in patients awaiting lung transplantation [53], although patients who have CF often require more intensive nutritional interventions, including supplemental nutrition administered through feeding tubes, to achieve this goal. Transplantation has been shown to lead to improved nutritional status in a cohort of patients, including those who have CF [54].

Operative considerations

Procedure type

As a result of the suppurative nature of CF-related lung disease and patient colonization with a variety of microbes, lung transplantation for patients who have CF requires bilateral pneumonectomy to prevent microbial contamination of the allograft. When lung transplantation was first performed for CF, recipients underwent combined heart–lung transplantation because of center familiarity with this technique for lung transplant recipients in general. This intervention limits the availability of cadaveric hearts for patients who medically require heart or heart–lung transplantation and increases the risk of rejection-related cardiac vasculopathy in patients who have CF with functioning hearts [55]. As experience with transplantation has increased, double lung transplantation via a bilateral, sequential procedure has become the operation of choice for patients who have CF, with or without the aid of cardiopulmonary bypass. Studies have demonstrated comparable short- and long-term outcomes to those of heart–lung transplantation [56–58]. Despite case reports of success with single lung transplantation and contralateral pneumonectomy [59], the benefits of double lung transplantation on pulmonary function in patients already undergoing bilateral thoracic interventions have led to the standard use of this procedure. Although pleural disease is an operative concern in patients who have CF, data show no increase in operative times, cardiopulmonary bypass length, or blood product requirements in patients who have CF as compared with other transplant recipients as a result of pleural abnormalities [60].

Living-donor lobar transplantation is an alternative for patients awaiting lung transplantation and is performed most commonly for patients who have CF as a result of their average smaller stature and more appropriate size matching for this procedure [61]. Although outcomes at 1, 3, and 5 years are comparable to those of cadaveric transplantation in limited reports [61], transplant centers typically pursue this procedure for patients unlikely to survive while awaiting cadaveric transplantation [62] primarily because of the low but not absent risk presented to the donor.

The living lobar transplantation procedure involves the removal of both diseased lungs from the recipient and the implantation of two lower lobes, each harvested from a separate donor. Donors undergo thorough assessments before acceptance. The medical evaluation includes a history and physical examination, chest radiograph, pulmonary function testing, and arterial blood gas assessment. An extensive psychologic evaluation is performed to ensure that the donor's decision is volitional and that no coercion is involved. Related and unrelated individuals can be considered for donation. Survival data for recipients are equivalent to those of cadaveric transplantation at transplant centers with extensive experience with this technique [61,62]. Although no donors have died as a result of lobar donation, complications after the procedure have been reported [61,62]. Studies are underway to assess the risk of living donor lung transplantation in comparison to that of other solid organ transplantation from living donors, but this procedure remains relatively infrequent.

Postoperative considerations

Outcomes

Various measures have been used to ascertain the benefits of lung transplantation in patients who have CF. Outcomes include survival data, quality of life evaluations, cost-effectiveness measures, and psychosocial outcomes. Retrospective studies of CF cohorts at individual institutions report survival statistics in patients who have CF comparable to those available for all transplant recipients nationally [63–65]. The 1- and 5-year survival data for these institutions range from 73% to 79% and up to 57%, respectively. Significant improvements in pulmonary function are noted in these studies. A subset of long-term survivors has been described, with a 38% 10-year survival rate noted at one institution [66]. In addition, in direct comparisons, CF survival statistics

for patients free of *B cepacia* are comparable to those of recipients who have other lung diseases [67], with no difference in the incidence of acute rejection or bronchiolitis obliterans syndrome seen [68]. In an analysis of data from the Joint United Network for Organ Sharing/International Society for Heart and Lung Transplantation Thoracic Registry, the clearest survival benefit from lung transplantation was observed in the CF cohort [69].

In addition to mortality benefits, lung transplant recipients who have CF experience improvements in measures of quality of life after transplantation. Patients who have CF who are awaiting lung transplantation are more likely to be employed, to have lower levels of anxiety, and to have stronger social support systems than lung transplant recipients who have other lung diseases [70], perhaps as a result of the extensive experience such patients have in living with chronic illness. Such coping skills benefit patients who have CF in the posttransplant period. Investigators have observed comparable changes in symptoms of anxiety and depression, assessments of well-being, and performance status in patients who have CF after transplantation to those with other lung diseases, with superior mobility and sleep assessments [71]. Thus, well selected patients who undergo lung transplantation seem to experience survival benefits and improvements to functioning and quality of life.

Despite these findings, individuals who have CF face significant challenges in approaching the prospect of lung transplantation. In addressing the psychosocial impact of lung transplantation on this population, Kurland and Orenstein [72] identify specific features of CF and its treatment that can act as obstacles to the transplant process. These include comanagement between CF and transplant physicians, with potentially conflicting goals and protocols; divergent approaches to noncompliance; and opposing viewpoints regarding end-of-life care. Such conflicts, according to the authors, can produce anxiety in patients, with potential distrust of one management team in comparison to another. As a result, adequate communication is paramount between the transplant team and the patient and between the transplant team and the CF physicians to ensure a successful outcome in the pre- and posttransplant periods. Indeed, patients who have CF have identified loss of control and disruptions to daily routine as some of the most detrimental aspects of life posttransplant [73]. Despite these

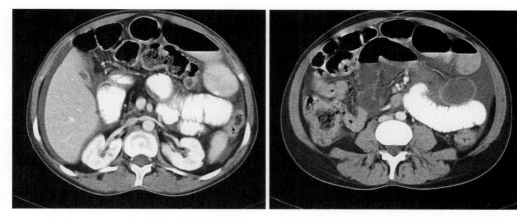

Fig. 4. High-grade small bowel obstruction with transition point in mid- to distal ileum in a patient who has CF after lung transplantation.

obstacles, patients who have CF describe positive outlooks and renewed interest in setting and achieving long-term goals after transplantation [74]. Finally, transplantation for CF seems to be cost-effective when assessing life-years, quality-adjusted life-years, and costs with and without transplantation [75].

Other considerations

Although transplantation for CF trades the consequences of the disease on lung function with the consequences of transplant itself, other complications of CF remain important and are potentially exacerbated in the postprocedure period. In particular, gastrointestinal complications and malabsorption continue to be significant factors in the posttransplant management of patients who have CF. Distal intestinal obstruction syndrome is common in patients who have CF and occurs as a result of inspissated secretions. This disorder occurs in 10% to 20% of patients who have CF after lung transplantation, most commonly in the immediate postoperative period (Fig. 4) [75,76]. Distal intestinal obstruction syndrome frequently necessitates laparotomy in this setting, with pretransplant abdominal surgery presenting the most significant risk factor for the development of obstruction [76]. Some institutions recommend prophylactic interventions, such as early enteral feeding and the introduction of pancreatic enzymes, along with institution of an aggressive bowel regimen and consideration of intestinal lavage with a balanced electrolyte solution, to prevent this complication [75,76].

Gastrointestinal disturbances can affect the level of immune suppression achieved in patients who have CF. Fat malabsorption, a common component of CF-related gastrointestinal disturbances, can affect calcineurin-inhibitor absorption. As a result, studies have shown lower bioavailability and greater inter- and intrasubject variability when measuring cyclosporine absorption in comparison to recipients who have other lung diseases [77]. Cyclosporine levels assessed at 2 hours postadministration seem to be more accurate than trough levels in assessing area under the curve for cyclosporine in this setting [77]. These findings remained unchanged despite medication administration in conjunction with pancreatic enzymes [78]. Some investigators suggest improved bioavailability with the use of a microemulsion formulation of cyclosporine, with beneficial effects on lung function observed at 3 months [79–81]. Similar, but less marked, abnormalities in drug absorption have been described with tacrolimus administration in patients who have CF, with monitoring of tacrolimus levels 3 hours after administration suggested as optimal [82,83]. Finally, cell cycle inhibitors, such as mycophenolic acid, which are used as a second arm in immune suppression postlung transplantation, are absorbed to lesser degrees in patients who have CF, and higher doses may be required to achieve optimal effect [84].

Other considerations in lung transplant recipients who have CF include vitamin deficiencies and osteoporosis prevention. Thus, posttransplantation management of patients who have CF requires a multidisciplinary, comprehensive approach to care. Continued attention to other end-organ dysfunction related to CF and communication between the transplant team and other specialized providers is necessary to ensure optimal outcomes.

Summary

Successful lung transplantation for patients who have CF is an attainable goal, and this therapeutic intervention should be considered in individuals who have advanced disease. The optimal timing of referral for consideration remains to be identified, particularly in light of new listing criteria, but discussion should be initiated when a comprehensive assessment of patient status indicates declining parameters. The decision to pursue transplantation is an individualized one, incorporating objective medical criteria and patient opinions and attitudes. A multidisciplinary approach should be used at all stages of the transplant process. Although outcomes similar to those of other recipients can be attained in patients who have CF, the unique challenges posed by this patient population require vigilance to achieve improvements in patient survival and quality of life.

References

[1] Cystic fibrosis foundation, patient registry 2004 annual report. Available at: http://www.cff.org/ID= 4573/TYPE=2676/2004PatientRegistryReport.pdf. Accessed November 22, 2006.

[2] Yankaskas JR, Mallory GB Jr. Lung transplantation in cystic fibrosis: consensus conference statement [review]. Chest 1998;113:217–26.

[3] Kerem E, Reisman J, Corey M, et al. Prediction of mortality in patients with cystic fibrosis [see comment]. N Engl J Med 1992;326:1187–91.

[4] Mayer-Hamblett N, Rosenfeld M, Emerson J, et al. Developing cystic fibrosis lung transplant referral criteria using predictors of 2-year mortality [see comment]. Am J Respir Crit Care Med 2002;166:1550–5.

[5] Augarten A, Akons H, Aviram M, et al. Prediction of mortality and timing of referral for lung transplantation in cystic fibrosis patients [see comment]. Pediatr Transplant 2001;5:339–42.

[6] Robinson W, Waltz DA. FEV(1) as a guide to lung transplant referral in young patients with cystic fibrosis. Pediatr Pulmonol 2000;30:198–202.

[7] Milla CE, Warwick WJ. Risk of death in cystic fibrosis patients with severely compromised lung function [see comment]. Chest 1998;113:1230–4.

[8] Rosenbluth DB, Wilson K, Ferkol T, et al. Lung function decline in cystic fibrosis patients and timing for lung transplantation referral [see comment]. Chest 2004;126:412–9.

[9] Doershuk CF, Stern RC. Timing of referral for lung transplantation for cystic fibrosis: overemphasis on FEV1 may adversely affect overall survival. Chest 1999;115:782–7.

[10] Belkin RA, Henig NR, Singer LG, et al. Risk factors for death of patients with cystic fibrosis awaiting lung transplantation. Am J Respir Crit Care Med 2006;173:659–66.

[11] Vizza CD, Yusen RD, Lynch JP, et al. Outcome of patients with cystic fibrosis awaiting lung transplantation. Am J Respir Crit Care Med 2000;162: 819–25.

[12] Kadikar A, Maurer J, Kesten S. The six-minute walk test: a guide to assessment for lung transplantation. J Heart Lung Transplant 1997;16:313–9.

[13] Fraser KL, Tullis DE, Sasson Z, et al. Pulmonary hypertension and cardiac function in adult cystic fibrosis: role of hypoxemia. Chest 1999;115:1321–8.

[14] Venuta F, Rendina EA, Rocca GD, et al. Pulmonary hemodynamics contribute to indicate priority for lung transplantation in patients with cystic fibrosis. J Thorac Cardiovasc Surg 2000;119:682–9.

[15] Stanchina ML, Tantisira KG, Aquino SL, et al. Association of lung perfusion disparity and mortality in patients with cystic fibrosis awaiting lung transplantation [see comment]. J Heart Lung Transplant 2002;21:217–25.

[16] Liou TG, Adler FR, Huang D. Use of lung transplantation survival models to refine patient selection in cystic fibrosis. Am J Respir Crit Care Med 2005; 171:1053–9.

[17] Aurora P, Gassas A, Ehtisham S, et al. The effect of prelung transplant clinical status on post-transplant survival of children with cystic fibrosis. Eur Respir J 2000;16:1061–4.

[18] Bartz RR, Love RB, Leverson GE, et al. Pre-transplant mechanical ventilation and outcome in patients with cystic fibrosis. J Heart Lung Transplant 2003;22:433–8.

[19] Information for transplant professionals about the lung allocation scoring system. Available at: http://www.unos.org/SharedContentDocuments/lung_ allocation.professionalv4.pdf. Accessed November 13, 2006.

[20] Steinbach S, Sun L, Jiang RZ, et al. Transmissibility of pseudomonas cepacia infection in clinic patients and lung-transplant recipients with cystic fibrosis [see comment]. N Engl J Med 1994;331:981–7.

[21] Heath DG, Hohneker K, Carriker C, et al. Six-year molecular analysis of burkholderia cepacia complex isolates among cystic fibrosis patients at a referral center for lung transplantation. J Clin Microbiol 2002;40:1188–93.

[22] Ramirez JC, Patterson GA, Winton TL, et al. Bilateral lung transplantation for cystic fibrosis. The Toronto Lung Transplant Group. J Thorac Cardiovasc Surg 1992;103:287–93.

[23] Snell GI, de Hoyos A, Krajden M, et al. Pseudomonas cepacia in lung transplant recipients with cystic fibrosis [see comment]. Chest 1993;103:466–71.

[24] Flume PA, Egan TM, Paradowski LJ, et al. Infectious complications of lung transplantation: impact of cystic fibrosis. Am J Respir Crit Care Med 1994; 149:1601–7.

[25] Egan JJ, McNeil K, Bookless B, et al. Post-transplantation survival of cystic fibrosis patients infected with pseudomonas cepacia. Lancet 1994; 344:552–3.

[26] Coenye T, Vandamme P, Govan JR, et al. Taxonomy and identification of the burkholderia cepacia complex. J Clin Microbiol 2001;39:3427–36.

[27] LiPuma JJ, Spilker T, Gill LH, et al. Disproportionate distribution of burkholderia cepacia complex species and transmissibility markers in cystic fibrosis. Am J Respir Crit Care Med 2001;164:92–6.

[28] Aris RM, Routh JC, LiPuma JJ, et al. Lung transplantation for cystic fibrosis patients with burkholderia cepacia complex: survival linked to genomovar type. Am J Respir Crit Care Med 2001; 164:2102–6.

[29] De Soyza A, McDowell A, Archer L, et al. Burkholderia cepacia complex genomovars and pulmonary transplantation outcomes in patients with cystic fibrosis. Lancet 2001;358:1780–1.

[30] De Soyza A, Morris K, McDowell A, et al. Prevalence and clonality of burkholderia cepacia complex genomovars in UK patients with cystic fibrosis referred for lung transplantation. Thorax 2004;59: 526–8.

[31] Manno G, Dalmastri C, Tabacchioni S, et al. Epidemiology and clinical course of burkholderia cepacia complex infections, particularly those caused by different burkholderia cenocepacia strains, among patients attending an Italian cystic fibrosis center. J Clin Microbiol 2004;42:1491–7.

[32] De Boeck K, Malfroot A, Van Schil L, et al. Epidemiology of burkholderia cepacia complex colonisation in cystic fibrosis patients. Eur Respir J 2004; 23:851–6.

[33] LiPuma JJ. Burkholderia cepacia complex: a contraindication to lung transplantation in cystic fibrosis? [review]. Transpl Infect Dis 2001;3:149–60.

[34] De Soyza A, Corris PA. Lung transplantation and the burkholderia cepacia complex [review]. J Heart Lung Transplant 2003;22:954–8.

[35] Chaparro C, Maurer J, Gutierrez C, et al. Infection with burkholderia cepacia in cystic fibrosis: outcome following lung transplantation. Am J Respir Crit Care Med 2001;163:43–8.

[36] Kanj SS, Tapson V, Davis RD, et al. Infections in patients with cystic fibrosis following lung transplantation [see comment]. Chest 1997;112:924–30.

[37] Khan SU, Arroglia AC, Gordon SM. Significance of airway colonization by burkholderia gladioli in lung transplant candidates [comment]. Chest 1998;114: 658.

[38] Walter S, Gudowius P, Bosshammer J, et al. Epidemiology of chronic pseudomonas aeruginosa infections in the airways of lung transplant recipients with cystic fibrosis. Thorax 1997;52:318–21.

[39] Nunley DR, Grgurich W, Iacono AT, et al. Allograft colonization and infections with pseudomonas in cystic fibrosis lung transplant recipients. Chest 1998;113:1235–43.

[40] Dobbin C, Maley M, Harkness J, et al. The impact of pan-resistant bacterial pathogens on survival after lung transplantation in cystic fibrosis: results from a single large referral centre. J Hosp Infect 2004;56: 277–82.

[41] Maurer JR, Frost AE, Estenne M, et al. International guidelines for the selection of lung transplant candidates. The International Society for Heart and Lung Transplantation, the American Thoracic Society, the American Society of Transplant Physicians, the European Respiratory Society. Transplantation 1998;66:951–6.

[42] Wise SK, Kingdom TT, McKean L, et al. Presence of fungus in sinus cultures of cystic fibrosis patients. Am J Rhinol 2005;19:47–51.

[43] Nunley DR, Ohori P, Grgurich WF, et al. Pulmonary aspergillosis in cystic fibrosis lung transplant recipients. Chest 1998;114:1321–9.

[44] Helmi M, Love RB, Welter D, et al. Aspergillus infection in lung transplant recipients with cystic fibrosis: risk factors and outcomes comparison to other types of transplant recipients. Chest 2003; 123:800–8.

[45] Saiman L, Siegel J. Cystic Fibrosis Foundation Consensus Conference on Infection Control. Infection control recommendations for patients with cystic fibrosis: microbiology, important pathogens, and infection control practices to prevent patient-to-patient transmission [review]. Am J Infect Control 2003;31:S1–62.

[46] Holzmann D, Speich R, Kaufmann T, et al. Effects of sinus surgery in patients with cystic fibrosis after lung transplantation: a 10-year experience. Transplantation 2004;77:134–6.

[47] Couetil JP, Houssin DP, Soubrane O, et al. Combined lung and liver transplantation in patients with cystic fibrosis: a 4 1/2-year experience. J Thorac Cardiovasc Surg 1995;110:1415–22.

[48] Schaedel C, de Monestrol I, Hjelte L, et al. Predictors of deterioration of lung function in cystic fibrosis. Pediatr Pulmonol 2002;33:483–91.

[49] Rosenecker J, Hofler R, Steinkamp G, et al. Diabetes mellitus in patients with cystic fibrosis: the impact of diabetes mellitus on pulmonary function and clinical outcome. Eur J Med Res 2001;6: 345–50.

[50] Moran A, Hardin D, Rodman D, et al. Diagnosis, screening and management of cystic fibrosis related diabetes mellitus: a consensus conference report [see comment]. Diabetes Res Clin Pract 1999;45: 61–73.

[51] Schwebel C, Pin I, Barnoud D, et al. Prevalence and consequences of nutritional depletion in lung transplant candidates. Eur Respir J 2000;16:1050–5.

[52] Plochl W, Pezawas L, Artemiou O, et al. Nutritional status, ICU duration and ICU mortality in lung transplant recipients. Intensive Care Med 1996;22: 1179–85.

[53] Forli L, Bjortuft O, Vatn M, et al. A study of intensified dietary support in underweight candidates for lung transplantation. Ann Nutr Metab 2001;45: 159–68.

[54] Madill J, Maurer JR, de Hoyos A. A comparison of preoperative and postoperative nutritional states of lung transplant recipients. Transplantation 1993; 56:347–50.

[55] Thomas P. Lung versus heart-lung transplantation for cystic fibrosis: is the debate still open? [comment]. Eur Respir J 2005;25:947–8.

[56] Ganesh JS, Rogers CA, Bonser RS, et al. Outcome of heart-lung and bilateral sequential lung transplantation for cystic fibrosis: a UK national study [see comment]. Eur Respir J 2005;25:964–9.

[57] Shennib H, Noirclerc M, Ernst P, et al. Double-lung transplantation for cystic fibrosis. The cystic fibrosis transplant study group. Ann Thorac Surg 1992;54: 27–31.

[58] Vricella LA, Karamichalis JM, Ahmad S, et al. Lung and heart-lung transplantation in patients with endstage cystic fibrosis: the Stanford experience. Ann Thorac Surg 2002;74:13–7.

[59] Shennib H, Massard G, Gauthier R, et al. Single lung transplantation for cystic fibrosis: is it an option? Cystic Fibrosis Transplant Study Group. J Heart Lung Transplant 1993;12:288–93.

[60] Bremner RM, Woo MS, Arroyo H, et al. The effect of pleural adhesions on pediatric cystic fibrosis patients undergoing lung transplantation. Am Surg 2001;67:1136–9.

[61] Barr ML, Baker CJ, Schenkel FA, et al. Living donor lung transplantation: selection, technique, and outcome [review]. Transplant Proc 2001;33:3527–32.

[62] Date H, Aoe M, Nagahiro I, et al. Living-donor lobar lung transplantation for various lung diseases. J Thorac Cardiovasc Surg 2003;126:476–81.

[63] Egan TM, Detterbeck FC, Mill MR, et al. Lung transplantation for cystic fibrosis: effective and durable therapy in a high-risk group. Ann Thorac Surg 1998;66:337–46.

[64] Aurora P, Whitehead B, Wade A, et al. Lung transplantation and life extension in children with cystic fibrosis. Lancet 1999;354:1591–3.

[65] Venuta F, Rendina EA, De Giacomo T, et al. Improved results with lung transplantation for cystic fibrosis. Transplant Proc 2001;33:1632–3.

[66] Egan TM, Detterbeck FC, Mill MR, et al. Long term results of lung transplantation for cystic fibrosis. Eur J Cardiothorac Surg 2002;22:602–9.

[67] de Perrot M, Chaparro C, McRae K, et al. Twentyyear experience of lung transplantation at a single center: influence of recipient diagnosis on longterm survival. J Thorac Cardiovasc Surg 2004;127: 1493–501.

[68] Lama R, Alvarez A, Santos F, et al. Long-term results of lung transplantation for cystic fibrosis. Transplant Proc 2001;33:1624–5.

[69] Hosenpud JD, Bennett LE, Keck BM, et al. Effect of diagnosis on survival benefit of lung transplantation for end-stage lung disease [see comment]. Lancet 1998;351:24–7.

[70] Burker EJ, Carels RA, Thompson LF, et al. Quality of life in patients awaiting lung transplant: cystic fibrosis versus other end-stage lung diseases. Pediatr Pulmonol 2000;30:453–60.

[71] Vermeulen KM, van der Bij W, Erasmus ME, et al. Improved quality of life after lung transplantation in individuals with cystic fibrosis. Pediatr Pulmonol 2004;37:419–26.

[72] Kurland G, Orenstein DM. Lung transplantation and cystic fibrosis: the psychosocial toll. Pediatrics 2001;107:1419–20.

[73] Durst CL, Horn MV, MacLaughlin EF, et al. Psychosocial responses of adolescent cystic fibrosis patients to lung transplantation. Pediatr Transplant 2001;5:27–31.

[74] Groen H, van der Bij W, Koeter GH, et al. Cost-effectiveness of lung transplantation in relation to type of end-stage pulmonary disease. Am J Transplant 2004;4:1155–62.

[75] Gilljam M, Chaparro C, Tullis E, et al. GI complications after lung transplantation in patients with cystic fibrosis [see comment]. Chest 2003;123:37–41.

[76] Minkes RK, Langer JC, Skinner MA, et al. Intestinal obstruction after lung transplantation in children with cystic fibrosis. J Pediatr Surg 1999;34: 1489–93.

[77] Knoop C, Vervier I, Thiry P, et al. Cyclosporine pharmacokinetics and dose monitoring after lung transplantation: comparison between cystic fibrosis and other conditions. Transplantation 2003;76: 683–8.

[78] Tsang VT, Johnston A, Heritier F, et al. Cyclosporin pharmacokinetics in heart-lung transplant recipients with cystic fibrosis: effects of pancreatic enzymes and ranitidine. Eur J Clin Pharmacol 1994;46: 261–5.

[79] Reynaud-Gaubert M, Viard L, Girault D, et al. Improved absorption and bioavailability of cyclosporine A from a microemulsion formulation in lung transplant recipients affected with cystic fibrosis. Transplant Proc 1997;29:2450–3.

[80] Mikhail G, Eadon H, Leaver N, et al. An investigation of the pharmacokinetics, toxicity, and clinical efficacy of neoral cyclosporin in cystic fibrosis patients. Transplant Proc 1997;29:599–601.

[81] Mikhail G, Eadon H, Leaver N, et al. Comparison of neoral and sandimmun cyclosporines for de novo lung transplantation in cystic fibrosis patients. Transplant Proc 1998;30:1510–1.

[82] Walker S, Habib S, Rose M, et al. Clinical use and bioavailability of tacrolimus in heart-lung and double lung transplant recipients with cystic fibrosis. Transplant Proc 1998;30:1519–20.

[83] Knoop C, Thiry P, Saint-Marcoux F, et al. Tacrolimus pharmacokinetics and dose monitoring after lung transplantation for cystic fibrosis and other conditions. Am J Transplant 2005;5: 1477–82.

[84] Gerbase MW, Fathi M, Spiliopoulos A, et al. Pharmacokinetics of mycophenolic acid associated with calcineurin inhibitors: long-term monitoring in stable lung recipients with and without cystic fibrosis. J Heart Lung Transplant 2003;22:587–90.

ELSEVIER
SAUNDERS

Clin Chest Med 28 (2007) 459–472

CLINICS
IN CHEST
MEDICINE

Current Issues in Quality Improvement in Cystic Fibrosis

Hebe B. Quinton, MS[a,*], Gerald T. O'Connor, PhD, DSc[b]
for the Northern New England CV Cystic Fibrosis Consortium

[a]*Clinical Research Section, Department of Medicine, Dartmouth Medical School,
One Medical Center Drive, Lebanon, NH 03756, USA*
[b]*Center for the Evaluative Clinical Sciences, Dartmouth Medical School,
Dartmouth-Hitchcock Medical Center, One Medical Center Drive, Lebanon, NH 03756, USA*

The modern history of cystic fibrosis (CF) is one of continuous improvement. When the US Cystic Fibrosis Foundation (CFF) was founded 50 years ago by parents of children who had CF, its stated mission was to find a cure for the disease and improve the quality of life for patients. In 1955, it was expected that a baby born with CF would not survive to attend school. By 1985, expected survival was 25 years, and in 2005 it was more than 36 years [1].

The central issue for quality improvement (QI) in healthcare is change—the need to change, the will to change, the directions in which to change, and the skill to make those changes. Like other sciences, however, QI science does not always get things right the first time but rather approaches truth (or improvement) through successive attempts.

Guidelines and evidence-based medicine provide a general roadmap for directing improvement efforts. Data and measurement are central to QI, a way of keeping score and staying on track. Training in QI methods, leadership, and management skills provides the tools for implementing change. Data transparency and public reporting

focus attention on the elements that the CF community considers important and keep responsibility and accountability for the processes and outcomes of healthcare in clear view.

This article describes the history and context of QI in CF, the use of guidelines and data with some examples from the work of one regional consortium, some approaches to developing QI skills with a view to implementing and managing desired changes in CF clinic settings, and the potential benefits and impact of public reporting and data transparency.

Challenges of quality improvement in cystic fibrosis clinics

Quality improvement in CF clinics poses a unique challenge in healthcare. A CFF-accredited CF care center must have a multidisciplinary pediatric team representing pulmonology, nursing, physical or respiratory therapy, nutrition, and social work. Improved survival means that, in 2005, more than 43% of the patients who had CF were over the age of 18 years [1], and additional clinicians providing care to adults are becoming vital members of the team. Some teams include other specialties such as endocrinology and gastroenterology. Although the number of patients who have CF in the United States may be around 30,000, almost half the certified CF centers and affiliates in the CFF network care for fewer than 100 patients. In the smaller centers, CF clinics may occur only twice a month, so the team really is a virtual team

Funding support was provided by Cystic Fibrosis Foundation grants: Measuring, Organizing, and Improving Cystic Fibrosis Care and Outcomes: Regional Organization to Get to Evidence-based Care for CF, OCONNO02C0QI.

* Corresponding author.
E-mail address: hebe.b.quinton@dartmouth.edu (H.B. Quinton).

than coalesces only episodically. Some important communication may occur through electronic mail, but the team does not have the bits and pieces of time available to more conventional clinic teams that allow the consistent application of attention and effort that can produce rapid changes and the development of the systematic factors that make those changes a permanent part of the clinic culture. Furthermore, as with other chronic diseases, most CF care occurs away from healthcare settings; the encounters with healthcare providers constitute a small percentage of the persistent efforts required to maintain health.

National quality improvement initiatives

The need for changes in the healthcare system is well understood in society at large. Many campaigns for elected office address the facts that more than 40 million of the United States population have no health insurance, that healthcare costs are rising, and that reimbursements are misaligned. In 1999, the Institute of Medicine (IOM) published *To Err is Human* [2], which asserts that tens of thousands of patients die each year from medical errors and puts "the issue of patient safety and quality on the radar screen of public and private policymakers." This first in a series of *Quality Chasm* reports described broad quality issues and defined six aims: care should be safe, effective, patient-centered, timely, efficient, and equitable [3].

A number of non-for-profit organizations are working nationally to improve or redesign the healthcare system. The Institute for Healthcare Improvement (IHI) [4] was founded in 1991 to "accelerate change in healthcare by cultivating promising concepts for improving patient care and turning those ideas into action." The IHI launched the 100,000 Lives Campaign [5] in 2004 in response to the IOM report as a nationwide effort to reduce morbidity and mortality significantly in healthcare organizations. IHI chose proven best practices to help participating hospitals save lives. The improvement initiatives focused on proven therapies for acute myocardial infarction and reductions in infections, and in adverse drug events.

The Chronic Care Model devised by Wagner [6] and the Improving Chronic Illness Care group [7] in Seattle provides a useful framework for integrating CF care into a larger picture of healthcare in the community with an "informed, activated" patient interacting with a "prepared, proactive,

practice team." Improving Chronic Illness Care is a national program supported by The Robert Wood Johnson Foundation. This conceptual framework dovetails well with the work of the Institute for Family-Centered Care [8], which has advocated during the last decade for healthcare that honors patient and family perspectives, in which providers share complete and unbiased information with patients who participate in their healthcare decisions at the level they choose, and in which patients are integrated into every level of the design of policies, programs, facilities, and the delivery of care at all healthcare institutions.

The Institute for Healthcare Delivery Research is affiliated with InterMountain Healthcare (IHC) [9]. IHC is an exemplar of a healthcare system that models the power of an information system embedded into healthcare delivery and an organization-wide dedication to QI as a culture and a business plan. The IHC has developed a multifaceted curriculum to train healthcare professionals in QI skills.

The Clinical Microsystems view of healthcare has been developed by a group at the Center for Evaluative Clinical Sciences at Dartmouth Medical School [10] as an empowering approach for the front-line care teams that provide healthcare. A Clinical Microsystem is a small group of people that regularly works together to provide care to a defined group of patients. It is the conceptual space where patients, families, and care teams meet, and it includes support staff and technology. Microsystems "evolve over time and are (often) embedded in larger organizations. As a type of complex adaptive system, they must: (1) do the work, (2) meet staff needs, (3) maintain themselves as a clinical unit." Microsystems thinking is a powerful tool for front-line care teams because it empowers them to adopt and test QI changes, to analyze their own processes and practices, and to adapt without relying on the larger healthcare organization in which they are embedded for direction.

In April 2002, Cincinnati Children's Hospital was one of seven healthcare organizations to receive a grant from the Robert Wood Johnson Foundation to collaborate closely with IHI. "Pursuing Perfection: Raising the Bar for Healthcare Performance" [11,12] is a hospital-wide effort with perfection defined using the IOM's measures of quality (timely, efficient, effective, patient-centered, equitable, and safe). The Cincinnati pediatric CF team was involved from the beginning, sharing data publicly with parents, and parents were members of all committees involved with redesigning care.

Data, measurement, and variation

Beginning in the early 1960s, the CFF collected demographic data on patients who had CF and started to organize and accredit CF clinics. The data were used mainly for descriptive statistics and to identify eligible patients for clinical trials of new therapies. In 1982, the Registry became computer based. The database now includes information on diagnosis, genotype, measures of height, weight, and lung function, complications such as liver disease and cystic fibrosis–related diabetes (CFRD), infections with common respiratory pathogens, and dates of birth, diagnosis, transplantation, and death. In 2003, the Registry moved to an Internet Web-based portal, PortCF, where information can be entered about patients on an encounter basis, including episodes of hospitalizations and courses of intravenous antibiotics. To improve outcomes, CF care teams (with patients and families at their core) need information at the point of care delivery, including current care guidelines, patient alerts, clinical reminders, and graphic displays of changes in key outcomes over time. PortCF continues to be developed with the goal that it will evolve into an information system that is fully integrated into clinical care and ultimately will give patients access to their own healthcare data.

Experience from the field

In 1995, the CF care centers of Northern New England (NNE) agreed to collaborate primarily for networking and education (Fig. 1). In 1997 a 2-year grant was obtained from the CFF to add analytical and organizational support, forming the Northern New England Cystic Fibrosis Consortium (NNECFC) [13] as a regional, voluntary, multidisciplinary, consortium of more than 80 clinicians and researchers from the CF care centers in Maine, New Hampshire, and Vermont. The mission of the group is to improve CF care and patient outcomes. Its goals are to develop and share information to improve the care and treatment of patients who have CF in the region and to develop a model for best practice. Several consortia formed around the same time. The Mountain West CF Consortium joined the CF centers in Utah, Colorado, Idaho, New Mexico,

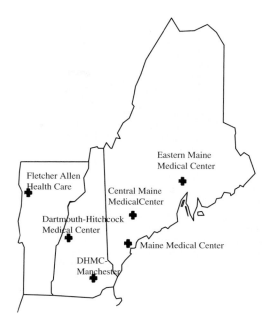

Fig. 1. The Northern New England Cystic Fibrosis Consortium.

and Arizona; others were formed by CF center directors in the southeastern and mid-Atlantic states and in Ohio.

The NNECFC received a dataset from the CFF that included all the Registry information on the more than 450 patients cared for by its centers. This dataset is updated annually. The late 1990s was a time of accelerated concern about infection control in CF, because person-to-person transmission of both *Burkholderia cepacia* in 1990 [14] and *Pseudomonas aeruginosa* in 1991 [15] had been established. The investigators wanted to compare infection control practices at different centers and began by comparing rates of mucoid *P aeruginosa* among those colonized with *P aeruginosa*. If there were true differences in infection rates among centers, investigators could learn about differences in infection control practices, the natural patterns of pathogens, and whether aggressive treatment through use of intravenous antibiotics and hospitalizations is effective and could start to understand the associations between infection and other outcomes in patients. The center rates of mucoid *P aeruginosa* varied from 0 to 97% of patients, as shown in Fig. 2. These improbably wide differences in rates of mucoid *P aeruginosa* led to a thorough review of laboratory practices at the different centers. A work group of microbiologists

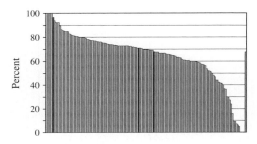

Fig. 2. Variation in rates of mucoid *P aeruginosa* by center, 1998. Each bar represents one CF care center or affiliate. The bar on the far right is the national rate, 66%. Bars corresponding to NNECFC centers are highlighted. The five centers of the NNECFC had rates of mucoid *P aeruginosa* that varied from 0 to 97% among patients culturing positive for *P aeruginosa*. Two centers sharing the same laboratory reported no mucoidy. (*Data from* The Cystic Fibrosis Foundation. Patient registry 1998. Bethesda (MD): Cystic Fibrosis Foundation; 1999.)

and clinicians from the five NNE centers shared center sputum protocols. The group uncovered multiple sources of variability between the centers: (1) differences in collection of sputum/bronchoscopy versus throat/nasal cultures (Fig. 3), (2) differences among laboratories in the use of selective media and incubation times, (3) different frequencies of culturing (some once a year, others at every clinic visit), (4) potential problems with laboratory results being reported into clinic charts and data from clinic charts being entered into the Registry, and (5) variability among NNE laboratories in reporting the mucoid phenotype for *P*

aeruginosa. The work group developed a standardized regional protocol for respiratory cultures in compliance with the Clinical Practice Guidelines for CF [16]. As of 2004 the rates of mucoidy range from 64% to 95% (the national rate is 66%) (Fig. 4) and have remained remarkably steady since 2000 [17,18]. The investigators now trust these differences and are comparing their infection control practices [19] and approaches to early, aggressive treatment of *P aeruginosa*.

Subsequent analyses have uncovered differences among centers in lung function (Fig. 5), nutritional status (Fig. 6) [20], prescribing patterns for Dornase Alfa (Pulmozyme) (Fig. 7), aerosolized tobramycin (TOBI) (Fig. 8), screening for CFRD (Fig. 9), and adherence to guidelines care [21]. The level of variation in the NNECFC centers for many measures closely reflected the range of variation in the national CF care center network.

In 1999 and 2002 the NNECFC was the recipient of 3-year QI grants from the CFF to develop strategies for improving patient care. A few guiding principles were followed. Required were multidisciplinary teams; buy-in and involvement from every center leader; an environment of trust and cooperation; and collection of data only with a clear purpose. Phase one of the QI journey focused on glucose screening for CFRD. QI interventions included (1) feedback of data to clinicians, including lists of those patients not screened, (2) patient education about CFRD, and (3) clinic system changes to trigger annual blood work and to track the results. Between 1998 and 2002,

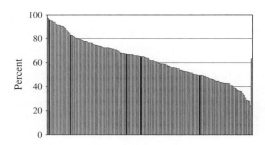

Fig. 3. Sputum plus bronchoscopy rates, 1998. Rates of sputum plus bronchoscopy versus throat swab for respiratory cultures. The bar on the far right is the national rate, 63%. Bars corresponding to NNECFC centers are highlighted. The five centers of the NNECFC had rates ranging from 48% to 96%. (*Data from* The Cystic Fibrosis Foundation. Patient registry 1998. Bethesda (MD): Cystic Fibrosis Foundation; 1999.)

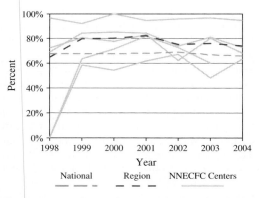

Fig. 4. Rates of mucoid *P aeruginosa* at the five NNECFC centers, 1998–2004. The rates of mucoid *P aeruginosa* in the NNECFC converged after the change in laboratory procedures and now range from 64% to 95%. In 2004 the national rate was 66%.

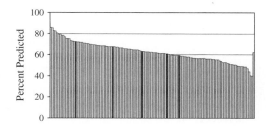

Fig. 5. Median forced expiratory volume in 1 second (FEV$_1$) percent of predicted by center for patients aged 18 to 30 years in 1999. Each bar represents the median FEV$_1$ for patients aged 18 to 30 years in 1999. The highlighted bars represent the NNECFC centers. The range of center medians is from 40% to 86%. The national median is 62%. The range in the NNECFC was 59% to 72%. (*Data from* The Cystic Fibrosis Foundation. Patient registry 1999. Bethesda (MD): Cystic Fibrosis Foundation; 2000.)

the CFRD screening rate in NNECFC centers improved at more than twice the national rate (Fig. 10) and became less variable among the centers (1998: NNECFC range, 16%–78%; NNE overall rate, 44%; national rate, 61%; 2002: NNECFC range, 71%–90%; NNE overall rate, 78%; national rate 74%). The improvement has been maintained and reflects both better data tracking and more screening driven by increased clinician and patient awareness. Data feedback has proven to be a strong incentive to improve and to identify and correct internal system problems.

The variation observed in all these different measures indicated an underlying variability in

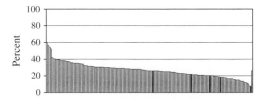

Fig. 6. Proportion of children below the tenth weight percentile of the Centers for Disease Control and Prevention (CDC), by center in 1999. Each bar represents the proportion of children below the tenth CDC weight percentile. The highlighted bars represent the NNECFC centers. The national rate is 26%; the range is 7% to 60%. The rates of low weight ranged from 7% to 26% in the NNECFC. (*Data from* The Cystic Fibrosis Foundation. Patient registry 1999. Bethesda (MD): Cystic Fibrosis Foundation; 2000.)

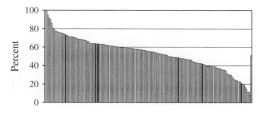

Fig. 7. Pulmozyme prescription by center in 1999. Each bar represents the proportion of patients prescribed Pulmozyme at a CF center. The highlighted bars represent the NNECFC centers with one adult center reporting separately. The national rate of Pulmozyme prescription in patients is 51%; the range is 8% to 100%. The range in the NNECFC centers is 21% to 73%. (*Data from* The Cystic Fibrosis Foundation. Patient registry 1999. Bethesda (MD): Cystic Fibrosis Foundation; 2000.)

clinic processes [22] and led NNECFC working groups to develop protocols for respiratory cultures, infection control, and outpatient nutrition screening and management.

The phase two goals for QI in the consortium were to (1) maintain the improvements in CFRD screening, (2) identify 100% of patients at risk of or in nutritional failure using the definitions laid out in the nutrition guidelines [23], (3) rationalize and track use of TOBI and Pulmozyme, and (4) understand patient-centered barriers to optimal care. A clinic encounter form was developed to collect data and shorten the delay in data feedback inherent in using annual Registry reports.

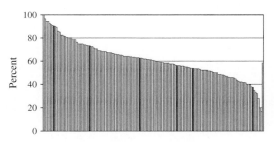

Fig. 8. Use of aerosolized tobramycin (TOBI) in *P aeruginosa*–positive patients, by center in 1999. Each bar represents the proportion of *P aeruginosa*–positive patients prescribed TOBI. The highlighted bars represent the NNECFC centers, with one adult center reporting separately. The national rate of TOBI use in patients positive for *P aeruginosa* is 59%; the range is 17% to 100%. The range at NNECFC centers is 37% to 90.5%. (*Data from* The Cystic Fibrosis Foundation. Patient registry 1999. Bethesda (MD): Cystic Fibrosis Foundation; 2000.)

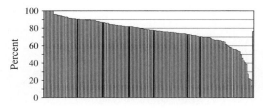

Fig. 9. Glucose screening in nondiabetic CF patients older than 13 years by center in 1999. Each bar represents the rate of glucose screening for CFRD (random, fasting, or oral glucose tolerance test). The national rate is 76%; the range is 14 to 100%. Seven centers report 100% screening. The highlighted bars represent the NNECFC centers; one adult center reports separately. (*Data from* The Cystic Fibrosis Foundation. Patient registry 1999. Bethesda (MD): Cystic Fibrosis Foundation; 2000.)

The clinic encounter form brought data collection into daily practice, provided an opportunity to create regular feedback reports so progress could be evaluated more quickly, and served as a reminder to trigger key clinical actions in a busy clinic. The encounter form included

Date of last CFRD screen
P aeruginosa status
Forced expiratory volume in 1 second (FEV_1)
Height, weight, and body mass index

Nutrition status per guideline definitions for failure and risk of failure
TOBI indications [24] and reasons why it was or was not prescribed
Pulmozyme indications [25] and reasons why it was or was not prescribed

The form was filled out partially in preclinic conferences and was completed at the time of the patients' appointments. During the 3 years of this work more than 4200 forms were completed and analyzed.

The NNECFC reduced the rates of nutritional failure in children younger than 18 years more quickly than the national rate of improvement, and the variation between the centers was reduced (Fig. 11). In 2002, the center rates ranged from 19% to 54%, the NNECFC overall rate was 30%, and the national rate was 35%. In 2004, rates in NNECFC centers ranged from 19% to 29%, the NNE overall rate was 23%, and the national rate was 32%.

The phase three effort centered on the respiratory therapies. Variation between centers was reduced, while rates of prescription of proven therapies increased (Figs. 12 and 13). This work revealed some interesting things about physician prescribing patterns. When the encounter form was first used, TOBI and Pulmozyme were prescribed for about 60% of eligible patients. The evidence from clinical trials for the use of both

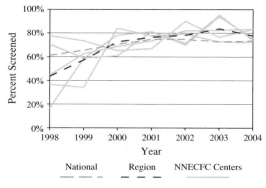

Fig. 10. Glucose screening in nondiabetics older than 13 years, 1998–2004. The rates of glucose screening in the NNECFC converged after the QI interventions. In 1998 the NNECFC range was 16% to 78%, the NNECFC overall rate was 44%, and the national overall rate was 61%. In 2002 the NNECFC range was 71% to 90%, the NNECFC overall rate was 78%, and the national rate was 74%. (*Data from* The Cystic Fibrosis Foundation. Patient registry 2005. Bethesda (MD): Cystic Fibrosis Foundation; 2006.)

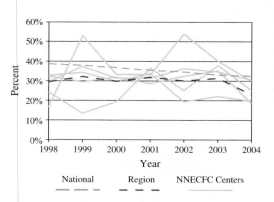

Fig. 11. Reduction in nutritional failure in patients younger than 18 years in the NNECFC. In 2002 the rates varied from 19% to 54%; the NNE overall rate was 30%, and the national overall rate was 35%. In 2004 variation as well as the overall rate was reduced: the range was 19% to 29%, the NNECFC overall rate was 23%, and the national rate was 32%. (*Data from* The Cystic Fibrosis Foundation. Patient registry 2005. Bethesda (MD): Cystic Fibrosis Foundation; 2006.)

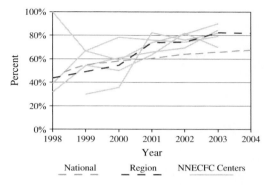

Fig. 12. Use of aerosolized tobramycin (TOBI) in *P aeruginosa*-positive patients more than 6 years old in the NNECFC. In 2000 the rates varied from 35% to 78%, the NNE overall rate was 55%, and the national rate was 58%. In 2004 variation as well as the overall rate was reduced: the range was 74% to 89%, the NNECFC overall rate was 82%, and the national rate was 67%. (*Data from* The Cystic Fibrosis Foundation. Patient registry 2005. Bethesda (MD): Cystic Fibrosis Foundation; 2006.)

therapies is for the prevention of pulmonary decline [26,27], but 45% of eligible patients not receiving TOBI did not receive a prescription because they were "well" (Fig. 14), whereas for the prescription of Pulmozyme, it was 51% (Fig. 15). Other reasons for not using these proven

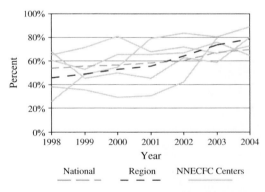

Fig. 13. Pulmozyme use in patients older than 6 years old with FEV$_1$ below 90% of predicted. In 2000 the rates of Pulmozyme use in the NNECFC varied from 29% to 81%. The NNE overall rate was 55%, and the national rate was 58%. In 2004 variation as well as the overall rate was reduced: the range was 65% to 89%, the NNECFC overall rate was 78%, and the national rate was 70%. (*Data from* The Cystic Fibrosis Foundation. Patient registry 2005. Bethesda (MD): Cystic Fibrosis Foundation; 2006.)

therapies resulted from patient factors—adverse reactions, nonadherence, and cost.

The value of the clinic encounter form was that it triggered a focus on few key processes that the investigators agreed were important for patient health every time a patient entered the healthcare system:

1. It improved team identification of patients in need of nutritional intervention.
2. It facilitated better decision making around TOBI and Pulmozyme prescription by providing accurate information at the time of clinic about which patients were or were not receiving these medications.
3. It fostered improvement in CFRD screening by displaying the date of the last glucose test.
4. It allowed the changes to be tracked and their effects to be measured.

Reasons for success were buy-in from all providers, open data sharing between centers, good communication, and the encounter form fitting neatly into the workflow of the clinic teams.

As a result of the years of collaboration, the NNECFC community has developed a sense of trust and has shared center outcomes openly within the consortium and, since 2003, with each center's patients and families at "Family Education Nights." In many cases this sharing of information has changed the conversations that clinicians have with their patients and has encouraged increased adherence by patients who want to "make the center look good."

More data: evidence for best practices from the Patient Registry

The IOM defines quality as "the degree to which health services for individuals and populations increase the likelihood of desired health outcomes and are consistent with current professional knowledge."

In 2002, the CFF convened a group of CF clinicians and QI leaders to develop strategies to start to identify what constitutes best practice in CF care and to enable all the centers in the care network to attain it. As the immediate result of this meeting, acknowledging what had been learned about effective but somewhat slow improvement from the regional consortia, the CFF launched an innovative QI initiative in 2002: "Accelerating the Rate of Improvement in CF Care."

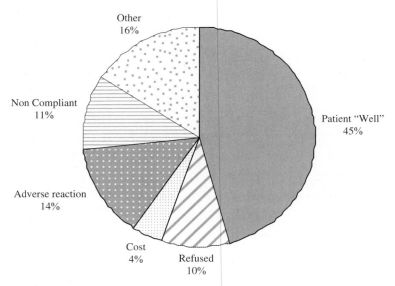

Fig. 14. Reasons clinicians do not prescribe TOBI. (*Data from* North American Cystic Fibrosis Conference Symposium presentation, 2003.)

An analysis of the Registry reveals wide variations in rates of pulmonary function and the percent of undernourished patients, children, and adults among the 117 CFF accredited care centers (see Figs. 5 and 6). Analyses also show wide differences in the use of pulmonary (see Figs. 7 and 8) and nutritional therapies, in screening for CF-related diabetes (see Fig. 9), and in other aspects of clinical care. The median age of death for patients at CF centers with documented best pulmonary and nutrition outcomes from 1999 through 2001 was 28 years; at all other centers that had more than 100 patients the median age of death was 22 years. It is unlikely that these differences are solely a consequence of differences in patient case mix. This variability in clinical outcomes is important: it represents an opportunity to identify best practices and to develop effective strategies to enable the rapid spread of these practices to all CF care centers. The results at the top centers represent care that has already been achieved, not breakthrough or new therapies. If

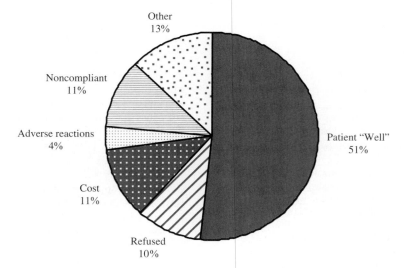

Fig. 15. Reasons clinicians do not prescribe Pulmozyme. (*Data from* North American Cystic Fibrosis Conference Symposium presentation, 2003.)

all centers were able to achieve care equal to that of the high-performing centers, years of life can be added for the CF population.

The "Accelerating the Rate of Improvement" initiative includes a vision statement: "We believe that, during the next 5 years, the life expectancy of CF patients can be extended by 5-10 years through the consistent implementation of existing evidence-based clinical care." There are five key strategies (Box 1): building a shared vision of exemplary care; developing leadership for change; identifying and enabling best practices through a benchmarking initiative; providing front-line decision support for clinical care teams; and increasing clinician partnerships with patients and parents. There are seven worthy goals (Box 2). The goals and strategies have been broadly shared throughout the CF community, and concurrent efforts are in place to implement them all.

The role of guidelines—directions for change

Guidelines provide the directions in which changes for QI should be made. Improvements in survival of patients who have CF have tracked with the development of better antibiotics, better pancreatic enzymes preparations, and the development of the CFF care center network [28]. In 1990, the CFF published a consensus document "to promote a uniform level of care and teaching services at CF Care Centers and to provide a general framework for good patient care" [29] and to provide the rationale and specifics of center care in the face of growing pressure from managed care organizations that tended to prevent patients who had CF from receiving the level of care they needed. The first nutrition guidelines were published in 1990, in rapid response to the insights of Corey and colleagues [30] about high-fat diets, and were updated in 2002 [23]. Microbiology and infection control guidelines were published in 1994 [16], the comprehensive guidelines were published in 1997 [31], adult care guidelines were published in 1999 [32], and bone health guidelines were published in 2002 [33]. Consensus guidelines, however, pose problems because they are the consensus of experts and are not necessarily supported by the criterion standard of evidence from multiple clinical trials.

Several organizations have developed rigorous methodologies for grading the evidence base of guidelines and recommendations [34,35]. Several groups have applied this methodology to their specialties (eg, coronary artery bypass surgery)

[36]. Developing evidence in CF can be difficult for many reasons: (1) there are relatively few patients, (2) it is not lucrative to care for patients who have chronic diseases, (3) clinical trials are expensive, and (4) enrolling children in clinical trials raises a set of ethical concerns. As a result many systematic reviews of evidence in CF conclude "insufficient evidence" [37]. Nevertheless, since 2004, the CFF has partnered with Johns Hopkins Evidence-based Practice Center to revise the Cystic Fibrosis Nutrition Clinical Care Consensus Guidelines and Pulmonary Clinical Care Consensus Guidelines using a the US Preventive Services Task Force grading system [35] to marshal the evidence that is available while acknowledging that expert opinion will continue to be critical for establishing care standards. The new nutrition guidelines set high goals for normal growth and nutrition based on analyses of the Registry that show what has been attained by some patients and how important nutrition is for maintaining lung health [38].

Guidelines alone do not produce change [39–41]. Guidelines must be disseminated effectively and persuasively by respected, credible agents. They must be presented objectively, and there must be a supportive local organization in place to implement them. Many experienced clinicians are somewhat dismissive of guidelines as "a record of the past." The current CF guidelines are available on PortCF. They are no longer a forgotten notebook on a shelf: the CFF has committed to updating them regularly.

The NNECFC used the clinic encounter form to reinforce the information about nutritional evaluation and the use of pulmonary therapies contained in the CFF guidelines. Protocols were developed for infection control and outpatient nutrition screening and management to tailor the guidelines to each local clinic setting.

Retrospective data feedback is an important component of improving the impact of guidelines. Since 1999, the CFF has provided annual reports from the Registry to CF center directors on outcomes and process measures for their center, with values from the top-performing centers in the care network and national averages.

Benchmarking

Benchmarking is the search for those best practices associated with superior performance. Benchmarking is a powerful tool because it opens

Box 1. Strategies for accelerating the improvement of care in cystic fibrosis

1. Building a shared vision of exemplary care:
    Include national reporting with an emphasis on center-related variability in both process and clinical outcomes and regular QI presentations at the national meeting.
    Encourage centers to share their center-specific CF Patient Registry data with patients and their families.
    Make a commitment to data transparency and public reporting.
    Report center data by the CFF publicly starting in December 2006.

2. Developing leadership for change:
    Empower change at CF care centers by recruit and educating leaders in all disciplines about state-of-the-art QI methodologies, including benchmarking, evidence-based medicine, systems thinking, and collaborative learning.
    The CFF will invest in developing leaders and provide mechanisms for the continued support and growth of these leaders.

3. Identifying and enabling best practices:
    Identify care centers with best practices.
    Understand the practices and care processes at these centers to establish the benchmark for excellence and enable best practices across all care centers.
    Recognize that best practices are actually "potentially better practices" that require adaptation and testing at each local care setting.
    Incorporate what is learned into the Clinical Practice Guidelines and Consensus Statements.
    Make QI tools developed within the learning collaborative sessions and at individual care centers available to all care centers.
    Foster communication, sharing, and collaboration among care centers

4. Providing front-line decision support for clinical care teams:
    Provide information at the point of care delivery, including current guideline recommendations, patient alerts, clinic reminders, and graphic displays of change in key outcomes over time. (PortCF is a Web-enabled database that deploys templates for the assessment and treatment of common conditions and access to timely reports.)
    Update practice guidelines updated based on expert interpretation of systematic, evidence-based reviews of the scientific literature and practical lessons learned through ongoing improvement work.
    Use recommendations derived from this work to guide the data collection and reports that are incorporated into PortCF

5. Increasing clinician partnerships with patients and parents:
    Deliver real patient and family-centered care, honoring the perspectives of people who have CF and their families at all times.
    A strong partnership between patients, families, and care providers is critical to achieve optimal outcomes for a chronic disease like CF. (This partnership will facilitate the customization of care to the needs and preferences of the individual who has CF. It also leads to the incorporation of self-management strategies and promotion of adherence into the daily medical regimen.)

Box 2. Seven worthy goals

1. Patients and families are full partners with the CF care team. Care will be respectful of individual patient preferences, needs, and values.
2. Children and adolescents will have normal growth and nutrition. Adults' nutrition will be maintained as near normal as possible.
3. All patients will receive appropriate therapies for maintaining lung function and reducing acute episodes of infection.
4. Clinicians and patients will be well-informed partners in reducing acquisition of respiratory pathogens, particularly *P aeruginosa* and *B cepacia*.
5. Patients will be screened and managed aggressively for complications of CF, particularly CFRD.
6. Severely affected patients will be well supported by their CF team in facing decisions about transplantation and end-of-life care.
7. Patients will have access to appropriate therapies, treatments, and supports regardless of race, age, education, or ability to pay.

---

organizations to new methods, ideas, and tools to improve effectiveness. It helps overcome resistance to change by demonstrating methods of solving problems other than the one currently used and by demonstrating that these methods work, because they are being used by others. Benchmarking has been used widely in business and industry (for example, Xerox visits LL Bean's mail order distribution center to benchmark) but is relatively rare in healthcare. Benchmarking is an important component of the CFF's strategic initiative to accelerate improvement. Some important attributes of high-quality care are not captured in Registry data or annual progress reports

from care centers and would be problematic to collect and report in a meaningful way. Benchmarking allows some of the subtleties of care at top-performing centers to be identified and learned. It is the intent of the CFF to document these qualitative findings of best practices (or potentially better practices) systematically in such a way that the information can be transmitted to all centers, patients, and families across the CF care center network. Centers with exemplary results have been identified, and a team of clinicians has begun visits.

Learning and leadership collaboratives: developing the skills for change

In 2002, the CFF awarded QI grants to the care centers at the University of Utah (for improving CFRD detection and treatment), the University of Wisconsin, Madison (for development of a computer-based CF QI care system), and to the NNECFC QI work. It also funded the first in a series of collaboratives: Sixteen CF care centers participated in the National Initiative for Children's Healthcare Quality CF Quality Improvement Collaborative (NICHQ) [42] based on the IHI model of a series of targeted interventions based on prescribed change packages and centralized measurement aimed at improving nutrition and reducing patient exposure to cigarette smoke. In 2003, another 10 care centers participated in the QI Learning and Leadership Collaborative I (LLC I) organized by IHC, and in 2004 12 more care centers participated in QI LLC II organized

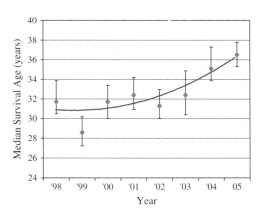

Fig. 16. Median predicted survival age, 1998–2005. Median predicted survival has increased from about 30 years in 1999 to 36 years in 2005. (*Data from* The Cystic Fibrosis Foundation. Patient registry 2005. Bethesda (MD): Cystic Fibrosis Foundation; 2006.)

by the Center for Evaluative Clinical Sciences using the Microsystems approach, which teaches front-line clinic teams the skills for effective change by focusing on professional formation, meeting skills, cause-and-effect diagrams, flowcharts, change processes, and statistical process control measurement. Local innovation and tests of change are essential features of rapid improvement and are an integral part of the training. The CFF continues to sponsor these collaboratives, and in the spring of 2007 the fifth LLC will combine the elements of the IHI, IHC, and Microsystems methodologies and focus on pulmonary care. Twenty-five quality coaches have been recruited from the collaboratives to participate in leadership training; they work closely with the new teams as they learn improvement science. To date, more than 60 clinicians managing the healthcare of more than 13,000 patients who have CF have been trained as part of these QI initiatives.

These QI collaboratives are binding the CF care center community ever more closely together and enabling clinicians to learn rapidly "what works" from each other.

Data transparency and public reporting

The 2001 IOM Report "Crossing the Quality Chasm: A New Healthcare System for the 21st Century" [3] stresses that "reform around the margins" is inadequate to address the problems of the healthcare system. The report said: 'The healthcare system should make information available to patients and their families that allows them to make informed decisions when selecting a health plan, hospital, or clinical practice. "The NNECFC centers have been sharing identified data internally since 2000 and with patients and families since 2003. A condition of participating in the LLCs was center-specific data transparency among participating centers. An informal survey of CF center directors meeting at the North American CF Conference in 2005 revealed that more than half were sharing their center reports from the Registry at "Family Education Night" presentations. By 2005, several CF centers published their center data on publicly accessible Web sites [20,42].

In 2004, a committee of CF clinicians, parents of children who have CF, biostatisticians, and leaders from the CFF convened to develop methods for case mix adjustment [43] and a format suitable for public reporting. The goal of the Web-based public reporting system is to provide accurate comparative data to accelerate centers' learning from one another and to inform the decision making of clinicians and people who have CF as to their joint responsibilities for care.

In December 2006, the CFF published center-specific data from all the accredited CF centers and affiliates on lung function and nutritional status in children and adults, screening for CFRD, and adherence to clinical guidelines care (ie, outpatient visits, pulmonary function tests, and sputum culture in children and adults). Two comparisons are reported also: the national average for each measure and the national CFF Clinical Care Center Network goals [45].

The argument has been made that public data reporting will drive improvement, if simply through embarrassment [46]. Public reporting makes clear that the interests of patients, not doctors, are paramount. It is the right thing to do because patients should be able to learn about anything that affects their healthcare. Many improvement leaders believe that public data reporting will help QI work by strengthening patient–provider partnerships and thereby facilitate improvement. Some have been concerned that patients will leave centers with average results, but this has not proved to be the case. Patients and families are not troubled that their CF center has average outcomes, as long as it is obvious that every effort is being made to improve.

Summary

A solid foundation for QI in CF has been built during the last decade. There are many remaining challenges: QI must become a habit and part of the workplace culture to retain the improvements that have been made. In the experience of many, if teams are not vigilant, old habits reassert themselves. QI must continue to be propagated to more aspects of healthcare and to all the CF clinics in the country. Healthcare disparities caused by socioeconomic factors must be assessed, understood, and mitigated [47–49]. Disadvantage is a complex construct that involves income, education, and the safety net provided by states. It is an important factor in the partnerships clinicians wish to build with patients and families, because it often reduces patient empowerment and the ability of patients and families to understand and adhere to the rigorous CF treatment regimens required for optimum health. The standardization of clinical care processes often meets resistance, but the customization of care to fit the needs of individual patients is vital to its success. Care providers must continue to learn from each other about best infection control practices and to learn from the best adult care clinics.

The CF care community has kept abreast of the national initiatives in QI and, in some cases, has influenced their creation and then tailored the lessons to local clinics. The CFF collaboratives build on the "all teach, all learn" atmosphere of trust and open data sharing pioneered by the NNECFC and have adapted for the CF community the most relevant elements from the IHI, NICHQ, IHC, and Clinical Microsystems curricula. Data feedback has been shown to produce accelerated improvement and is a way of keeping score, and PortCF is being developed to provide better decision support for front-line teams. Benchmarking is helping identify best practices (or potentially better practices). Guidelines are being updated rapidly using the best evidence available and are becoming integrated into the flow of clinics as part of the "shared vision of exemplary care." Quality coaches are part of the strategic plan for developing leadership for QI across the CF care network. Public reporting and data transparency are increasing the accountability of the healthcare community to patients and families. Quality improvement training aimed at organizing front-line CF clinics into teams that have the will, the direction, and the skills for change will continue to accelerate the improvement in survival for patients who have CF (Fig. 16).

Acknowledgments

This work was possible because of the vision, persistence, and hard work of all the clinicians and providers of the Northern New England Cystic Fibrosis Consortium, particularly William Boyle, MD, Edgar Caldwell, MD, H. Worth Parker, MD, Donald Schwartz, MD, Thomas Lever, MD, Ana Cairns, DO, Ralph Harder, MD, and Terry Kneeland, MPH.

References

[1] Cystic Fibrosis Foundation. Patient registry 2005. Bethesda (MD): Cystic Fibrosis Foundation; 2006.

[2] Kohn LT, Corrigan JM, Donaldson MS, editors. Committee on Quality of Healthcare in America, Institute of Medicine. To err is human: building a safer health system. Washington, DC: National Academy Press; 1999.

[3] Institute of Medicine. In: Briere R, editor. Crossing the quality chasm: a new health system for the 21st century. Washington, DC: National Academy Press; 2001. p. 1–5.

[4] Institute for Healthcare Improvement. Available at: http://www.ihi.org/ihi. Accessed January 15, 2007.

[5] Berwick DM, Calkins DR, McCannon CJ, et al. The 100,000 lives campaign: setting a goal and a deadline for improving healthcare quality. JAMA 2006; 295(3):324–7.

[6] Wagner EH. Chronic disease management: what will it take to improve care for chronic illness? Eff Clin Pract 1998;1:2–4.

[7] Improving chronic illness care. Available at: http://www.improvingchroniccare.org/. Accessed January 15, 2007.

[8] Institute for Family Centered Care. Available at: http://www.familycenteredcare.org/. Accessed January 15, 2007.

[9] Intermountain Healthcare. Available at: http://intermountainhealthcare.org/xp/public/. Accessed January 15, 2007.

[10] Clinical Microsystems. Available at: http://www.clinicalmicrosystem.org/. Accessed January 15, 2007.

[11] Pursuing perfection. Available at: http://www.ihi.org/IHI/Programs/PursuingPerfection/. Accessed January 15, 2007.

[12] Cincinnati children's hospital quality measures. Available at: http://www.cincinnatichildrens.org/about/measures/perfect.htm. Accessed January 15, 2007.

[13] The Northern New England Cystic Fibrosis Consortium. Available at: http://www.nnecfc.org/. Accessed January 15, 2007.

[14] LiPuma JJ, Dasen SE, Nielson DW, et al. Person-to-person transmission of Pseudomonas cepacia between patients with cystic fibrosis. Lancet 1990; 336(8723):1094–6.

[15] Tummler B, Koopman U, Grothues D, et al. Nosocomial acquisition of Pseudomonas aeruginosa by cystic fibrosis patients. J Clin Microbiol 1991;29(6):1265–7.

[16] Cystic Fibrosis Foundation. Consensus conference: microbiology and infectious diseases in cystic fibrosis. Bethesda (MD): Cystic Fibrosis Foundation; 1994. p. 1–26.

[17] Boyle W, Caldwell E, Cogswell L, et al. Evaluation of regional variation in respiratory infection rates. Pediatr Pulmonol 1998;A440(Suppl):328.

[18] Doing K, Boyle W, Caldwell E, et al. Sources of variability in rates of positive respiratory cultures. Pediatr Pulmonol 1999;A383(Suppl 19):273.

[19] Caldwell E, Maddock J, Buteyn M, et al. Regional variation in nutritional status, assessment, and treatment. Pediatr Pulmonol 1998;A578(Suppl 17):371.

[20] University of Minnesota Cystic Fibrosis Care Center. Available at: http://www.med.umn.edu/peds/cfcenter/outcomes/home.html. Accessed January 15, 2007.

[21] Parker HW, Leiter J, Harder R, et al. Evaluation of regional variation in guidelines compliance using

CFF registry data. Pediatr Pulmonol 1998; A701(Suppl 17):408.

[22] Zuckerman JB, Prato S, Zuaro D, et al. Measurement of bacterial shedding in CF clinics. Pediatr Pulmonol 2005;(Suppl 28):301.

[23] Borowitz D, Baker RD, Stallings V. Consensus report on nutrition for pediatric patients with cystic fibrosis. J Pediatr Gastroenterol Nutr 2002;35: 246–59.

[24] Steinkamp G, Tummler B, Gappa M, et al. Long-term tobramycin therapy in cystic fibrosis. Pediatr Pulmonol 1989;6(2):91–8.

[25] MacLusky IB, Gold R, Corey M, et al. Long-term effects of inhaled tobramycin in patients with cystic fibrosis colonized with *Pseudomonas aeruginosa*. Pediatr Pulmonol 1989;7(1):42–8.

[26] Fuchs HJ, Borowitz DS, Christiansen DH, et al. Effect of aerosolized recombinant human DNase on exacerbations of respiratory symptoms and on pulmonary function in patients with cystic fibrosis. The Pulmozyne Study Group. N Engl J Med 1994; 331(10):672–3.

[27] Ramsey BW, Pepe MS, Quan JM, et al. Intermittent administration of inhaled tobramycin in patients with cystic fibrosis. Cystic Fibrosis Inhaled Tobramycib Study Group. N Engl J Med 1999;340(1):23–30.

[28] Mahadeva R, Webb K, Westerbeck RC, et al. Clinical outcome in relation to care in centres specialising in cystic fibrosis: cross sectional study. BMJ 1998; 316(7147):1771–5.

[29] The Cystic Fibrosis Foundation Center Committee and Guidelines Subcommittee. Cystic fibrosis foundation guidelines for patient services, evaluation, and monitoring in cystic fibrosis centers. Am J Dis Child 1990;144:1311–2.

[30] Corey M, McLaughlin FJ, Williams M, et al. A comparison of survival, growth and pulmonary function in patients with cystic fibrosis in Boston and Toronto. J Clin Epidemiol 1988;41:588–91.

[31] Cystic Fibrosis Foundation. Clinical practice guidelines for cystic fibrosis. Bethesda (MD): Cystic Fibrosis Foundation; 1997.

[32] Yankaskas JR, Marshall BC, Sufian B, et al. Cystic fibrosis adult care: consensus conference report. Chest 2004;125:1–39.

[33] Aris RM, Merkel PA, Bachrach LK, et al. Consensus statement: guide to bone health and disease in cystic fibrosis. J Clin Endocrinol Metab 2004;90(3):1888– 1896.

[34] American Dietetic Association. ADA evidence analysis guide. 2nd edition. American Dietetic Association, Scientific Affairs and Research. Chicago (IL): American Dietetic Association; 2003.

[35] United States Preventive Services Task Force. The guide to clinical preventive services 2005. Rockville (MD): Department of Health and Human Services AHRQ Pub. No. 05–0570; 2005.

[36] Eagle KA, Guyton RA, Davidoff R, et al. ACC/AHA guidelines for coronary artery bypass graft surgery. J Am Coll Cardiol 1999;34(4): 1262–347.

[37] Wood DM, Smyth AR. Antibiotic strategies for eradicating Pseudomonas aeruginosa in people with cystic fibrosis. Cochrane Database Syst Rev 2006;1:CD004197.

[38] Stallings VA, Stark LJ, Robinson KA, et al. Evidence-based recommendations for energy intake and pancreatic enzyme therapy and update on nutritional status monitoring for cystic fibrosis, submitted for publication.

[39] Eagle KA, Lee TH, Brennan TA, et al. Task force 2: guideline implementation. J Am Coll Cardiol 1997; 29(4):1141–8.

[40] Wise CG, Billi JE. A model for practice guideline adaptation and implementation: empowerment of the physician. Jt Comm J Qual Improv 1995;21(9): 465–76.

[41] Kibbe DC, Kaluzny AD, McLaughlin CP. Integrating guidelines with continuous quality improvement: doing the right thing the right way to achieve the right goals. Jt Comm J Qual Improv 1994;20(4): 181–91.

[42] National Initiative for Children's Healthcare Quality. Available at: http://www.nichq.org/nichq. Accessed January 15, 2007.

[43] Dartmouth-Hitchcock Medical Center CF Center. Available at: http://www.dhmc.org/qualityreports/ list.cfm?metrics=CF. Accessed January 15, 2007.

[44] O'Connor G, Quinton H, Kahn R, et al. Case-mix adjustment in cystic fibrosis—a model for predicting survival based on patient and disease characteristics present at diagnosis. Pediatr Pulmonol 2002;33: 99–105.

[45] Cystic Fibrosis Foundation. Available at: http:// www.cff.org/LivingWithCF/CareCenterNetwork/ CareCenterData/. Accessed January 15, 2007.

[46] Gawande A. The bell curve. The New Yorker. June 12, 2004. Available at: http://www.newyorker.com/ online/content/articles/041206on_onlineonly01?041 206on_onlineonly01. Accessed January 15, 2007.

[47] O'Connor GT, Quninton HB, Kneeland T, et al. Median household income and mortality rate in cystic fibrosis. Pediatrics 2003;111(4 Pt 1):e333–9.

[48] Marmot M. The status syndrome: how social standing affects out health and longevity. New York: Times Books; 2004.

[49] Swartz DR, Quinton HB, Maddock J, et al. Relationship of income to outcome and treatment in CF patients. Pediatr Pulmonol 2002; A424(Suppl 24):324.

ELSEVIER
SAUNDERS

Clin Chest Med 28 (2007) 473–477

CLINICS
IN CHEST
MEDICINE

Index

Note: Page numbers of article titles are in **boldface** type.

0272-5231/07/$ - see front matter © 2007 Elsevier Inc. All rights reserved.
doi:10.1016/S0272-5231(07)00045-7

Moving?

Make sure your subscription moves with you!

To notify us of your new address, find your **Clinics Account Number** (located on your mailing label above your name), and contact customer service at:

E-mail: elspcs@elsevier.com

800-654-2452 (subscribers in the U.S. & Canada)
407-345-4000 (subscribers outside of the U.S. & Canada)

Fax number: 407-363-9661

Elsevier Periodicals Customer Service
6277 Sea Harbor Drive
Orlando, FL 32887-4800

*To ensure uninterrupted delivery of your subscription, please notify us at least 4 weeks in advance of move.